STUDENT WORKBOOK FOR

UNDERSTANDING
Medical Surgical
Nursing

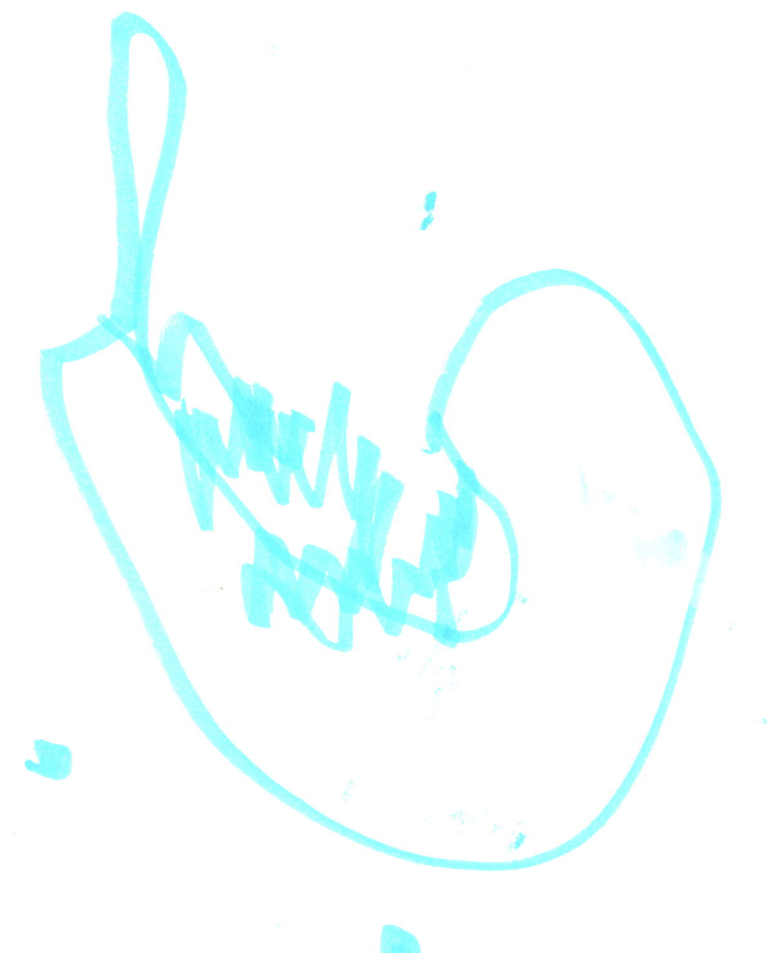

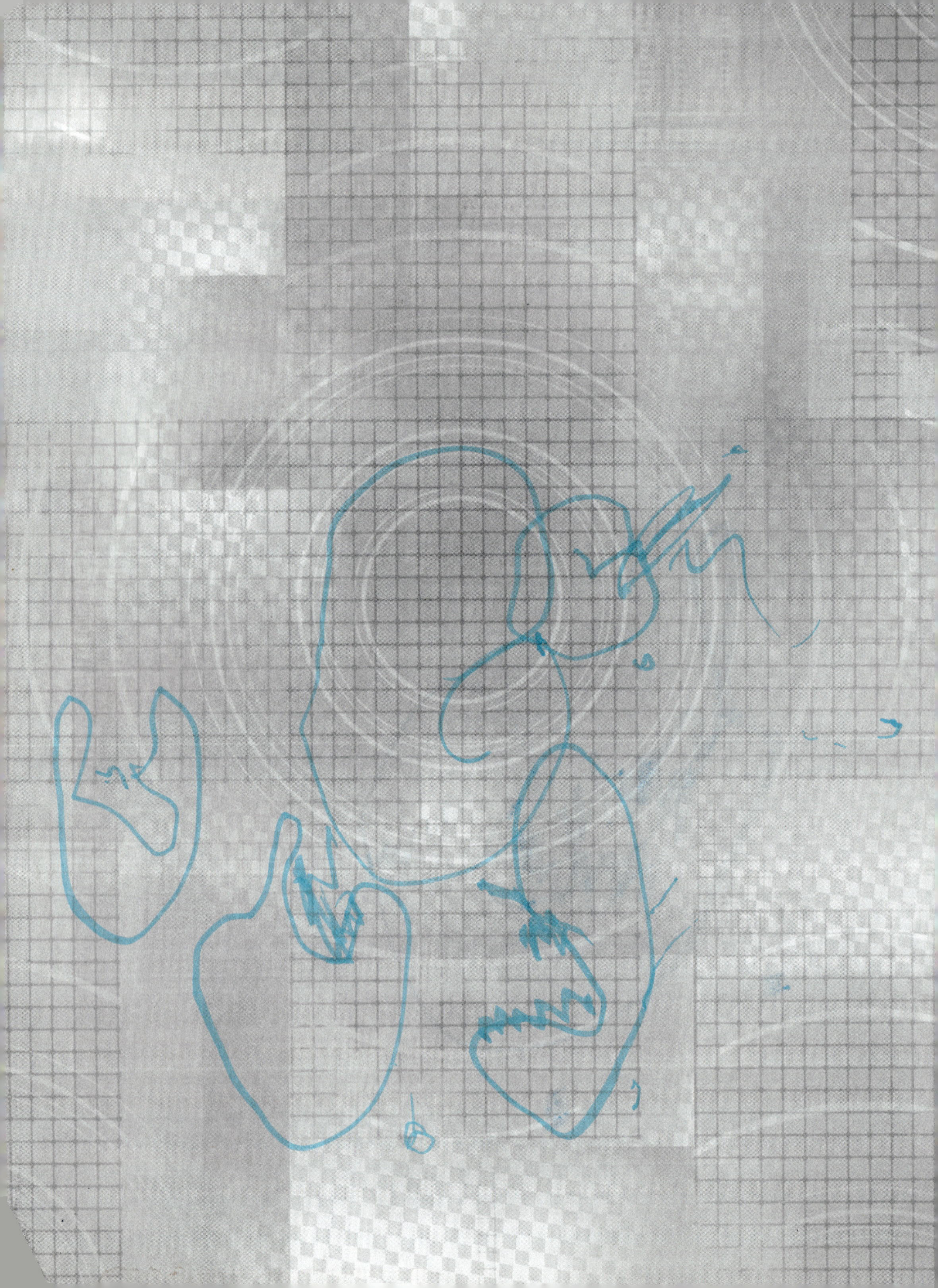

UNDERSTANDING Medical Surgical Nursing

THIRD EDITION

PAULA D. HOPPER, MSN, RN
Professor of Nursing
Jackson Community College
Jackson, Michigan

LINDA S. WILLIAMS, MSN, RNBC
Professor of Nursing
Jackson Community College
Jackson, Michigan

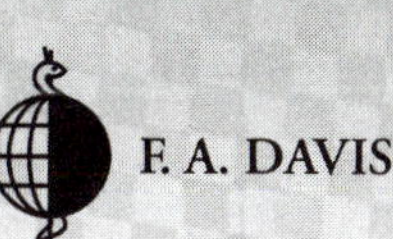

F. A. DAVIS COMPANY · Philadelphia

F. A. Davis Company
1915 Arch Street
Philadelphia, PA 19103
www.fadavis.com

Printed in the United States of America

Last digit indicates print number: 10 9 8 7 6 5 4 3

Acquisitions Editor: Lisa B. Deitch/Jonathan Joyce
Director of Content Development: Darlene D. Pederson
Special Projects Editor: Shirley A. Kuhn
Senior Project Editor: Ilysa H. Richman

As new scientific information becomes available through basic and clinical research, recommended treatments
and drug therapies undergo changes. The author(s) and publisher have done everything possible to make
this book accurate, up to date, and in accord with accepted standards at the time of publication. The authors,
editors, and publisher are not responsible for errors or omissions or for consequences from application of
the book, and make no warranty, expressed or implied, in regard to the contents of the book. Any practice
described in this book should be applied by the reader in accordance with professional standards of care used
in regard to the unique circumstances that may apply in each situation. The reader is advised always to check
product information (package inserts) for changes and new information regarding dose and contraindications
before administering any drug. Caution is especially urged when using new or infrequently ordered drugs.

ISBN 13: 978-0-8036-1591-5
ISBN 10: 0-8036-1591-4

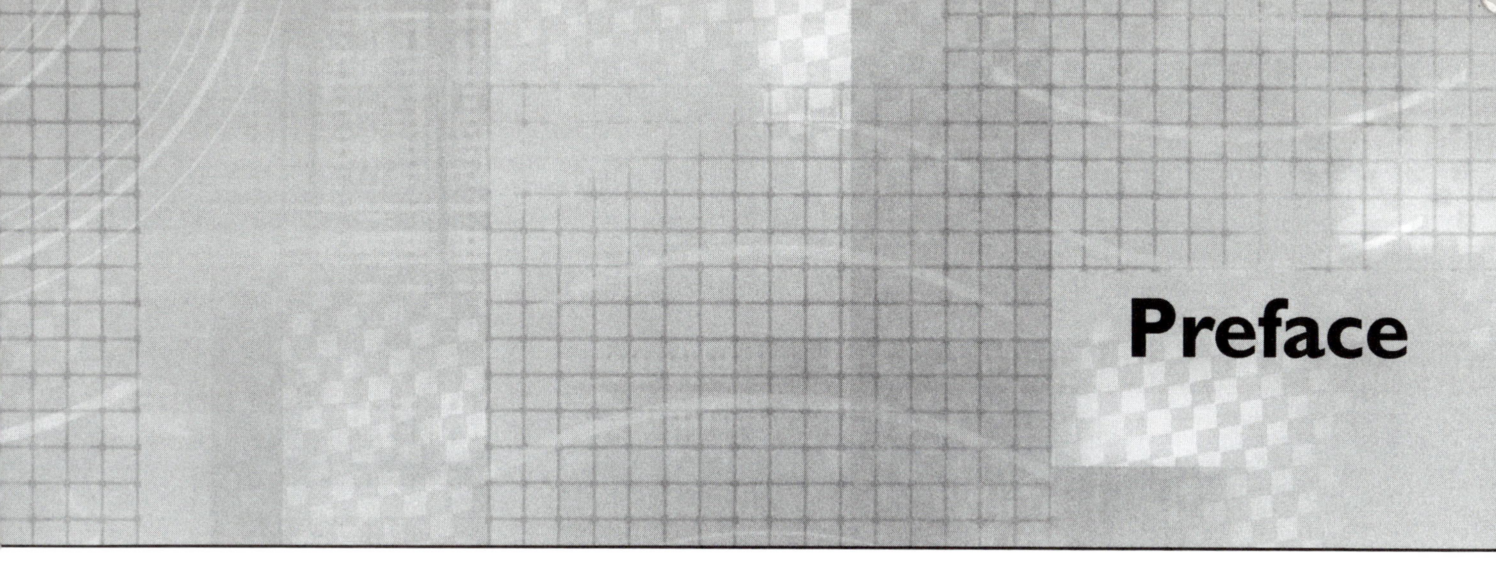

Preface

NOTE TO THE STUDENT:

The *Student Workbook for Understanding Medical Surgical Nursing* has been written and edited by the authors to accompany the third edition of Understanding Medical-Surgical Nursing. Many of the exercises included have been used by our own licensed practical nurse/licensed vocational nurse (LPN/LVN) students. We have included exercises that will help you develop your critical thinking abilities. We feel this is an important part of understanding the material and will also help you as you prepare for the NCLEX-PN. Most of the items in this paperback Student Workbook are different from the items in the Electronic Study Guide, except for the labeling exercises. We hope you find both formats helpful in your studies.

SUGGESTIONS FOR USING THE STUDY GUIDE:

Checklists for Learning Success are provided at the beginning of each unit. You can use these checklists to track your study of the major topics.

Each chapter includes:

- An exercise to help you practice chapter vocabulary items. It is important to understand the underlying vocabulary before attempting to apply the terms to understand the remainder of the information in each chapter.
- Basic matching, true/false, word scramble, and other exercises to allow you to practice and understand medical-surgical nursing information. These exercises are most helpful for developing knowledge and recall of material.
- Critical thinking exercises (in most chapters) to help you practice your new knowledge in patient situations. We feel strongly that you must learn to think critically, rather than just memorize facts. The answers we give for the critical thinking exercises are just some of the possibilities. You will come up with additional answers of your own as your knowledge base expands.
- NCLEX-PN style questions to give you practice in applying your new knowledge. Rationale for why an answer is correct or incorrect has been included to strengthen your critical thinking abilities for test taking.
- Function and Assessment chapters also include a labeling exercise to help you review basic anatomy.

We hope you find this study guide useful. Happy studying!

PAULA D. HOPPER and LINDA S. WILLIAMS

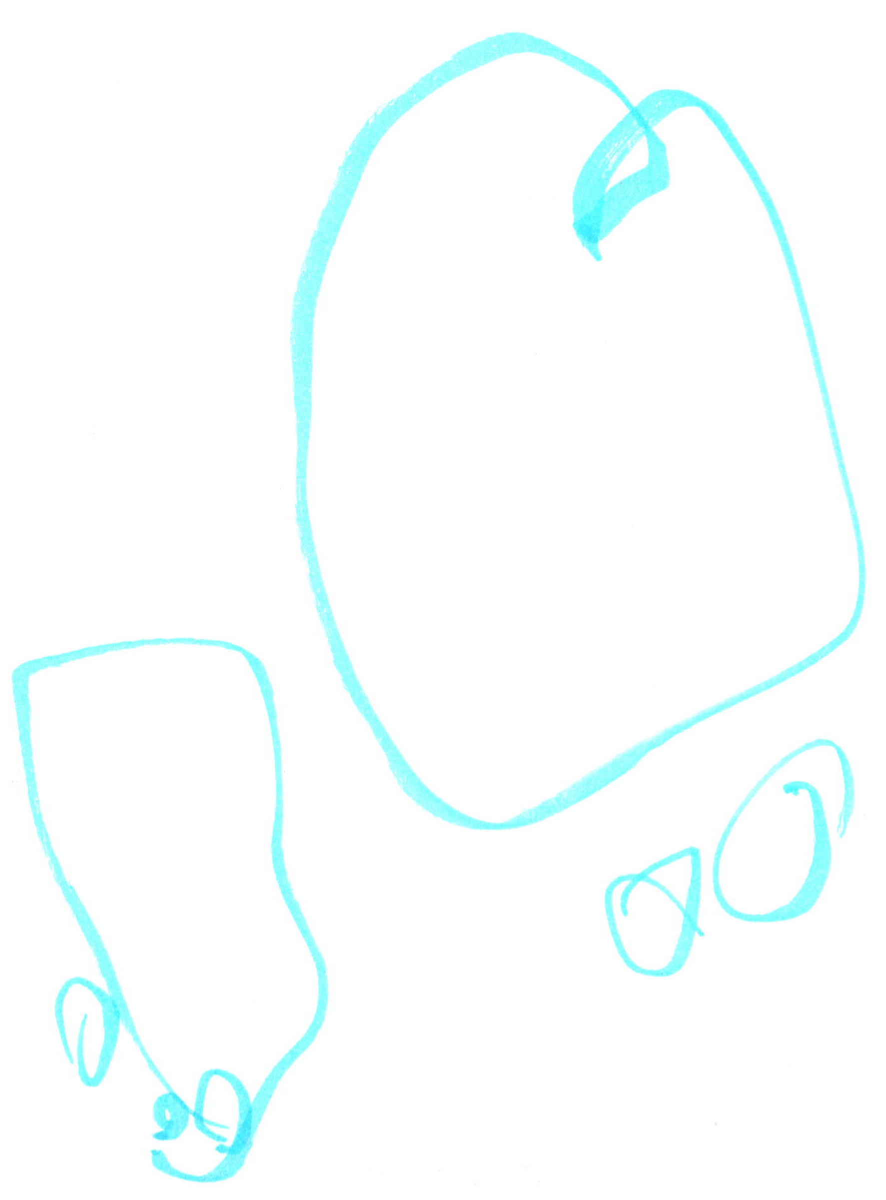

Contents

UNDERSTANDING HEALTH CARE ISSUES

CHECKLIST FOR LEARNING SUCCESS

Critical Thinking

Critical thinking attitudes
- ❑ Knowledge base
- ❑ Patient safety
- ❑ Critical thinking skills
- ❑ Problem solving
- ❑ Role of the licensed practical nurse/licensed vocational nurse (LPN/LVN)
- ❑ Nursing process
- ❑ Data collection
- ❑ Documentation of data
- ❑ Nursing diagnosis
- ❑ Plan of care
- ❑ Implementation
- ❑ Identifying interventions
- ❑ Evaluation

Issues

- ❑ Health care delivery
- ❑ Economic issues
- ❑ Nursing/health team
- ❑ Leadership in nursing practice
- ❑ Career opportunities
- ❑ Ethics and values
- ❑ Ethical obligations and nursing
- ❑ Building blocks of ethics
- ❑ Ethical principles
- ❑ Ethical theories
- ❑ Ethical decision-making
- ❑ Legal concepts
- ❑ HIPAA
- ❑ Nursing liability and the law

Cultural Influences

- ❑ Cultural diversity
- ❑ Communication
- ❑ Space
- ❑ Time orientation
- ❑ Social organization
- ❑ Environmental control
- ❑ Health beliefs
- ❑ Biological variations
- ❑ Death & dying
- ❑ Health practitioners
- ❑ Cultural groups

Alternative/Complementary

- ❑ Alternative vs. complementary therapies
- ❑ Allopathy
- ❑ Ayurveda
- ❑ Chinese medicine
- ❑ Chiropractic
- ❑ Homeopathy
- ❑ Naturopathy
- ❑ Native-American medicine
- ❑ Osteopathy
- ❑ Herbal therapy
- ❑ Relaxation therapies
- ❑ Massage therapy
- ❑ Aquatherapy
- ❑ Heat and cold
- ❑ Safety/effectiveness
- ❑ Role of LPN/LVN

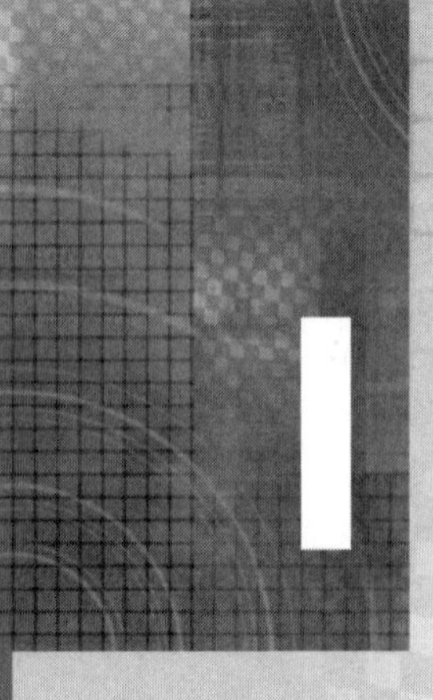

Critical Thinking and the Nursing Process

VOCABULARY

Define the following terms and use them in sentences.

Nursing process

Definition: ____

Sentence: ____

Critical thinking

Definition: ____

Sentence: ____

Assessment

Definition: ____

Sentence: ____

Objective data

Definition: ____

Sentence: ____

Subjective data

Definition: ____

Sentence: ____

Evaluation

Definition: ____

Sentence: ____

SUBJECTIVE AND OBJECTIVE DATA

Identify the following data as subjective (symptom) or objective (sign).

1. Pain ____________________________________
2. Dyspnea ________________________________
3. Edema __________________________________
4. Capillary refill 2 seconds _______________
5. Nausea _________________________________
6. Vomiting _______________________________
7. Dizziness _______________________________
8. Cyanosis ________________________________
9. Numbness _______________________________
10. Indigestion ____________________________
11. Pale ___________________________________
12. Serum potassium 3.6 mEq/L ____________
13. Palpitations ___________________________
14. Blood pressure 130/82 _________________
15. White blood cell count 7000/mm^3 _______

CRITICAL THINKING

Sometimes cognitive maps are used to organize thinking. Look at samples in any of the Function and Assessment chapters under Aging Changes. Some of the workbook chapters will ask you to make a cognitive map—so here is an opportunity to practice. Consider a time when you have had a headache. Fill in the spaces with information related to the WHAT'S UP? questions. See Chapter 1 Answers for one patient's responses. Once you have the questions answered, you could go even further and make links with possible interventions. There is no one right way to make a cognitive map—use your imagination!

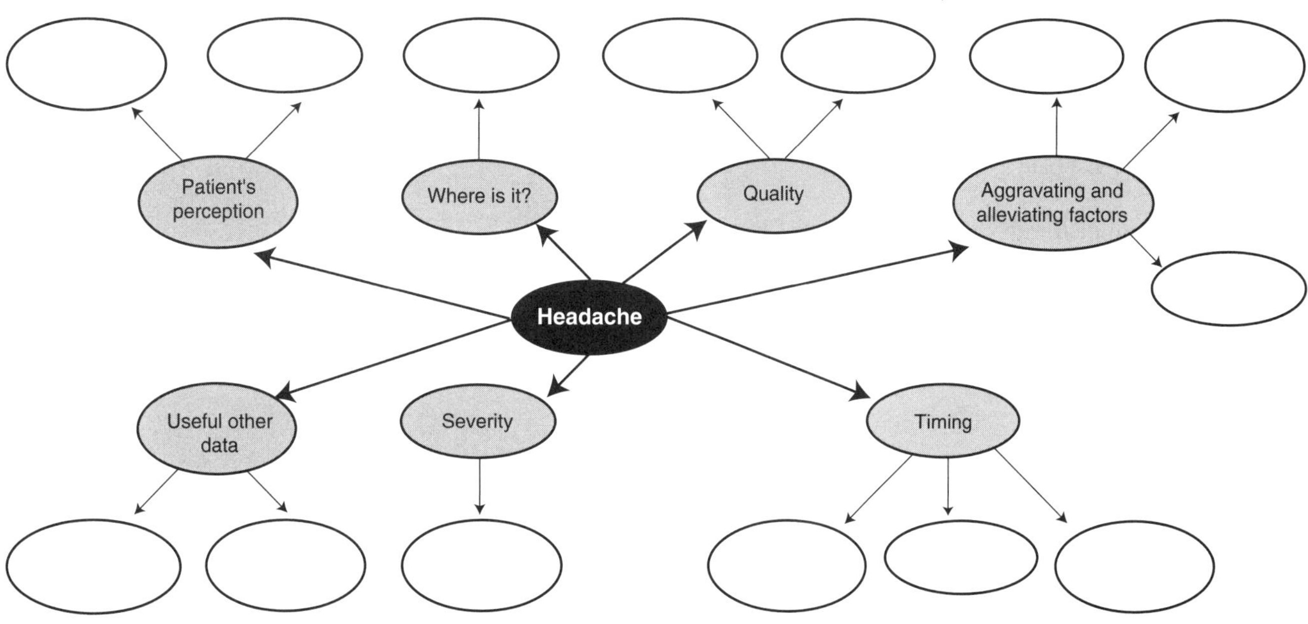

REVIEW QUESTIONS

Choose the best answer unless directed otherwise.

1. Which one of the following is a nursing diagnosis?
   a. Peptic ulcer
   b. Pneumonia
   c. Ineffective airway clearance
   d. Myocardial infarction

2. Which one of the following is a medical diagnosis?
   a. Hiatal hernia
   b. Impaired mobility
   c. Powerlessness
   d. Anxiety

3. An LPN desires to learn about why a patient's lung sounds have crackles, and questions the physician during morning rounds. Which critical thinking attitude is the nurse exhibiting?
   a. Intellectual humility
   b. Intellectual sense of justice
   c. Intellectual empathy
   d. Intellectual integrity

4. The LVN is caring for a patient with diabetes. In what order should the nurse carry out the nursing process? Place all steps in correct sequential order.
   a. Implement plan of care
   b. Assist with evaluation
   c. Collect data
   d. Assist with development of nursing diagnoses
   e. Assist with planning of outcomes and interventions

5. Which of the following statements best defines *critical thinking*?
   a. Goal-focused directed thinking
   b. Clear thinking during critical situations
   c. Constructive feedback about nursing actions
   d. Critical evaluation of patient response to care

6. The LPN is reviewing the nursing care plan of a patient with a fractured ankle. Which of the following steps in the nursing process does the nurse use to determine the effectiveness of the plan of care?
   a. Assessment
   b. Diagnosis
   c. Implementation
   d. Evaluation

7. Which of the following is one role of the LPN/LVN in using the nursing process?
   a. Collect data
   b. Formulate nursing diagnoses
   c. Determine outcomes
   d. Plan interventions

8. The LPN/ is documenting patient data. Which of the following should the nurse document under objective data?
   a. Denies nausea
   b. Shortness of breath
   c. Heart rate 72 beats per minute
   d. Midsternal chest pain

9. A patient is admitted with chest pain, which has been resolved. The patient states, "I hope I can live a normal life." According to Maslow's hierarchy of needs, at which of the following levels does this statement indicate the patient to be?
   a. Physiological needs
   b. Safety and security
   c. Love and belonging
   d. Self-esteem

10. A patient has a nursing diagnosis of impaired swallowing related to muscle weakness as evidenced by drooling, coughing, and choking. Which of the following outcomes is appropriate for this patient's nursing diagnosis?
    a. Improved airway clearance within 8 hours as evidenced by clear lung sounds and productive cough
    b. Baseline body weight maintained as evidenced by no weight loss
    c. Improved muscle strength as evidenced by ability to sit up while eating
    d. Improved swallowing within 48 hours as evidenced by no coughing or choking

Issues in Nursing Practice

VOCABULARY

Match the following legal terms and definitions.

1. _______ Assault
2. _______ Battery
3. _______ Defamation
4. _______ False imprisonment
5. _______ Outrage
6. _______ Invasion of privacy and wrongful disclosure of confidential information

A. Unlawful touching of another
B. Unlawful conduct that places another in the immediate fear of unlawful touching or battery; the real threat of bodily harm
C. Unlawful restriction of a person's freedom
D. Extreme and outrageous conduct by a defendant relating to the care of the patient or the body of a deceased individual
E. Wrongful injury to another's reputation or standing in a community; may be written (libel) or spoken (slander)
F. Liability when a patient's privacy is invaded physically or if records are released without authority

NURSING PRACTICE, ETHICAL AND LEGAL PRINCIPLES

1. The health-illness continuum represents the potential shifting between _______-_______ health and poor health throughout the _______ span.
2. Nurses must be _______-licensed to practice to _______ the public and maintain the _______ of health care services.
3. _______ is a central virtue in nursing.
4. Nursing care uses the following principles: ensuring _______ and respect, _______ confidentiality, respecting the patient's right to make care choices, and maintaining a professional relationship with the patient.
5. Effective leaders are _______ in management process, _______ _______, positive thinkers, use _______ and earn of _______ their co-workers.

VALUES CLARIFICATION

Complete the following sentences.

1. The one thing I have always wanted to do is

   _______________________________________.

2. If I inherited 5 million dollars, I would

   _______________________________________.

3. As President of the United States, I would

   _______________________________________.

4. If I died today, I would like my obituary to say

   _______________________________________.

5. If I could control the world and its destiny, I would

   _______________________________________.

Complete this list of things people value with items you believe should be included, then rank the value you believe each item has, with 1 being the highest value.

________ Family		________ Professionalism	
________ Career		_______	___________
________ Religion		_______	___________
________ Honor		_______	___________
________ Material possessions		_______	___________
________ Health		_______	___________
________ Recreation		_______	___________

What have you learned about yourself by doing this exercise? What do the rankings signify? Can you identify yourself as more utilitarian, or more deontological? (There are no answers to this section because this is an exercise requiring personal responses.)

CRITICAL THINKING

Read the following case study and answer the questions.

Mrs. Reo, a 5 foot 3 inch, 105-lb, 86-year-old retired cleaning lady, was admitted to a general medical-surgical unit in a small rural hospital. She had been diagnosed 3 months previously as having metastatic cancer that had spread from her liver to her lungs and bone marrow. She received chemotherapy and radiation therapy for several weeks, but the treatment was not effective. She was admitted to the hospital because she became too weak to walk or care for herself at home. The cancer returned, and the large doses of oral narcotic medications taken at home were having little effect on her pain while increasing her confusion and weakness.

Her oncologist decided that further chemotherapy or radiation therapy would not be effective, and she ordered Mrs. Reo to be kept comfortable with medications. A continuous morphine intravenous drip was started to help control the pain. Even with this medication, Mrs. Reo cried out in pain, particularly when morning care was given, and begged the nurses not to move her. Because she was severely underweight, the skin over her bony prominences quickly became reddened and showed the beginning signs of breakdown.

The hospital standards of care for immobile patients require that they be turned from side to side at least every 2 hours. Mrs. Reo yelled so loudly when she was turned that the nursing staff wondered if they were helping or hurting her.

To help decide what should be done, a patient care conference was called by the nurses who gave care to Mrs. Reo. The manager of the unit stated very clearly that the hospital standards of care required that she be turned at least every 2 hours to prevent skin breakdown, infections, and perhaps sepsis. In her already weakened condition, an infection or sepsis would most likely be fatal. Betsy, who had been a licensed practical nurse for some 15 years, disagreed with the manager. Her feeling was that causing this obviously terminal patient so much pain by turning her was cruel and violated her dignity as a human being. She stated that she could not stand to hear Mrs. Reo yell anymore and refused to take care of her until some other decision was made about her nursing care. Sally, a new graduate nurse, felt that the patient should have some say in her own care and that perhaps some type of compromise could be reached about turning her, perhaps turning her less frequently. Monica, a registered nurse who had worked on the unit for 2 years, felt that the physician should make the decision about turning this patient, and then the nurses should follow the order. This last suggestion was met with strong negative comments by the other nurses present. They felt that patient comfort and turning were nursing measures.

1. What are the important ethical principles in this dilemma? _____________________________________

2. How does the Code of Ethics apply to this situation? ____

3. What are the legal issues? _____________________

4. Are there ever any situations when a nurse might legally and ethically violate a standard of care? ____

5. What are some other possible solutions to this dilemma? What types of consequences might they have? ____

(There are no right answers to this section because this is an ethical exercise that has many choices to be considered for the best outcome for the patient. Discuss your options with classmates.)

REVIEW QUESTIONS

Choose the best answer unless directed otherwise.

1. A client with emphysema is being seen by the home health nurse. The client is on oxygen, lives alone, and is able to perform activities of daily living, prepare meals, and do light household tasks with rest periods. The client is unable to perform yard work, which was a favorite hobby. Which of the following would describe the client's location on the health-illness continuum?
   a. Near death
   b. High-level wellness
   c. Poor health
   d. Moderate-level wellness

2. One nurses' Code of Ethics states, "The nurse safeguards the patient's right to privacy by judiciously protecting information of a confidential nature." This statement is based on which of the following principles?
   a. The right to privacy is an inalienable right of all persons.
   b. The nurse-patient relationship is based on trust.
   c. A breach of confidentiality may expose the nurse to liability.
   d. Nurses know what is best for patients' health care.

3. The ethical principle that the primary goal of health care and nursing is to do good for others is called which of the following?
   a. Autonomy
   b. Fidelity
   c. Beneficence
   d. Veracity

4. The ethical principle of nonmaleficence is defined as which of the following?
   a. Health-care workers avoiding harm to patients
   b. Telling the truth to patients in all matters
   c. Being faithful to commitments made to patients
   d. The right of self-determination of patients

5. Which of the following is the term used to describe an ethical situation that arises in which there is a choice between two equally unfavorable alternatives?
   a. A tort
   b. Ethical antagonism
   c. Contraindication
   d. Ethical dilemma

6. Which of the following is the first step in the ethical decision-making process?
   a. Analyze the alternatives.
   b. Gather and verify the information.
   c. Consider the consequences of the actions.
   d. Make a decision.

7. Ethical dilemmas most often involve which of the following situations?
   a. A conflict of basic human rights
   b. Violations of the Nurses' Code of Ethics
   c. Nurses who do not understand the ethical code
   d. Patients who wish to die

8. When applying the ethical principle of autonomy to patient care, the nurse should understand that which of the following is applicable to autonomy?
   a. Autonomy is an absolute principle that has no exceptions.
   b. Only patients who are awake and oriented have the right to autonomy.
   c. Under certain conditions, autonomy can be limited.
   d. Autonomy is the same as the principle of nonmaleficence.

9. A patient asks the nurse why he is taking a new medication. The nurse tells the patient that the medication will help him feel better, and not to worry about it. The nurse's response demonstrates which of the following conditions?
   a. Therapeutic communication
   b. Paternalism
   c. Lack of knowledge
   d. Legal obligations

10. The nurse attempts to apply the standard of best interest to a patient who has had a cardiac arrest and is now unconscious. Which of the following conditions is the most important factor for the nurse to consider?
    a. The patient's wishes as expressed before he became unconscious
    b. The family's wishes now that the patient can no longer communicate
    c. The patient's chances for survival after the cardiac arrest
    d. The physician's orders regarding future arrest situations

11. Which of the following punishments distinguishes criminal liability from civil liability?
    a. Personal liability
    b. Financial recovery
    c. Loss of license
    d. Potential loss of freedom

12. Which of the following is an unintentional tort?
    a. Negligence
    b. Outrage
    c. Assault
    d. Privacy invasion

13. The nurse is administering medication to a patient who has tuberculosis. The patient refuses the medication. The nurse understands that which of the following is true regarding the patient's autonomous rights?
    a. Patients can refuse any or all treatments.
    b. Patient's Self-Determination Act guarantees the right to refuse all treatments.
    c. Legal systems can force patients to take medication for contagious diseases.
    d. Health-care systems cannot force patients to take medications for contagious diseases.

Multiple response item. Select all that apply.

14. The LPN is considering if the task of taking a blood pressure on a 78-year-old resident with hypertension can be delegated to a nursing assistant. Which of the following steps should the nurse consider in this decision-making process for delegation?
    a. Right task
    b. Right circumstances
    c. Right patient
    d. Right communication
    e. Right supervision
    f. Right route

Cultural Influences on Nursing Care

3

VOCABULARY

Match the words on the left with the definitions on the right.

1. _______ Belief
2. _______ Cultural awareness
3. _______ Cultural competence
4. _______ Ethnic
5. _______ Ethnocentrism
6. _______ Generalization
7. _______ Stereotype
8. _______ Value
9. _______ Worldview
10. _______ Custom
11. _______ Cultural sensitivity
12. _______ Assimilation

A. A usual way of acting in a given situation

B. Accepted as true, need not be proven

C. Focuses on history and ancestry

D. Avoiding actions that may offend another person's cultural beliefs

E. Belief that "my way is the only right way"

F. An assumption that needs validation

G. An opinion or belief about someone because of ethnic background

H. Belonging to a subgroup of a larger cultural group

I. Way a person perceives the world

J. The process of taking on a dominant culture's values, sometimes with risk of losing own cultural heritage

K. Having knowledge and skills about another culture

L. A principle or belief that has worth to an individual or group

CULTURAL CHARACTERISTICS

Answer the following questions. Discuss with a classmate.

1. What are some examples of primary characteristics of culture? _______________________________________
   ____
   ____

2. What are some examples of secondary characteristics of culture? _______________________________________
   ____
   ____

3. What is meant by traditional health care practitioners? Give an example. _____________________________
   ____
   ____

4. What are some characteristics of people who are primarily present oriented? Past oriented? Future oriented?
   ____
   ____
   ____

CRITICAL THINKING: IMMIGRANTS

There are no right or wrong answers to the following questions. Share your thoughts with your classmates.

1. Are immigrants taking away from the United States, or are they adding to its richness? Give specific examples and share your reasons for your position.

2. Identify difficulties that new immigrants must overcome in the United States. How might you, as a nurse, help immigrants overcome these difficulties?

PERSONAL INSIGHTS

Answer the following questions. Consider how people from other cultures might answer differently.

1. What do you personally do to prevent illness?

2. What home remedies do you use when you have a minor illness such as a cold or flu? Do you use over-the-counter medications to treat yourself? How might these over-the-counter medicines cause a problem with prescription medications?

3. What significance does food have to you besides satisfying hunger?

4. Are you usually on time for social events? For appointments? Why or why not?

CRITICAL THINKING: BATHING

Read the following case study and answer the questions.

An elderly male Arab American patient refuses to be bathed by a female nurse's aide. He has not been bathed for 3 days, and today he really needs a bath. His family is at his bedside.

1. Why do you think he is refusing his bath?

2. What alternatives do you have?

3. What is the best solution to the problem?

REVIEW QUESTIONS

Choose the best answer.

1. A 26-year-old Pueblo Native American mother arrives at the health clinic to receive treatment for a laceration on her leg. Accompanying her are her two children, who missed their immunization appointments last month because she did not have transportation. As the clinic nurse, what is the best approach to ensure that the children get their immunizations?
   a. Give the immunizations today.
   b. Reschedule the appointment for next month at the regular hours for the immunization clinic.
   c. Reschedule the immunizations when she returns to have her stitches removed.
   d. Ask the community health nurse to go to the home to give the immunizations.

2. A Guatemalan patient died after a cardiac arrest. His wife is uncontrollably wailing and shouting "Vaya con dios," and is lying on the floor shaking. What action should the nurse take?
   a. Call a cardiac arrest team.
   b. Immediately call for a stretcher and get her off the floor.
   c. Calmly remain beside her and talk to her.
   d. Call the house physician to order a tranquilizer.

3. A Laotian child is brought to the emergency department by the school nurse. She wants the child examined for the possibility of child abuse because he has several circular ecchymotic areas 2 inches in diameter on his back. What action should the intake nurse perform?

a. Call the child welfare authorities to intervene.
b. Explain to the school nurse that the bruised areas are consistent with the traditional Chinese practice of cupping.
c. Inform the child's mother that he is in the emergency department.
d. Report the school nurse for not getting consent from the mother to bring the child to the emergency department.

4. A 42-year-old Arab American patient has chronic renal failure. He asks the nurse where he can purchase a kidney for transplantation. Which response is best?
a. Organs cannot be purchased in the United States.
b. Explain the ethical dilemma in purchasing organs.
c. Call the unit supervisor.
d. Give him the area organ procurement telephone number.

5. A 12-year-old child from a traditional Korean American family is newly diagnosed with diabetes mellitus. His home health nurse is to teach the patient and family diabetes care. Both parents and the child can administer his insulin and recite the signs and symptoms of hypoglycemia and hyperglycemia. They are highly educated and read and speak English well. Which is the best first step in teaching them about nutrition therapy for diabetes?
a. Give them a food exchange list for a diabetic diet.
b. Determine whether they can calculate calories in a sample meal.
c. Assess current dietary food practices.
d. Have them make an appointment with a consulting dietitian.

6. A 46-year-old Cuban American high school teacher has been admitted for cancer of the breast. She wants her religious counselor, a Santero, to visit. Which action should the nurse take?
a. Ask the nursing supervisor to see if it is permitted.
b. Tell her Santeros are not permitted in the hospital.
c. Suggest that she see a priest instead.
d. Tell her it is okay, but for safety reasons the Santero cannot perform animal sacrifice in the hospital.

7. A 62-year-old Peruvian woman is in the operating room having bypass surgery. Eighteen to 20 family members arrive on the unit and wait in her room, which is shared by two other patients. Which is the best solution to this problem?
a. Allow two family members to wait in the room and send the rest of them to the cafeteria.
b. Send all of them to the lobby and tell them they will be notified when the patient returns to her room.
c. Allow only her husband and elderly mother to visit.
d. Assign the patient to a private room and allow the family to wait there.

8. A 42-year-old African American patient is 40 pounds overweight. She admits to baking pies with lard and frying in bacon grease, practices she does not wish to stop. To reduce fat and calories, what can the home health nurse encourage her to do?
a. Do not purchase lard.
b. Reduce the portion size when she cuts her pies.
c. Bake two separate pies, one for her and one for her family.
d. Continue baking with lard, but reduce calories she receives from other foods in her diet.

9. A 41-year-old Hispanic woman has had a mastectomy for cancer of the breast. Her physician recommends radiation therapy. She says, "What is the use? My life is in God's hands anyway." Which of the following responses is appropriate?
a. Agree with her, but tell her she must accept the radiation or she will die.
b. Assure that she understands all the implications of her decision before accepting it.
c. Keep encouraging her to think about the radiation, and ask all the other staff to do the same.
d. Have her ask her physician to prescribe chemotherapy instead of radiation therapy.

10. A 72-year-old Iranian patient refuses his morning antibiotic, which is scheduled every 8 hours because he is celebrating Ramadan and has to fast from sunup to sundown. Which of the following actions should the nurse take?
a. Explain that the medicine must be taken now to maintain the blood level of the drug.
b. Rearrange his medication schedule so he can take all his medicines between sundown and sunup.
c. Omit the medicine and record his refusal on the medication administration record.
d. Ask his family to encourage him to take the medicine.

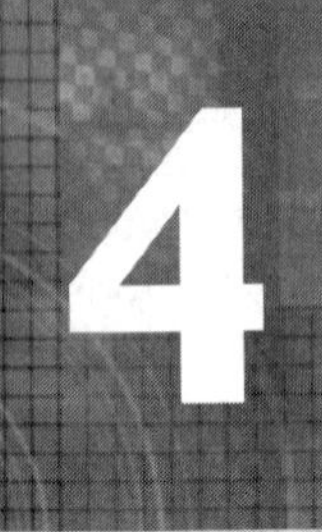

4 Alternative and Complementary Therapies

VOCABULARY

Match the term with the appropriate definition or statement.

1. _______ Alternative therapy
2. _______ Complementary therapy
3. _______ Homeopathy
4. _______ Naturopathy
5. _______ Ayurvedic
6. _______ Chiropractic

A. Illness is falling out of balance with nature
B. Uses nutrition, herbs, and hydrotherapy
C. Illness is a result of nerve dysfunction
D. Added to a conventional therapy
E. Unconventional therapy
F. "Like cures like"

COMPLEMENTARY THERAPY: GUIDED IMAGERY

Describe the purpose of guided imagery. Write a teaching plan on how to do guided imagery. Try teaching it to a family member or friend.

Purpose: ____________________________________
____
____

Teaching Plan: ________________________________
____
____

CRITICAL THINKING

Mrs. Lawless is admitted to your unit with heart failure and fluid overload. As you collect admission data, you find that she is taking feverfew and capsaicin regularly in addition to her prescribed medications for heart failure. When you question her, she says that the salesperson at the health food store told her these herbs were safe to use with her other medications.

1. What is feverfew used for? ____________________

2. What is capsaicin used for? ___________________

3. Where can you get information about the safety of taking these herbs with heart failure or with heart failure medications? _______________________________
____

4. What should you tell Mrs. Lawless?
____

REVIEW QUESTIONS

Choose the best answer.

1. Which of the following therapies would be considered a complementary therapy?
   a. Using both inhalers and oral medications for asthma
   b. Participating in a cardiac rehabilitation program after having a heart attack
   c. Using echinacea instead of antibiotics for an upper respiratory infection
   d. Using progressive muscle relaxation in addition to muscle relaxants for back pain

2. Which of the following therapies would be considered an alternative therapy?
   a. Using hydrotherapy in place of nonsteroidal anti-inflammatory drugs for arthritis
   b. Visiting a spiritual healer in addition to chemotherapy for cancer treatment
   c. Using antibiotics and bronchodilators for acute bronchitis
   d. Using aspirin for a headache

3. Which of the following statements would indicate to the nurse that the patient needs additional teaching on the use of guided imagery?
   a. "I will focus on my breathing."
   b. "I imagine the ocean, including the smell, the sound, and the feel of the air."
   c. "I will relax all parts of my body."
   d. "I will keep my eyes open until the exercise is complete."

4. Which of the following terms describes traditional Western medicine?
   a. Homeopathy
   b. Naturopathy
   c. Allopathy
   d. Ayurveda

5. A patient tells a nurse that a chiropractor is going to do minor surgery to remove a small superficial lump on her neck. Which response by the nurse is best?
   a. "The lump is probably pressing against a nerve; that is why it needs to be removed."
   b. "You need to question your chiropractor's qualifications. Chiropractors do not perform surgery."
   c. "Chiropractors specialize in nerve function; removing the lump will restore normal nerve function."
   d. "Surgery might not be necessary; usually a simple chiropractic adjustment will relieve pressure on a nerve."

6. Which of the following herbal remedies might be effective against viruses and colds?
   a. Echinacea
   b. Feverfew
   c. Chamomile
   d. Ginger

7. A client admitted with chronic pain says he is interested in pursuing an alternative therapy for his pain, but he is unsure how to determine whether it is safe. Which of the following responses by the nurse is best?
   a. "As long as the therapy does not include medication, it should be safe."
   b. "You should talk with your primary care practitioner before trying anything new."
   c. "Be careful, because most alternative therapies have dangerous side effects."
   d. "Traditional analgesics are always the safest bet for chronic pain."

8. A nurse is interested in providing therapeutic touch therapy for her home care patient with severe pain. This will be her first experience with therapeutic touch. Which of the following steps is least appropriate before beginning to provide this new service?
   a. Obtain permission from the patient's physician and home care agency.
   b. Take classes on how to administer therapeutic touch.
   c. Tell the patient he will be able to reduce the number of medications he takes.
   d. Read current research on the use of therapeutic touch.

UNDERSTANDING HEALTH AND ILLNESS

CHECKLIST FOR LEARNING SUCCESS

Fluid, Electrolyte, and Acid-Base Balance and Imbalance
- ❑ Fluid balance
- ❑ Dehydration
- ❑ Fluid overload
- ❑ Electrolyte balance
- ❑ Sodium imbalances
- ❑ Potassium imbalances
- ❑ Calcium imbalances
- ❑ Magnesium imbalances
- ❑ Acid-base balance
- ❑ Respiratory acidosis
- ❑ Metabolic acidosis
- ❑ Respiratory alkalosis
- ❑ Metabolic alkalosis

Nursing Care of Patients Receiving Intravenous Therapy
- ❑ Indications for intravenous (IV) therapy
- ❑ Venipuncture steps
- ❑ Types of infusions
- ❑ Methods of infusion
- ❑ Types of fluids (tonicity)
- ❑ IV access
- ❑ Peripheral IV therapy
- ❑ Complications of IV therapy
- ❑ Central catheters
- ❑ Nutrition support

Nursing Care of Patients with Infections
- ❑ Infectious process
- ❑ Body's defense mechanisms
- ❑ Infectious disease
- ❑ Community infection control
- ❑ Health-care agency infection control
- ❑ Antibiotic-resistant infections
- ❑ Infectious disease interventions
- ❑ Nursing process for infection

Nursing Care of Patients in Shock
- ❑ Pathophysiology of shock
- ❑ Complications from shock
- ❑ Hypovolemic shock
- ❑ Cardiogenic shock
- ❑ Obstructive shock
- ❑ Distributive shock
- ❑ Shock therapeutic interventions
- ❑ Nursing process

Nursing Care of Patients in Pain
- ❑ Definitions of pain
- ❑ Mechanisms of pain transmission
- ❑ Types of pain
- ❑ Nonopioid analgesics
- ❑ Opioid analgesics
- ❑ Adjuvants
- ❑ Routes for analgesic administration
- ❑ Nondrug therapies
- ❑ Pain assessment
- ❑ Patient education

Nursing Care of Patients with Cancer
- ❑ Review of normal anatomy and physiology
- ❑ Cancer classification
- ❑ Risk factors for cancer
- ❑ Diagnostic tests
- ❑ Staging and grading
- ❑ Surgery
- ❑ Radiation therapy
- ❑ Chemotherapy
- ❑ Side effects of therapies
- ❑ Nursing care of patients with cancer
- ❑ Hospice care
- ❑ Superior vena cava syndrome
- ❑ Spinal cord compression
- ❑ Hypercalcemia
- ❑ Pericardial effusion
- ❑ Disseminated intravascular coagulation (DIC)

Nursing Care of Patients Having Surgery
- ❑ Surgery urgency/purpose
- ❑ Preoperative phase
- ❑ Preoperative assessment/admission
- ❑ Nursing process: preoperative
- ❑ Intraoperative phase
- ❑ Postoperative phase
- ❑ Postanesthesia Care Unit (PACU)
- ❑ Postoperative nursing care
- ❑ Respiratory
- ❑ Circulatory
- ❑ Pain
- ❑ Urinary
- ❑ Wound care
- ❑ Gastrointestinal (GI)
- ❑ Mobility
- ❑ Patient discharge
- ❑ Home health care

Nursing Care of Patients with Emergent Conditions
- ❑ Primary survey
- ❑ Secondary survey
- ❑ Shock
- ❑ Anaphylaxis
- ❑ Major trauma
- ❑ Hypothermia
- ❑ Frostbite
- ❑ Hyperthermia
- ❑ Poisoning and drug overdose
- ❑ Near-drowning
- ❑ Psychiatric emergencies
- ❑ Disaster response
- ❑ Bioterrorism

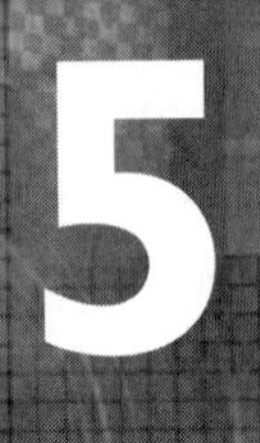

Nursing Care of Patients with Fluid, Electrolyte, and Acid-Base Imbalances

VOCABULARY

Fill in the blanks with key words from the chapter.

1. The process by which a solute moves across a membrane from an area of higher to an area of lower concentration is _____________.

2. A fluid that has the same osmolarity as blood is said to be _____________.

3. A fluid that has a higher osmolarity than blood is said to be _____________.

4. A decrease in blood volume is called _____________.

5. Electrolytes in the blood that have a positive charge are called _____________.

6. The patient with an excess of sodium in the blood has _____________.

7. The patient with not enough potassium in the blood has _____________.

8. The patient with not enough calcium in the blood has _____________.

9. _____________ occurs when the serum pH falls below 7.35.

10. If the serum pH is too high, the condition is called _____________.

DEHYDRATION

Circle the errors in the following paragraph and write the correct information in the space provided.

Mrs. White is a 78-year-old woman admitted to the hospital with a diagnosis of severe dehydration. The licensed practical nurse/licensed vocational nurse (LPN/LVN) assigned to Mrs. White is asked to collect data related to fluid status. The LPN expects Mrs. White's blood pressure to be elevated because of the shift of fluid from tissues to her bloodstream. The nurse also finds Mrs. White's skin to be taut and firm, and notes that the urine is copious and dark amber. The nurse asks Mrs. White if she knows where she is and what day it is because severe dehydration may cause confusion. In addition, the nurse initiates intake and output measurements because this is the most accurate way to monitor fluid balance.

ELECTROLYTE IMBALANCES

Match the electrolyte imbalance with its signs and symptoms.

1. _________ Hyponatremia
2. _________ Hyperkalemia
3. _________ Hypokalemia
4. _________ Hypercalcemia
5. _________ Hypocalcemia

A. Osteoporosis, hyperactive reflexes
B. Muscle weakness, weak pulse
C. Muscle weakness, impaired clotting
D. Fluid balance and mental status changes
E. Muscle cramps, irregular heart rate

CRITICAL THINKING

Read the following case study and answer the questions.

Mr. James is an 89-year-old man admitted to your unit with worsening chronic bronchitis. On admission he is short of breath, but he is able to walk to the bathroom without difficulty. The physician orders bronchodilators, antibiotics, and an intravenous infusion of normal saline at 150 mL per hour. The next day when you return to work, you find Mr. James gasping for breath, coughing, and panicky. You quickly listen to his lungs and hear an increase in moist crackles since yesterday.

1. What additional data do you collect to confirm your suspicion of fluid overload? _________________
   ____
   ____

2. You report your findings to the registered nurse (RN) and collaborate on quickly developing a nursing diagnosis of fluid overload. What factors contributed to this problem? _________________________________
   ____
   ____

3. The RN pages the physician while you return to check on the patient. What nursing interventions can help until orders are received? _________________________
   ____
   ____

4. How will you know when the problem has been resolved? _______________________________________
   ____
   ____

REVIEW QUESTIONS

Choose the best answer.

1. Which of the following intravenous solutions is hypotonic?
   a. Normal saline
   b. 0.45% saline
   c. Ringer's lactate
   d. 5% dextrose in normal saline

2. Which of the following hormones retains sodium in the body?
   a. Antidiuretic hormone
   b. Thyroid hormone
   c. Aldosterone
   d. Insulin

3. Which patient is most at risk for fluid volume overload?
   a. The 40-year-old with meningitis
   b. The 35-year-old with kidney failure
   c. The 60-year-old with psoriasis
   d. The 2-year-old with influenza

4. Which patient should be monitored most closely for dehydration?
   a. The 50-year-old with an ileostomy
   b. The 19-year-old with chronic asthma
   c. The 72-year-old with diabetes mellitus
   d. The 28-year-old with a broken femur

5. Which food should be avoided by the patient on a low-sodium diet?
   a. Apples
   b. Cheese
   c. Chicken
   d. Broccoli

6. Which food is recommended for the patient who must increase intake of potassium?
   a. Bread
   b. Egg
   c. Potato
   d. Cereal

7. Which is the most reliable method for monitoring fluid balance?
   a. Daily intake and output
   b. Daily weight
   c. Vital signs
   d. Skin turgor

8. An elderly nursing home resident who has always been alert and oriented is now showing signs of dehydration and has become confused. Which electrolyte imbalance is most likely involved?
   a. Hyponatremia
   b. Hyperkalemia
   c. Hypercalcemia
   d. Hypomagnesemia

9. Which nursing action is most appropriate for the weak patient with osteoporosis?
   a. Maintain bedrest.
   b. Encourage fluids.
   c. Ambulate with assistance.
   d. Provide a high-protein diet.

10. Which organ(s) is/are most at risk for dysfunction in a patient with a potassium level of 6.2 mEq/L?
    a. Lungs
    b. Kidneys
    c. Liver
    d. Heart

11. A 19-year-old student develops symptoms of respiratory alkalosis related to an anxiety attack. Which nursing intervention is appropriate?
    a. Make sure his oxygen is being administered as ordered.
    b. Have him breathe into a paper bag.
    c. Place him in a semi-Fowler's position.
    d. Have him do coughing and deep breathing exercises.

12. A patient has chronic respiratory acidosis related to long-standing lung disease. Which of the following problems is the cause?
    a. Hyperventilation
    b. Hypoventilation
    c. Loss of acid by kidneys
    d. Loss of base by kidneys

Nursing Care of Patients Receiving Intravenous Therapy

6

VOCABULARY

Match the following words to their definitions.

1. _________ Intravenous (IV)
2. _________ Cannula
3. _________ Venipuncture
4. _________ Bolus
5. _________ Peripherally inserted central catheter (PICC)
6. _________ Central line
7. _________ Phlebitis
8. _________ Infiltration

A. Inserting a needle into a vein
B. Seepage of IV fluid into tissues
C. Catheter inserted into a centrally located vein with the tip residing in the vena cava
D. Inflammation of a vein
E. Access device inserted into a superficial peripheral vein and advanced into the central system (usually the superior vena cava)
F. An IV needle or catheter
G. Volume of medication injected into a vein
H. Inside the vein

PERIPHERAL VEINS

Label the veins that can be used for IV therapy.

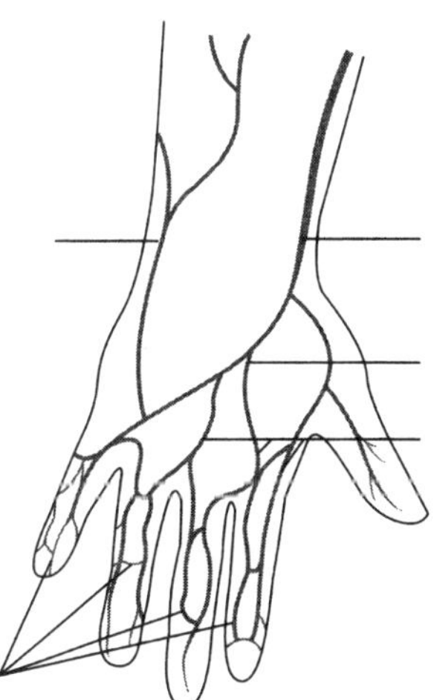

COMPLICATIONS OF IV THERAPY

Fill in the blank with the correct complication.

1. Pain and inflammation at the IV insertion site is called

    ____________.

2. Redness and exudate at the IV insertion site indicate presence of ____________.

3. Infiltration of tissue by a vesicant drug is called

    ____________.

4. Dyspnea and crackles can be a sign of ____________

    ____.

5. A cool, puffy insertion site indicates ____________.

6. Fever, chills, and tachycardia indicate a systemic infection called ____________.

7. Chest pain and sharp pain at the IV site might be present if a _________ _________ has occurred.

8. If the patient develops cyanosis, hypotension, and loss of consciousness, the nurse should suspect ____________ ____________.

CRITICAL THINKING

Read the following case study and answer the questions.

Mr. Livesay is admitted with cellulitis and is receiving IV fluids by gravity drip. When you check his IV, you find it is not dripping. What assessment can you do to determine the cause of the problem? What is the role of the licensed practical nurse (LPN)? When must the registered nurse (RN) be consulted? ____
____
____
____
____

CALCULATION PRACTICE

Calculate the answers to the following problems.

1. June has an IV of 5% dextrose and water to run at 83 mL/hr. How many drops per minute should be set if the tubing delivers 15 drops per milliliter?

2. Frank has a piggyback antibiotic of 500 mg in 50 mL of 5% dextrose and water. The medication must infuse over 20 minutes. The tubing drip factor is 10. How many drops per minute?

3. Dave has an IV of normal saline ordered at 1 L over 12 hours. How many milliliters per hour should he receive?

4. Lucy has an order to administer 800 units of heparin per hour. You have heparin 50,000 units in 500 mL of D5W. You will run it on a controller. How many milliliters should be administered per hour?

5. Jack has an order for 1000 mL of normal saline over 24 hours. You use minidrip tubing. How many drops should be administered per minute?

REVIEW QUESTIONS

Choose the best answer.

1. Which patient would benefit most from a capped IV catheter that is used intermittently rather than continuously?
   a. The patient with pneumonia who needs fluids and antibiotics
   b. The patient who has had major blood loss after a motor vehicle accident
   c. The young child who is dehydrated
   d. The elderly patient who is receiving a diuretic for fluid overload

2. The physician orders furosemide (Lasix) 40 mg IV STAT for an acutely fluid-overloaded patient. Why was the IV route likely chosen?
   a. Furosemide can be administered only by the IV route.
   b. IV is the route of choice for rapid administration.
   c. IV dosing is more accurate.
   d. IV furosemide has fewer side effects than oral.

3. Which vein should be used first when initiating IV therapy?
   a. Jugular
   b. Basilic
   c. Brachiocephalic
   d. Axillary

4. When preparing a site for venipuncture with alcohol, how long must the area be cleaned?
   a. 5 seconds
   b. 10 seconds
   c. 30 seconds
   d. 60 seconds

5. Which of the following complications can occur if a clotted cannula is aggressively flushed?
   a. A clot can enter the circulation.
   b. An air embolism can enter the circulation.
   c. A painful arterial spasm can occur.
   d. Fluid extravasation into surrounding tissue can occur.

6. Which of the following symptoms most likely indicates that an infusion is infiltrated?
   a. Redness at the site
   b. Pain at the site
   c. Puffiness at the site
   d. Exudate at the site

7. A patient has orders to receive 1 L (1000 mL) of 5% dextrose and lactated Ringer's solution to be infused over 8 hours. How many milliliters will be infused per hour?
   a. 80
   b. 100
   c. 125
   d. 150

8. A patient is receiving an IV piggyback antibiotic in 50 mL of 5% dextrose and water to run over 1 hour. The tubing has a drip factor of 60. How many drops per minute should be delivered?
   a. 6
   b. 17
   c. 50
   d. 100

9. Which of the following IV solutions is hypertonic?
   a. Normal saline
   b. 5% dextrose in 0.9 % NaCl
   c. 0.45% NaCl
   d. 0.225% NaCl

10. What is the last step when inserting an IV cannula?
   a. Secure the cannula with tape.
   b. Document the insertion site, date, and type of cannula used.
   c. Assess the site.
   d. Place a sterile dressing over the insertion site.

7

Nursing Care of Patients with Infections

VOCABULARY

Define the following terms and use them in a sentence.

Antigen

Definition: ____

Sentence: ____

Asepsis

Definition: ____

Sentence: ____

Bacteria

Definition: ____

Sentence: ____

Hand Hygiene

Definition: ____

Sentence: ____

Nosocomial Infection

Definition: ____

Sentence: ____

Pathogens

Definition: ____

Sentence: ____

Personal Protective Equipment

Definition: ____

Sentence: ____

Phagocytosis

Definition: ____

Sentence: ____

Sepsis

Definition: ____

Sentence: ____

Virulence

Definition: ____

Sentence: ____

Viruses

Definition: ____

Sentence: ____

PATHOGEN TRANSMISSION

Match the pathogen with its mode of transmission.

1. _______ Chickenpox
2. _______ Malaria
3. _______ Tuberculosis
4. _______ Rocky Mountain spotted fever
5. _______ Meningitis
6. _______ Pneumonia
7. _______ Measles
8. _______ Influenza
9. _______ Pneumonic plague
10. _______ Hepatitis A

A. Common vehicle
B. Droplet
C. Airborne
D. Vectorborne

PATHOGENS AND INFECTIOUS DISEASE

Fill in the word for the definition of pathogens and infectious diseases.

1. _______________ Gram-positive bacteria clusters that can cause pneumonia, cellulitis, peritonitis, and toxic shock
2. _______________ Group of plantlike organisms that includes yeast, molds, and mushrooms; rarely pathogenic
3. _______________ A fungi that can cause thrush
4. _______________ The virus that causes infectious mononucleosis
5. _______________ A systemic fungal respiratory disease caused by *Histoplasma capsulatum*
6. _______________ A disease caused by infection with the protozoan *Toxoplasma gondii*
7. _______________ Single-celled parasitic organisms that move and live mainly in the soil
8. _______________ Small intracellular parasites that can only live inside cells; may produce disease when they enter a cell
9. _______________ A bacterium that must be inside living cells to reproduce and cause disease and causes Rocky Mountain spotted fever
10. _______________ Bleach is used to kill its spores

CRITICAL THINKING

Read the following case study and answer the questions.

A 72-year-old patient is admitted to a private room with an antibiotic-resistant respiratory tract infection.

1. What equipment is needed for isolation? _______________
____
____

2. What type of equipment would be used to do assessments and nursing interventions? _______________

____

____

3. Describe the psychosocial effects on a patient in isolation. _________________________________

____

____

4. What can the nurse include in the plan of care for a patient in isolation to reduce social isolation? _______

____

____

REVIEW QUESTIONS

Choose the best answer unless directed otherwise.

1. The nurse is assisting the patient with a urinary catheter with bathing. The urinary bag has 300 mL of clear pale yellow urine, and is placed below the level of the bladder. The nurse notes the catheter moves freely when the patient turns. Which of the following actions is required by the nurse to decrease risk for urinary infection?
   a. Raise the level of the urinary bag.
   b. Report urine color.
   c. Encourage fluids.
   d. Secure catheter per agency policy.

2. Which of these actions would be most appropriate for the nurse to take while providing patient care to help prevent the spread of infection?
   a. Sterilizing hands with a germicide once a day
   b. Washing hands at the beginning of patient rounds
   c. Washing hands before and after each patient contact
   d. Wearing gloves for all patient care

3. In planning care for a patient, the nurse understands that surgical asepsis is based on which of the following principles?
   a. Destroying organisms before they enter the body
   b. Isolating all patients who have infectious diseases
   c. Destroying bacteria as they leave the body
   d. Maintaining basic cleanliness

Multiple response item. Select all that apply.
4. Which of the following does the nurse understand is needed by all pathogenic organisms to multiply?
   a. Moisture
   b. Light
   c. A host
   d. Oxygen
   e. Warmth
   f. Food

Multiple response item. Select all that apply.
5. A patient is to have a sterile urine specimen collected. Which of the following techniques is used to collect this specimen?
   a. Cleansing the patient's external genitalia before the patient voids
   b. Having the patient void into a sterile container
   c. Straight catheterizing the patient
   d. Obtaining a midstream voided specimen
   e. Obtaining a second voiding specimen

6. Which of the following actions can the nurse take to help prevent nosocomial infections in an incontinent patient?
   a. Avoid requesting urinary catheter
   b. Applying absorbent briefs
   c. Toileting patient every four hours
   d. Restricting fluids

7. A patient has been diagnosed recently as having an upper respiratory infection. Which of the following symptoms would indicate to the nurse that the patient is developing a complication?
   a. Scratchy throat
   b. Clear, watery drainage from the nose
   c. Dry cough
   d. High fever

8. The nurse is collecting a culture of wound drainage, and the patient asks what a culture is. Which of the following is the best response by the nurse to explain what a culture is?
   a. A culture identifies presence of pathogens.
   b. A culture measures antibiotic levels.
   c. A culture identifies an antibiotic's effect on a pathogen.
   d. A culture determines the appropriate medication dosage.

9. Which of the following would the nurse recognize as a sign of a local infection during data collection?
   a. Warm skin
   b. Clammy skin
   c. Anorexia
   d. Paleness

10. Which of the following does the nurse understand is a method of sterile technique?
    a. Use of antiseptics
    b. Use of autoclaves
    c. Frequent hand washing
    d. Use of gloves when coming in contact with body fluids

11. Which of the following infections would the nurse recognize as being a nosocomial infection?
    a. Chronic urinary tract infection
    b. A sexually transmitted infection
    c. Pneumonia in postoperative patient
    d. Hospitalization for cellulitis

12. Which of the following antibiotics would the nurse anticipate would be used to treat methicillin-resistant *Staphylococcus aureus?*
    a. Gentamicin
    b. Tobramycin
    c. Penicillin
    d. Vancomycin

Multiple response item. Select all that apply.

13. Which of the following data collection findings should the nurse recognize and report as a possible sign of infection in the older adult?
    a. Edema
    b. Irritability
    c. Headache
    d. Bradycardia
    e. Pacing behavior

14. The nurse observes a nursing assistant providing oral care to an immunocompromised patient. Which of the following actions by the nursing assistant would require further instruction for patient safety?
    a. Use of sterile water
    b. Use of tap water
    c. Use of a fluoride toothpaste
    d. Use of a soft toothbrush

8

Nursing Care of Patients in Shock

VOCABULARY

Fill in the blank with the word formed by word building.

1. _________________ acid—sour + osis—condition
2. _________________ an—without + aerobic—presence of oxygen
3. _________________ an—without + phylaxis—protection
4. _________________ anti—against + a—not + rhythmic—rhythm
5. _________________ coagulo—clotting + pathies—diseases
6. _________________ cyan—blue coloring + osis—condition
7. _________________ tachy—fast + pnea—breathing
8. _________________ olig—few + uria—urine condition
9. _________________ tachy—fast + cardia—heart condition

MATCHING

Match the area of the cardiovascular system that contributes to the development of shock with each type of shock.

1. _______ Hypovolemic shock
2. _______ Cardiogenic shock
3. _______ Anaphylactic shock
4. _______ Septic shock
5. _______ Neurogenic shock
6. _______ Obstructive shock

A. Heart
B. Blood vessels
C. Fluid volume

Nursing Care of Patients in Pain

9

VOCABULARY

Match the word to its definition.

1. _______ Addiction
2. _______ Tolerance
3. _______ Ceiling effect
4. _______ Pain
5. _______ Prostaglandin
6. _______ Adjuvants
7. _______ Opioid
8. _______ Patient-controlled anesthesia (PCA)
9. _______ Endorphins
10. _______ Analgesics

A. Whatever the experiencing person says it is
B. Endogenous chemicals that act like opioids
C. Larger dose of analgesic required to relieve same pain
D. Psychological dependence
E. Self-administered analgesics
F. Dose of analgesic limited by side effects
G. Medications that relieve pain
H. Drugs that are used to potentiate analgesics
I. Neurotransmitter released during pain
J. A morphinelike drug

CULTURAL COMPETENCE

You are working on a medical unit in a large metropolitan area. Your patients come from varied cultural backgrounds. What differences in pain expressions might you expect to see in patients from the following cultures?

Native American ____________________________________

European American __________________________________

African American ___________________________________

Hispanic American __________________________________

Asian American _____________________________________

CRITICAL THINKING

Read the following case study and answer the questions.

Miss Murphy is a 32-year-old admitted to your unit following an emergency appendectomy at 8:00 a.m. When you enter her room at 2 p.m., she is sitting up in bed smiling and visiting with her family. She tells you she is hurting and asks for a pain shot. You check her medication record and find orders for morphine 5 to 10 mg IM q4hr as needed (PRN) for pain.

1. List at least seven areas you will assess related to her pain. ____
____
____
____

2. Based on your assessment, you decide to administer 10 mg of morphine. What class of drugs does morphine belong to? What is its mechanism of action?
____
____
____
____

3. What is the most effective medication schedule you can implement today? ____

4. What side effects will you watch for? ____

5. How will you know if the medication has been effective? ____

6. The next morning you decide to administer Tylenol No. 3 for Miss Murphy's pain, but it is not effective. Why do you think it did not help? ____

7. What nondrug therapies might be appropriate for Miss Murphy? What technique has already been effective for her? ____

REVIEW QUESTIONS

Choose the best answer.

1. Which of the following definitions of pain is most appropriate?
   a. Knifelike sensation along a nerve pathway
   b. Burning sensation that accompanies severe injury or trauma
   c. Injured tissues responding with release of neurotransmitters that cause a sensation of pressure or discomfort
   d. Whatever the experiencing person says it is, occurring whenever the experiencing person says it does

2. Which of the following terms describes a feeling of threat to one's self-image or life that may accompany pain?
   a. Fear
   b. Anxiety
   c. Suffering
   d. Panic

3. Which of the following is a common side effect of opioid administration?
   a. Constipation
   b. Respiratory depression
   c. Tachycardia
   d. Addiction

4. Which is the most accurate way to assess the severity of a patient's pain?
   a. Observe for moaning or other physical signs.
   b. Watch for elevated blood pressure and pulse.
   c. Have the patient rate pain on a standard pain scale.
   d. Monitor the frequency with which the patient requests pain medication.

5. Which of the following statements best explains why a patient can be laughing and talking and yet still be in pain?
   a. Most patients try to deny their pain because pain is socially unacceptable.
   b. Distraction can help relieve pain when used in conjunction with analgesics.
   c. Most patients who are laughing and talking are not in pain.
   d. Laughing prolongs the effects of opioids in the body.

6. Which type of pain may be accompanied by changes in vital signs?
   a. Acute pain
   b. Chronic nonmalignant pain
   c. Cancer pain

7. An 82-year-old male patient has been receiving meperidine (Demerol) IM for chronic back pain. After several weeks he becomes very irritable, which is unlike him. Which response by the nurse is best?
   a. Understand that chronic pain can cause a patient to become irritable.
   b. Obtain an order for an adjuvant sedative to administer with the meperidine.
   c. Ask him if there is something bothering him that he would like to talk about.
   d. Consult with the registered nurse or physician about possible toxic effects of normeperidine.

8. Which of the following should be assessed and documented before administering an opioid analgesic?
   a. Liver and kidney function studies
   b. Blood glucose level
   c. Pain level and respiratory rate
   d. Physical cause of pain

9. Which drug can be given to reverse the effects of an opioid overdose?
   a. Naloxone (Narcan)
   b. Methadone (Dolophine)
   c. Hydrocodone with acetaminophen (Vicodin)
   d. Phenytoin (Dilantin)

10. A 42-year-old woman has chronic pain for which no cause can be found. Her physician orders a placebo. Which response by the nurse to the physician is best?
   a. "I will give the placebo and document her response."
   b. "I know if the placebo helps her pain, then her pain is not real."
   c. "I am not comfortable administering this placebo without the patient's consent."
   d. "May we alternate the placebo with her opioid order?"

11. A patient has a PCA pump following surgery on his spine. He appears to be in pain, but is too drowsy to push the button on the pump. Which response by the nurse is correct?
   a. Push the button for the patient.
   b. Instruct the patient's wife to push the button, not to exceed every 10 minutes.
   c. Assess the patient's vital signs.
   d. Increase the dose of medication delivered in each injection.

12. A known cocaine abuser is admitted following a motorcycle accident. He calls you into his room and says, "I need something for this pain. Now." Which assumption by the nurse is best?
   a. The patient is withdrawing from cocaine and needs an opioid to prevent withdrawal symptoms.
   b. The patient is in pain and needs an analgesic.
   c. The patient is trying to establish control over his situation.
   d. The patient is faking pain to gain access to opioids.

Nursing Care of Patients with Cancer

VOCABULARY

Fill in the blank.

1. Loss of hair is called _alopecia_.
2. Loss of appetite is called _anorexia_.
3. Leuko_penia_ places the patient at risk of infection.
4. Dry mouth is called _xerostomia_.
5. Treatment aimed at maintaining comfort is called _palliative_ therapy.
6. _Chemo_ is the use of drugs to combat cancer.
7. Substances that poison cells are called _cytotoxic_.
8. _Neoplasm_ is the term used to describe new growth.
9. When cancer _meta_, it travels to a new site.
10. A tumor that is not cancerous is called _benign_.

CELLS

Label each statement as true or false.

1. _F_ Chromosomes are made of DNA and protein.
2. _F_ A gene is the code for one DNA molecule.
3. _F_ Messenger RNA carries the genetic code to the cell membrane.
4. _____ A genetic change in a cell is called a mutation.
5. _T_ Transfer RNA brings amino acids to the proper sites on the DNA. msr RNA
6. _T_ Cells become malignant by mutating.
7. _____ In any human cell, most of the genes are always active.
8. _____ The chromosome number for a human cell is 48.
9. _____ The process of mitosis produces two identical cells with 23 chromosomes each.
10. _____ Mitosis is necessary only for growth of the body.

BENIGN VERSUS MALIGNANT TUMORS

Compare the characteristics of benign and malignant tumors. List as many characteristics as you can remember.

____
____
____
____
____

CRITICAL THINKING

Delmae is a 48-year-old restaurant worker undergoing chemotherapy following a right modified mastectomy. List two or three nursing interventions for each of the side effects she can expect to experience.

1. Leukopenia: ____
____

2. Thrombocytopenia: ____
____

3. Anemia: ____
____

4. Stomatitis: ____
____

5. Nausea and vomiting: ____
____

6. Alopecia: ____
____

REVIEW QUESTIONS

Choose the best answer.

1. Genes are made of which of the following?
   a. Chromosomes
   b. DNA
   c. RNA
   d. Protein

2. Which is the correct term used for a group of similar cells found on an external or internal body surface?
   a. Skin
   b. Mucous membrane
   c. Epithelial tissue
   d. Connective tissue

3. Which of the following foods can increase cancer risk?
   a. Broccoli, cauliflower
   b. Butter, ice cream
   c. Chicken, fish
   d. Cakes, breads

4. A patient is admitted with suspected lung cancer and asks, "How will my physician know for sure if I have cancer?" Which of the following responses is correct?
   a. "Your physician will do cultures of your sputum."
   b. "An x-ray examination will be done to confirm the diagnosis."
   c. "A biopsy is the only way to know for sure."
   d. "Your physician will do a bronchoscopy to look at the cancer."

5. A 47-year-old woman has mucositis related to radiation therapy. Which of the following nursing interventions will help relieve her symptoms?
   a. Provide frequent mouth care.
   b. Offer cold liquids often.
   c. Provide high-carbohydrate foods.
   d. Offer juices frequently.

6. A nurse is caring for a patient with a radioactive implant. How can the nurse avoid unnecessary radiation exposure?
   a. Avoid entering the patient's room for 24 hours.
   b. Limit the amount of time spent with the patient.
   c. Avoid touching the patient.
   d. Place a "contaminated" sign on the patient's bed.

7. A male patient is receiving chemotherapy following surgery for prostate cancer. Which of the following signs or symptoms indicates that he is experiencing thrombocytopenia?
   a. Fever
   b. Petechiae
   c. Pain
   d. Vomiting

8. How can the nurse best prevent complications in the patient with leukopenia?
   a. Wash hands frequently.
   b. Avoid injections.
   c. Allow no visitors.
   d. Offer fresh fruits and vegetables.

9. A patient has severe pain related to bone cancer. The nurse notes that the patient does not ask for pain medication while watching television. Which of the following statements best explains this?
   a. Distraction is a good pain relief method and can prevent the need for analgesics.
   b. The patient may ask for pain medication when the television is not on because of boredom.
   c. The pain must be psychosomatic because it is relieved by television.
   d. Distraction can be a helpful intervention when used in addition to analgesics.

10. A patient with terminal cancer is referred to hospice for support. How can hospice help the patient and family?
    a. Hospice nurses can help administer curative chemotherapy.
    b. Hospice supports research efforts in finding cancer cures.
    c. Hospice can help the patient's family keep the patient comfortable until his death.
    d. Hospice can help the patient find financial resources for cancer treatment.

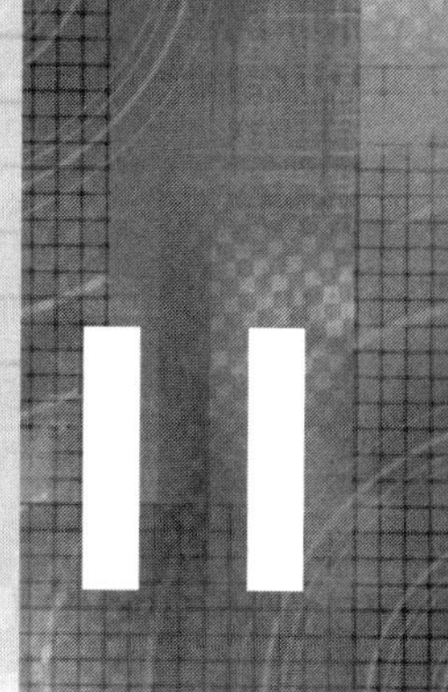

Nursing Care of Patients Having Surgery

VOCABULARY

Fill in the blank.

1. _____________ are physicians who perform surgical procedures.
2. The three surgical phases are referred to collectively by the term _____________.
3. The _____________ phase begins with the admission of the patient to the postanesthesia care unit (PACU) and continues until the patient's recovery is completed.
4. _____________ is the period when an anesthetic is first given until full anesthesia is reached.
5. The _____________ phase begins with the decision to have surgery and ends with transfer of the patient to the operating room.
6. The _____________ phase begins when the patient is transferred to the operating room and ends when the patient is admitted to the PACU.
7. An _____________ agent is medication (such as narcotics, muscle relaxants, or antiemetics) used with the primary anesthetic agents.
8. The sudden bursting open of a wound's edges that may be preceded by an increase in serosanguineous drainage is referred to as _____________.
9. _____________ are physicians who administer anesthesia.
10. _____________ causes a loss of sensation and allows the surgical procedure to be done safely.
11. _____________ occurs from hypoventilation or mucous obstruction that prevents some alveoli from opening and being fully ventilated.
12. _____________ is the removal of necrotic and infected tissue.
13. _____________ is a body temperature that is below normal range.
14. _____________ is the viscera spilling out of the abdomen.

SURGERY URGENCY LEVELS

Match the surgery urgency level to the appropriate definition or example. The level may be used more than once.

1. _______ Surgery needed when any delay jeopardizes the patient's life or limb
2. _______ Fracture repair
3. _______ Surgery needed within 24 to 30 hours
4. _______ Extremity emboli
5. _______ Surgery planned and scheduled without immediate time constraints
6. _______ Surgery done at request of patient
7. _______ Hernia repair
8. _______ Rhinoplasty
9. _______ Infected gallbladder
10. _______ Cosmetic surgery

A. Optional surgery
B. Elective surgery
C. Urgent surgery
D. Emergency surgery

NOURISHING THE SURGICAL PATIENT

Find the seven errors and insert the correct information.

Healing requires increased vitamin A for collagen formation, vitamin B_{12} for blood clotting, and magnesium for tissue growth, skin integrity, and cell-mediated immunity. Carbohydrates are essential for controlling fluid balance and manufacturing antibodies and white blood cells. Hypoalbuminemia, low urine albumin, impedes the return of interstitial fluid to the venous return system, decreasing the risk of shock. A serum zinc level is a useful measure of protein status.

MEDICATIONS

Indicate whether the statement is true or false and correct the false statement.

1. ___________ All medications that patients are taking must be reviewed preoperatively.
2. ___________ Most anticoagulants, such as warfarin (Coumadin), do not need to be stopped before surgery.
3. ___________ Diabetic patients on insulin are told to increase their normal insulin dose the day of surgery.
4. ___________ Blood glucose monitoring for diabetic patients is ordered on admission.
5. ___________ If a patient is on chronic oral steroid therapy it cannot be abruptly stopped when nil per os (NPO).
6. ___________ Surgery is not a great stressor for the body.
7. ___________ Chronic oral steroid therapy should be continued via the parenteral route if the patient is NPO.
8. ___________ Circulatory collapse can develop if steroids are not stopped abruptly.

INTRAOPERATIVE NURSING DIAGNOSES AND OUTCOMES

Write a patient objective (goal) for each nursing diagnosis.

1. Risk for injury related to pressure points from positioning, chemicals, electrical equipment, and effect of being anesthetized ____

2. Risk for impaired skin integrity related to chemicals, pressure points from positioning, and immobility ____

3. Risk for deficient fluid volume related to being NPO and blood loss ____

4. Risk for infection related to incision and invasive procedures ____

5. Pain related to pressure points from positioning, incision, and surgical procedure ____

WOUND HEALING PHASES

Complete the table.

Phase	Time Frame	Wound Healing	Patient Effect
Phase I	__________	__________	Fever, malaise
Phase II	__________	Granulation tissue forms	__________
Phase III	__________	Collagen deposited	__________
Phase IV	Months to 1 year	__________	__________

CRITICAL THINKING

Read the case study and answer the questions.

Mrs. Vell, 74, is scheduled for a total hip replacement because of osteoarthritis. She is seen in the preadmission testing department 1 week before surgery.

1. Why is Mrs. Vell being seen in preadmission testing?
   ____
   ____

2. What testing may be done in preadmission testing?
   ____
   ____

3. What teaching should the nurse do in preadmission testing? __________________________
   ____

4. What are the responsibilities of the admitting nurse to prepare Mrs. Vell for surgery? ________________
   ____

5. What is the role of the holding area nurse?
   ____
   ____

6. What is a role of the licensed practical nurse/licensed vocational nurse (LPN/LVN) in the operating room?
   ____
   ____

7. What are the two prioritized primary responsibilities of the postanesthesia care nurse? ________________
   ____

8. Explain why postoperative care for this patient must include pain control, deep breathing and coughing, leg exercises, activity, leg abduction, and drain care.
   ____
   ____
   ____
   ____
   ____
   ____

Choose the best answer unless directed otherwise.

1. Which of the following is an LPN/LVN patient care role in the preoperative phase?
   a. Obtaining preoperative orders
   b. Explaining the surgical procedure
   c. Offering emotional support
   d. Providing informed consent

2. The LPN/LVN is caring for a patient in the preoperative period who, even after verbalizing concerns and having questions answered, states, "I know I am not going to wake up after surgery." Which of the following actions should the LPN/LVN take?
   a. Reassure patient everything will be all right.
   b. Inform the registered nurse.
   c. Explain national surgery death rate.
   d. Ask family to comfort the patient.

3. The nurse is reviewing the medication history of a new preoperative patient who is nil by mouth (NPO). The nurse notes that the patient has been on long-term oral steroid therapy. The nurse understands that which of the following is the reason that steroids cannot be abruptly stopped?
   a. Higher steroid levels are needed during stress.
   b. Malignant hyperthermia will result.
   c. Malignant hypertension will occur.
   d. Respiratory failure will result.

4. When teaching a preoperative older patient, which of the following is a teaching technique to improve learning?
   a. Sit in front of window in bright sunlight.
   b. Use small, white-on-black printed materials.
   c. Speak in high tone.
   d. Eliminate background noise.

5. When the patient's signature is witnessed by the nurse on the surgical consent, which of the following does the nurse's signature indicate?
   a. The nurse obtained informed consent.
   b. The nurse provided informed consent.
   c. The nurse answered all surgical procedure questions.
   d. The nurse verified that the patient signed the consent.

6. Which of the following is an intraoperative outcome for a patient undergoing an inguinal hernia repair?
   a. Verbalizes fears
   b. Maintains skin integrity
   c. Demonstrates leg exercises
   d. Explains deep breathing exercises

7. Which of the following is a discharge criterion from the PACU for a patient following surgery?
   a. Oxygen saturation above 90%
   b. Oxygen saturation below 90%
   c. Intravenous (IV) narcotics given less than 15 minutes ago
   d. IV narcotics given less than 30 minutes ago

8. Which of the following is one of the discharge criteria from ambulatory surgery for patients following surgery?
   a. Able to drive self home
   b. Has home telephone
   c. Understands discharge instructions
   d. IV narcotics given less than 30 minutes before discharge

9. Several hours after returning from surgery, the nurse tells the patient that she is ordered to be ambulated. The patient asks, "Why?" Which of the following complications would the nurse correctly explain can be prevented by early postoperative ambulation?
   a. Increased peristalsis
   b. Coughing
   c. Pneumonia
   d. Wound healing

10. Which of the following actions should the nurse take to maintain patient safety when ambulating a patient for the first time postoperatively?
    a. Use one person to assist patient.
    b. Use two people to assist patient.
    c. Encourage patient to "dangle" self 1 hour before ambulation.
    d. Give narcotic 15 minutes before ambulation.

11. The nurse is caring for a patient with a bowel resection. Which of the following would indicate that the patient's gastrointestinal tract is resuming normal function?
    a. Firm abdomen
    b. Excessive thirst
    c. Presence of flatus
    d. Absent bowel sounds

12. The patient is dangling at the bedside and states, "Oh, my stomach is tearing open." Which of the following actions should the nurse immediately take when dehiscence occurs?
    a. Have patient sit upright in a chair.
    b. Slow intravenous fluids.
    c. Have patient lie down.
    d. Obtain a sterile suture set.

13. When the LPN/LVN is assisting the patient to use an incentive spirometer, which of the following actions by the patient indicates that the patient needs further teaching on how to use the spirometer?
    a. Taking two normal breaths before use
    b. Inhaling deeply to reach target
    c. Sitting upright before use
    d. Exhaling deeply to reach target

14. After surgery the nurse notes that the patient's urine is dark amber and concentrated. Which of the following does the nurse understand may be the reason for this?
    a. The sympathetic nervous system saves fluid in response to stress of surgery.
    b. The sympathetic nervous system diureses fluid in response to stress of surgery.
    c. The parasympathetic nervous system saves fluid in response to stress of surgery.
    d. The parasympathetic nervous system diureses fluid in response to stress of surgery.

Multiple response item. Select all that apply.
15. The patient develops a low-grade fever 18 hours postoperatively and has diminished breath sounds. Which of the following actions is most appropriate for the nurse to take to prevent complications?
    a. Administer antibiotics.
    b. Encourage coughing and deep breathing.
    c. Administer acetaminophen (Tylenol).
    d. Decrease fluid intake.
    e. Ambulate patient as ordered.

Nursing Care of Patients with Emergent Conditions and Disaster/Bioterrorism Response

12

VOCABULARY

Match the word with its definition.

1. _______ Skin scraped away because of injury
2. _______ Disease caused by organism entering body through an open wound resulting in convulsions, muscle spasms, stiffness of the jaw, coma, and death
3. _______ Insufficient intake of oxygen
4. _______ Inadequate and progressively failing tissue perfusion that can result in cellular death
5. _______ Irregular tear of the skin
6. _______ Loss of water and electrolytes through heavy sweating, causing hypovolemia
7. _______ Tearing away or crushing of body limbs
8. _______ Frozen body parts that are white or yellow-white
9. _______ A biological weapon that may occur in three forms: inhalational, cutaneous, and gastrointestinal
10. _______ A biological weapon that can result in a severe febrile illness with hemoptysis as a classic sign

A. Asphyxia
B. Tetanus
C. Abrasion
D. Laceration
E. Shock
F. Amputation
G. Heat exhaustion
H. Frostbite
I. Anthrax
J. Plague

PRINCIPLES FOR TREATING SHOCK

Indicate whether the statement is true or false, and correct the false statement.

1. Maintain an open airway and give oxygen as ordered. _______________________
2. Control external bleeding by indirect pressure. _______________________
3. Apply cooling blanket to keep patient cool. _______________________
4. If possible, keep the patient supine. _______________________
5. Take hourly vital signs. _______________________
6. Give the patient oral fluids. _______________________
7. Administer intravenous fluids as ordered. _______________________

SIGNS AND SYMPTOMS OF INCREASED INTRACRANIAL PRESSURE

Indicate whether the sign is an early sign or a late sign of increased intracranial pressure.

1. _______ Abnormal posturing
2. _______ Altered level of consciousness
3. _______ Amnesia
4. _______ Changes in respiratory pattern
5. _______ Changes in speech
6. _______ Decreased pulse rate
7. _______ Dilated nonreactive pupils
8. _______ Drowsiness
9. _______ Headache
10. _______ Nausea and vomiting
11. _______ Unresponsiveness
12. _______ Widening pulse pressure

A. Early sign
B. Late sign

ASSESSMENT OF MOTOR FUNCTION

Complete the table.

If the patient is unable to	The lesion is above the level of
_____________	C-5 to C-7
Extend and flex legs	_____________
Flex foot, extend toes	_____________
_____________	S-3 to S-5

HYPERTHERMIA

Indicate whether the sign is an early sign or a late sign of hyperthermia caused by exposure to a hot environment.

1. _______ Core body temperature 100.4°F to 102.2°F (38°C to 39°C)
2. _______ Diaphoresis
3. _______ Hot, dry, flushed skin
4. _______ Hypotension
5. _______ Pulse rate more than 100
6. _______ Increasing body core temperature of 106°F (41°C) or more
7. _______ Cool, clammy skin
8. _______ Altered mental status
9. _______ Coma or seizures
10. _______ Dizziness

A. Early sign
B. Late sign

PRINCIPLES FOR DISASTER OR BIOTERRORISM RESPONSE

Fill in the blank.

1. A disaster _____________ existing personnel, facilities, and equipment

2. Hospitals activate _____________ _____________ in a disaster.

3. In a disaster, off-duty staff are _____________ _____ and noncritical patients are _____________.

4. The emergency department serves as the _____________ and _____________ area.

5. Those treated first are the most ___________ injuried but have the greatest chance for __________ recovery.

6. Disaster ____________ are conducted on a regular basis.

7. You should be ____________ with your ____________ in a disaster.

8. Clinical illness from a biological weapon may differ from ____________ infections.

CRITICAL THINKING

Read the case study and answer the questions.

Mr. Ricks, age 66, retired 1 year ago and made plans to travel with his wife. His wife unexpectedly died from a myocardial infarction 2 months ago. Mr. Ricks now lives alone. He has been withdrawn and rarely leaves the house since his wife's funeral. His son, Ted, who lives in another state, arrives for a weekend visit and is concerned about his father's behavior. Mr. Ricks has not bathed and is wearing soiled clothing. The refrigerator is bare and he keeps the curtains drawn. He continually paces and says, "I want to die." Ted takes his father to the local emergency room.

1. Why might Mr. Ricks be exhibiting this behavior change? _________________________________

2. What symptoms of an acute psychiatric episode is Mr. Ricks exhibiting? ____________________

3. Why should Mr. Ricks be referred for treatment?

4. What nursing diagnoses apply to Mr. Ricks?

5. What nursing interventions are appropriate for Mr. Ricks initially? _______________________

REVIEW QUESTIONS

Choose the best answer unless directed otherwise.

1. A patient who experiences anaphylactic shock after receiving a medication is most likely to experience which of the following symptoms?
   a. Chest pain
   b. Hot, dry skin
   c. Difficulty breathing
   d. Fever

2. The nurse is assessing a patient's extremity, which may be fractured. Which of the following is the nurse's purpose in checking capillary refill during the assessment?
   a. To evaluate arterial blood flow in an extremity
   b. To assess venous blood flow in an extremity
   c. To measure oxygen saturation of the blood
   d. To assess peripheral edema

3. The nurse anticipates that treatment for a semiconscious patient who has ingested 50 tablets of alprazolam (Xanax), a noncaustic substance, would include which of the following?
   a. Administering an antiemetic
   b. Activated charcoal
   c. Forced vomiting
   d. Forcing fluids

4. The nurse is planning care for a patient who has hyperthermia. Which of the following is an outcome criterion for hyperthermia?
   a. Core body temperature less than 94°F (34.4°C)
   b. Patient alert and oriented
   c. Skin cool and moist to touch
   d. Core body temperature greater than 101°F (38.3°C)

5. The physician orders haloperidol (Haldol) 3 mg intramuscularly for a patient who is experiencing a psychiatric crisis. Haloperidol 5 mg/mL is available. How many milliliters should the nurse give?
   a. 0.3 mL
   b. 0.5 mL
   c. 0.6 mL
   d. 1.3 mL

6. The nurse is assessing a patient who has lost a large volume of blood from a laceration. Which of the following pulse findings would indicate to the nurse that the patient requires immediate treatment?
   a. Normal, bounding pulse
   b. Slow, strong pulse
   c. Rapid, thready pulse
   d. Slow, bounding pulse

7. The nurse is admitting a trauma patient to the emergency department. Place in order of priority the areas on which data is collected as the nurse performs the primary survey. Use all options.
   a. Circulation
   b. Breathing
   c. Airway
   d. Disability

8. The nurse is caring for a patient who is bleeding from the radial artery and has lost a large volume of blood from a laceration. The nurse is applying direct pressure to the radial artery and has elevated the arm, but the wound continues to bleed. Which of the following actions should the nurse take now?
   a. Apply pressure to the carotid artery.
   b. Apply pressure to the brachial artery.
   c. Apply pressure to the femoral artery.
   d. Apply pressure to the temporal artery.

Multiple response item. Select all that apply.

9. The nurse is caring for a patient with a painful rash on the face and forearms who is febrile. Which of the following items is important for the unvaccinated nurse to use while providing care to the patient?
   a. Mask
   b. Gown
   c. Gloves
   d. Fit-tested N95 respirator
   e. Shoe covers

10. Which of the following monitoring is a priority for the nurse when caring for a patient with botulism exposure?
    a. Gag reflex
    b. Pupil response
    c. Corneal reflex
    d. Babinski's response

UNDERSTANDING LIFE SPAN INFLUENCES ON HEALTH AND ILLNESS

CHECKLIST FOR LEARNING SUCCESS

Influences on Health and Illness

- ❏ Health, wellness, illness
- ❏ Nurse's role in supporting and promoting wellness
- ❏ Young adult
- ❏ Middle-aged adult
- ❏ Older adult
- ❏ Chronic illness
- ❏ Nursing care

Nursing Care of Older Adult Patients

- ❏ Physiological aging changes
- ❏ Cognitive and psychological aging changes
- ❏ Health promotion for older patients
- ❏ Nursing implications for older patients

Nursing Care of Patient at Home

- ❏ Introduction to home health nursing
- ❏ History of home health nursing
- ❏ Home health eligibility
- ❏ Home health care team
- ❏ Transition from hospital based nursing to home health care
- ❏ The role of the LPN/LVN in home health
- ❏ Steps in the home health visit
- ❏ Nursing process: the home health patient
- ❏ Other types of home health nursing

End of Life

- ❏ Advance directive
- ❏ Living wills
- ❏ Durable medical power of attorney
- ❏ End-of-life choices
- ❏ Communicating with dying patients
- ❏ The dying process

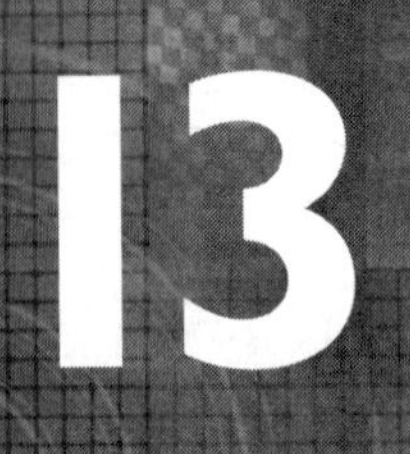

Developmental Considerations in the Nursing Care of Adults

VOCABULARY

Unscramble the word that fits the definition.

1. Short-term intermittent rest provided to care givers—*serptei crea* ______________

2. Perception that one's own actions will not affect an outcome—*wporelsesesns* ______________

3. Condition of long duration—*rhcnoic* ______________

4. Life principles that pervade one's being—*sitrpiauilty* ______________

5. State in which person sees no alternatives or choices—*pohelesnsses* ______________

6. A certain life time frame containing tasks an individual needs to accomplish for high-level wellness—
   evdlepoemnatl taseg ______________ ______________

CHRONIC ILLNESS AND THE OLDER ADULT

Find and correct the seven errors.

Older adults constitute one of the smallest age groups living with chronic illness. Older adult spouses or older family members rarely have to care for a chronically ill family member. Children of older adults who themselves are reaching their 40s are being expected to care for their parents. These older adult caregivers do not experience chronic illness themselves. For older adult spouses, it is usually the less ill spouse who provides care to the other spouse. The older adult family unit is at great risk for ineffective coping or further development of health problems. Nurses should assess ill members of the older adult family to ensure that their health needs are being met.

Older adults are not concerned about becoming dependent and a burden to others. They may become depressed and give up hope if they feel that they are a burden to others. Establishing long-term goals or self-care activities that allow them to participate or have small suc-cesses are important nursing actions that can decrease their self-esteem.

CRITICAL THINKING

Read the case study and answer the questions.

Mrs. Martin is hospitalized for an exacerbation of her multiple sclerosis. She tells the nurse she is tired of being ill and is not getting any better. She says, "When I am in the hospital, I cannot attend church, which is my only enjoyment." Later in the day, Mrs. Martin is tearful and withdrawn when the nurse makes rounds.

1. What further data collection should the nurse obtain to meet Mrs. Martin's needs? ______________

2. What possible nursing diagnoses would be appropriate for Mrs. Martin? ______________

3. What interventions could the nurse use to meet Mrs. Martin's goal? _______________

4. How would the nurse know that Mrs. Martin's goal has been met? _______________

Choose the best answer.

1. As the nurse assesses a patient's developmental stage, which of the following does the nurse understand is Erikson's developmental stage for the older adult?
   a. Generativity versus self-absorption
   b. Identity versus role confusion
   c. Intimacy versus isolation
   d. Integrity versus despair

2. The nurse is developing a plan of care for a patient, age 68, focusing on preventive health care. While planning the care, the nurse understands that aging processes are most affected by which of the following factors?
   a. Stress management
   b. Financial issues
   c. Age at retirement
   d. Hobbies

3. A patient, age 64, is active and wants to learn how to promote her health. Which of the following actions by the nurse supports the patient's desire to actively promote her health?
   a. Assign responsibilities for the patient's care to her family.
   b. Select a family physician for the patient.
   c. List health-care activities for the patient to carry out.
   d. Ask the patient to select desired health-care activities.

4. The home care nurse is caring for a patient with emphysema who seems depressed. Which of the following nursing interventions increases the patient's participation in self-care and assists with improving the patient's depression?
   a. Being a caretaker instead of a partner
   b. Assisting the patient instead of doing everything for the patient
   c. Performing activities of daily living (ADLs) for the patient instead of empowering the patient
   d. Doing everything for the patient instead of assisting the patient

5. The nurse is caring for a patient who is recovering from a stroke. Which of the following nursing interventions during rehabilitation will most increase the patient's self-esteem?
   a. Offering praise for small patient efforts
   b. Offering praise for major patient efforts
   c. Performing ADLs for the patient
   d. Assisting patient at first sign of difficulty with ADLs

6. Which of the following nursing actions might be most helpful for psychosocial intervention for the patient who is withdrawn, depressed, or tense because of isolation resulting from a chronic illness?
   a. Avoiding the use of humor
   b. Reading comics or jokes from magazines
   c. Maintaining a serious demeanor
   d. Limiting conversation to a minimum

7. Which of the following can result for caregivers of chronically ill patients when respite care is not available?
   a. Personal time increases.
   b. Rest time increases.
   c. Financial costs decrease.
   d. Stress increases.

8. Which of the following is a health promotion method useful for the chronically ill patient?
   a. Making the choices for the patient
   b. Setting the goals for the family
   c. Setting the goals for the patient
   d. Allowing the patient to make informed decisions

9. In contributing to the chronically ill patient's plan of care, which of the following is an appropriate nursing intervention for the nurse to include to empower the patient?
   a. Provide educational information.
   b. Limit visiting hours for family members.
   c. Ask family members to provide care.
   d. Set goals for the patient and family.

10. Which of the following does the nurse understand is an example of a chronic illness?
    a. Peripheral vascular disease
    b. Cellulitis
    c. Peritonitis
    d. Bowel obstruction

11. Which of the following is a primary task that patients who are chronically ill need to perform?
    a. Being willing and able to carry out the medical regimen
    b. Reducing social activities to compensate for limitations
    c. Learning how to play the sick role
    d. Refusing to accept negative changes

12. Which of the following does the nurse understand is a congenital chronic illness?
    a. Head injury
    b. Malabsorption syndrome
    c. Chronic obstructive pulmonary disease
    d. Arthritis

13. The nurse is caring for a patient with Huntington's disease. The family asks what the cause of the illness is. Which of the following responses is most appropriate by the nurse?
    a. Genetic
    b. Congenital
    c. Acquired

Nursing Care of Older Adult Patients

VOCABULARY

Fill in the blank with the word for the definition.

1. _______________ Behaviors that are performed in the care and maintenance of self and surroundings
2. _______________ Irregular heart rhythm
3. _______________ Opacity of the lens of the eye, its capsule, or both
4. _______________ State of feeling or mind
5. _______________ Accidental drawing of foreign substances into the airway
6. _______________ Collection of excess fluid in body tissues
7. _______________ A group of eye diseases characterized by increased intraocular pressure
8. _______________ The act or process of coughing up materials from the air passageways leading to the lungs
9. _______________ A condition of sluggish or difficult bowel action/evacuation
10. _______________ The body's attempts to maintain a balance whenever a change occurs
11. _______________ Abnormal accumulation of fibrosis connective tissue in skin, muscle, or joint capsule that prevents normal mobility
12. _______________ An open sore or lesion of the skin that develops because of prolonged pressure against an area
13. _______________ Excessive urination at night
14. _______________ External variables that determine the occurrence and rate of structural and functional declines in the human body over time
15. _______________ Age-related breakdown of the macular area of the retina of the eye, disrupting central vision
16. _______________ A condition in which there is a reduction in the mass of bone per unit volume
17. _______________ None or minimal stimulation of senses that creates potential for maladaptive coping
18. _______________ Highest level of patient activity considering the patient's condition
19. _______________ A process to orient a person to names, dates, time, and other pertinent information through use of repeating messages
20. _______________ Excessive stimulation of the senses that creates the potential for maladaptive coping

AGING CHANGES

Match the aging change with the effect of the change.

1. __A__ Increased conduction time
2. __C__ Decreased blood vessel elasticity
3. __E__ Leg veins dilate, valves less efficient
4. __F__ Basal metabolic rate slows
5. __B__ Decreased cardiac output
6. __H__ Decreased insulin release
7. __D__ Irregular heartbeats
8. __G__ Altered adrenal hormone production
9. __K__ Decreased gag reflex
10. __N__ Decreased peristalsis
11. __M__ Reduced liver enzymes
12. __J__ Decreased saliva
13. __I__ Delayed gastric emptying
14. __L__ Decreased bladder size and tone, changes from pear to funnel shaped
15. __O__ Decreased kidney concentrating ability
16. __P__ Less sodium saved
17. __Q__ Reduced renal blood flow
18. __R__ Decreased immune function
19. __T__ Body content water loss
20. __U__ Decreased sebaceous/sweat gland
21. __S__ Reduced cell replacement
22. __V__ Muscle responses slowed
23. __W__ Decreased brain blood flow
24. __Z__ Less vaginal lubrication
25. __X__ Decreased sensation
26. __Y__ Decreased lung capacity

A. Heart rate slows, unable to increase quickly
B. Less oxygen delivered to tissues
C. Increased blood pressure and cardiac workload
D. Poor heart oxygenation
E. Varicose veins, fluid accumulation in tissues
F. Possible weight gain
G. Decreased ability to respond to stress
H. Hyperglycemia
I. Appetite may be reduced
J. Dry mouth, altered taste
K. Increased aspiration risk
L. Frequency of urination
M. Reduced drug metabolism/detoxification
N. Reduced appetite, constipation
O. Nocturia
P. Risk of dehydration
Q. Decreased renal clearance of all medications
R. Greater infection and cancer risk
S. Slower healing process
T. Dryness of the skin
U. Decreased temperature regulation
V. Response time increased
W. Short-term memory loss
X. Risk of injury, burns
Y. Dyspnea with activity
Z. Painful intercourse

COMMUNICATING WITH THE HEARING IMPAIRED

Indicate whether the statement is true or false, and correct false statements.

1. __T__ Ensure that hearing aids are turned on and have working batteries.
2. __F__ The speaker should turn to the side so the speaker's profile is visible to patient.
3. __F__ Speak toward the patient's impaired side of hearing.
4. __T__ Speak in a clear, moderate-volume, low-pitched tone.
5. __T__ Do not shout because doing so distorts sounds.
6. __F__ Recognize that high-frequency tones and consonant sounds are lost last—*s, z, sh, ch, d, g.*
7. __T__ Eliminate background noise because it distorts sounds.

MEDICATIONS

Find the six errors and correct them.

Older patients are less susceptible to drug-induced illness and adverse medication side effects for various reasons. They take few medicines for the one chronic illness that they have. Different medications interact and produce side effects that can be dangerous. Over-the-counter medicines that older patients take, as well as the self-prescribed extracts, elixirs, herbal teas, cultural healing substances, and other home remedies commonly used by individuals of their age cohort, do not influence other medications.

If an older patient crushes a large enteric-coated pill so it can be taken in food and is easily swallowed, it enhances the enteric protection and can inadvertently cause damage to the stomach and intestinal system. Some patients unintentionally skip prescribed doses in an effort to save money. When prescribed doses are not being taken as expected, problems do not clear up as quickly and new problems may result. The nurse should educate the older patient and the patient's family. Patients need to know what each prescribed pill is for, when it is prescribed to be taken, and how it should be taken.

CRITICAL THINKING

Read the following case study and answer the questions. This is a values clarification exercise.

While making 10 p.m. rounds in the extended-care facility, the nurse looks into Mr. B's room to find Mr. B and a female resident from down the hall together, sleeping soundly in Mr. B's bed with the side rails up. Mr. B and the female resident are both 63 years of age. Mr. S, who is Mr. B's roommate, is sound asleep alone in his own bed.

1. What are your initial feelings about this situation?
   ____
   ____

2. What influences your feelings? _______________
   ____

3. What is the first thing that you would do after this discovery? ___________________________________

4. What issues did you consider before making this decision? ____

5. How will you interact with these patients in the future?
   ____

REVIEW QUESTIONS

Choose the best answer.

1. A 72-year-old patient has been seeing a doctor for treatment of glaucoma for the last 5 years. Which of the following symptoms does the nurse expect the patient to relate when discussing the symptoms?
   a. Headaches more severe in the evening
   b. Blurred vision when attempting to focus
   c. Morning headaches that disappear after rising
   d. Increased sensitivity to light in the early morning

2. As the nurse performs an oral assessment on an 84-year-old patient, which of the following is an expected finding within the patient's mouth caused by advancing age?
   a. Loss of teeth
   b. Hardness of the gums
   c. Increased production of saliva
   d. Decreased taste sensitivity for salt

3. As the nurse collects data on a 79-year-old patient, which of the following does the nurse recognize as an aging change in the cardiovascular system?
   a. Increased cardiac output
   b. Increased peripheral vascular resistance
   c. Increased resting heart rate
   d. Increased cardiac reserve

4. Which of the following does the nurse understand is the rationale for dangling a 70-year-old patient at the bedside before helping the patient to stand upright?
   a. To provide a heightened awareness of body position
   b. To accommodate a less efficient circulatory system
   c. To strengthen legs
   d. To reduce anxiety about getting up

5. As the nurse provides care to an 80-year-old patient with an intravenous (IV) infusion, the nurse understands that it is essential for older patients who are receiving IV fluids to be monitored closely to prevent which of the following?
   a. Circulatory distress
   b. Dislodging of the IV
   c. Venous distention
   d. Increased urinary output

6. The nurse is talking with a patient who is hard of hearing and is having the most difficulty with high-pitched tones. To increase the patient's hearing, which of the following should the nurse do when speaking with the patient?
   a. Speak slowly with emphasis on important words.
   b. Double the voice volume.
   c. Whisper responses in close proximity to the patient's ear.
   d. Use a modulated voice and talk normally in either ear.

7. The nurse understands that wax build-up in an older patient's ears can cause which type of hearing loss?
   a. Sensorineural
   b. Bone conduction
   c. Perceptive
   d. Neural

8. The nurse understands that which of the following factors is most often the cause of sexual dysfunction for older people?
   a. Physical factors
   b. Psychological factors
   c. Social factors
   d. Environmental factors

9. A nurse is working in an extended care facility. Which of the following nursing behaviors demonstrates the nurse's respect for the older patient's sexuality?
   a. Providing privacy time for a patient by enclosing the bed with the curtain and ensuring that the patient is undisturbed for an hour
   b. Entering a patient's room without knocking when a visitor is present
   c. Walking in on a patient and visitor during an embrace to prepare medications
   d. Changing the subject when a patient expresses feelings toward a friend

10. Which of the following actions should be taken to help an older person prevent osteoporosis?
    a. Decrease dietary intake of calcium.
    b. Encourage regular exercise.
    c. Increase dietary intake of salt.
    d. Increase dietary protein intake.

Nursing Care of the Patient at Home

15

VOCABULARY

Match the term to the correct definition.

1. _______ Autonomous
2. _______ Case management
3. _______ Certified
4. _______ Collaborative care
5. _______ Community resources
6. _______ Homebound
7. _______ Private duty
8. _______ Respite care
9. _______ Skilled nursing
10. _______ Start of care

A. Care that can only be delivered by a licensed professional nurse
B. Occurs when a patient is unable to leave his or her home to obtain necessary health services
C. To work together to achieve a goal
D. Coordinates care between patient, physician, and caregivers
E. A physician's order that allows home health services to care for a patient for 60 days
F. To work independently
G. Available to a home health patient to improve his or her quality of care; usually coordinated by a social service worker
H. Scheduled care to assist the patient with personnel and homemaking needs
I. Begins on the first day of nursing services
J. Provides family members and caregivers time to take care of themselves

HOME HEALTH SERVICES

Match the home health services/roles to the appropriate definition.

1. _______ Social services
2. _______ Physical therapy
3. _______ Occupational therapy
4. _______ Registered nurse
5. _______ Certified nursing assistant

A. Assists the patient with activities of daily living
B. Develops the plan of care and manages the care of the patient during home health services
C. Assists the patient with developing independence with activities of daily living
D. Assists the patient with access to community resources
E. Assists the patient with strength and gait training

CRITICAL THINKING

Mrs. Thompson was just discharged from the hospital following an exacerbation of her respiratory disease. Her health history includes chronic obstructive pulmonary disease (COPD), type II diabetes, and coronary artery disease (CAD). She is receiving O_2 therapy at 2 L/min via nasal cannula. She has a skin tear on her right lower extremity requiring dressing changes every other day for 4 weeks. The physician increased her heart medications to include a beta blocker for heart rate control.

Mrs. Thompson lives alone and has verbalized to the RN, on admission, that it is difficult for her to prepare meals and "get around the house." She has one married daughter who lives locally and works full time.

1. How often will Mrs. Thompson require skilled nursing services? _______________________________

____

____

____

2. What services will the home health nurse be performing? _______________________________

____

____

____

3. What are some safety considerations for Mrs. Thompson? _______________________________

____

____

____

4. Would Mrs. Thompson benefit from any other home health services? _______________________________

____

____

____

Choose the best answer unless directed otherwise.

1. Which of the following nursing leaders demonstrated the impact nurses can have with the care and improvement of patients in the home?
   a. Florence Nightingale
   b. Clara Barton
   c. Lillian Wald
   d. Jean Watson

2. The nurse is making a first-time visit to a patient at home. Which of the following techniques could the home health nurse use to develop trust with the patient?
   a. Review patient's history to plan patient needs before visit.
   b. Call the night before the visit to set a time for the visit.
   c. Acknowledge patient's fears that are expressed.
   d. Discuss treatment plans with the patient only.

Multiple response item. Select all that apply.

3. The nurse collects safety data on an initial visit to a patient's home who has returned home from the hospital and has an infected abdominal wound requiring dressing changes. Which of the following interventions should the nurse include in the plan of care to promote safety in the home?
   a. Explain to the patient never to get out of bed without assistance.
   b. Instruct a family member to be available at all times to assist with ambulation.
   c. Clean the patient's home each visit to maintain asepsis.
   d. Instruct the family to remove all scatter rugs.
   e. Ask family to install handrails in the hallway for ambulation.
   f. Clear walkways of all clutter.

4. A patient has just been discharged from the hospital following open heart surgery. The patient's spouse is the primary caregiver and confides that handling all the finances, the patient's complex medication regime, assistance with activities of daily living (ADLs), and general household management is a concern. Which of the following would be an appropriate nursing diagnosis for the patient's spouse?
   a. Ineffective coping
   b. Powerlessness
   c. Ineffective health maintenance
   d. Risk for caregiver role strain

5. The nurse arrives at a patient's home. Which of the following interventions performed by the nurse would demonstrate understanding of the importance of following infection control principles in the home?
   a. Setting the nurse's home health bag on the floor
   b. Cleaning supplies after each home health visit
   c. Hand washing in the patient's kitchen sink
   d. Using dressing supplies sitting opened on table

Fill in the blank (Calculation)
6. The nurse is to give a patient morphine 8 mg IM for pain. The nurse has available 10 mg of morphine/mL . How many mL will the nurse give?
   _______________ mL

Multiple response item. Select all that apply.
7. The nurse is making a home visit to a 68-year-old patient and is reinforcing medication teaching that was done in the hospital setting. The nurse understands that the teaching will be more effective with which of the following techniques?
   a. Provide a long teaching session.
   b. Include a support person.
   c. Make instructions simple.
   d. Provide demonstration.
   e. Repeat instructions often.

8. When providing care to a patient in the patient's home, the nurse understands that which of the following persons is in control of the home care environment?
   a. Family
   b. Physician
   c. Nurse
   d. Patient

9. The LPN is visiting a patient to check blood glucose and administer insulin. As the LPN obtains the insulin from the refrigerator where the patient stores it, the LPN observes that dirty dishes are stacked in the kitchen sink, and there is only a moldy opened can of soup, a sandwich, and cat food in the refrigerator. Which of the following actions should the LPN take regarding the visit findings?
   a. Inform the RN of the moldy and sparse food.
   b. Tell the patient to wash the dishes.
   c. Notify the RN that the patient is eating cat food.
   d. Wash the dirty dishes.

Multiple response item. Select all that apply.
10. Which of the following could the nurse do to prepare for a home health visit and ensure that it is a safe and effective visit?
    a. Give the patient a time range for arrival.
    b. Provide an exact time for arrival.
    c. Obtain driving directions to the patient's home.
    d. Park in the patient's driveway.
    e. Keep gas tank filled.

Nursing Care of Patients at the End of Life

VOCABULARY

Fill in the blank.

1. Documents instructing caregivers in patients' medical preferences at end of life are called

   _____________ _____________.

2. A _____________ _____________ _____________ _____________ document specifies who can make

   decisions for a patient when he can no longer make his own decisions.

3. Patients qualify for _____________ care when their prognosis is 6 months or less.

4. Care of the body after death is called _____________ _____________.

5. The nurse who communicates patients' and families' wishes to the health team is acting as a

   patient _____________.

TRUE OR FALSE?

Answer True or False after each statement.

1. Elderly patients usually gain weight while undergoing treatment in a hospital. _______

2. Only a few health insurance companies provide a hospice benefit. _______

3. Insomnia, headaches, and fatigue can be a sign of grief in nurses. _______

4. Dehydration in dying patients causes endorphins to be released that will enhance comfort. _______

5. Patients who live longer than 6 months while on hospice will be discharged from the hospice

   program. _______

6. Terminal illness is experienced by the whole family. _______

7. To improve the chance of success for patients receiving cardiopulmonary resuscitation (CPR) at the

   time of cardiac arrest, CPR must be started within 8 minutes. _______

8. One benefit of withholding artificial fluids in patients who are actively dying is fewer pharyngeal and

   lung secretions. _______

9. Eighty percent of communication with terminal patients and their families is nonverbal. _______

10. Confusion and agitation are two common indicators that elderly patients are approaching the end of

    life. _______

CRITICAL THINKING

Read the case study and answer the questions.

Your patient, Mrs. Brown is actively dying from end-stage lung cancer. List at least two nursing interventions that may be helpful to treat each symptom she is experiencing:

Dyspnea _______________________________

____

Bowel and bladder incontinence _________

____

Copious oral secretions _________________

Body temperature changes _______________

____

Restlessless __________________________

____

REVIEW QUESTIONS

Choose the best answer.

1. Research on patients with dementia who received tube feedings revealed which of the following risks?
   a. The risk of aspiration was decreased.
   b. The risk of aspiration was increased.
   c. The patients gained excess weight.
   d. Pressure ulcers healed more quickly.

2. A family member asks why a dying patient is receiving morphine when he doesn't appear to be in any pain. Which response by the nurse is best?
   a. "Morphine will make him less aware of his surroundings."
   b. "Morphine will make his breathing more comfortable."
   c. "Morphine helps keep his temperature under control."
   d. "Morphine helps him sleep."

3. What should the nurse do first after a patient has been pronounced dead?
   a. Contact the nursing supervisor.
   b. Remove the patient's tubes and create a clean, peaceful impression for the family.
   c. Make sure the patient gets to the funeral home within 12 hours for embalming.
   d. Move the patient out of the hospital room to the morgue.

4. A dying patient appears confused and keeps saying he sees his wife who died 10 years earlier. The family appears upset by this. What teaching should the nurse provide?
   a. Teach them to redirect the patient and gently remind him that his wife died long ago.
   b. Explain that this happens because of the medications that the patient is receiving.
   c. Explain that this is a common occurrence and encourage them to allow him to talk about his experience.
   d. Explain that this can occur when the brain is deprived of oxygen, and then get an order for oxygen if the patient does not already have it.

5. A dying patient's family members are upset and crying. Which action by the nurse is best?
   a. Sustain eye contact and encourage them to talk about their concerns.
   b. Ask them to speak quietly so as not to disturb the other patients.
   c. Tell them for the sake of their loved one, they need to compose themselves.
   d. Move them to another room away from the patient.

6. An older patient with chronic disease is very weak and chokes when he tries to eat. His wife is upset and wants a feeding tube inserted. The physician has told her that the patient is dying and that a tube will not make him live longer. The wife is now crying in the hallway. Which response by the nurse is best?
   a. Reiterate what the doctor said about him not living any longer with a tube.
   b. Tell her that a tube is uncomfortable for the patient.
   c. Tell her you will feed him more slowly to prevent choking.
   d. Acknowledge how hard this is for her, as she has taken such good care of feeding him throughout the course of his illness.

7. A patient being discharged from the hospital has decided she does not want to be resuscitated should she experience a cardiopulmonary arrest. What document will she need signed and in place to assure this will not happen upon her return home?
   a. A Living Will
   b. An Advance Medical Directive
   c. A Durable Medical Power of Attorney
   d. A Durable Do Not Resuscitate (DNR) document

8. What question can be most effective in finding out the patient's understanding of the severity of his or her illness?
   a. How do you feel about your illness?
   b. How is your family coping with your illness?
   c. What has the doctor told you about your illness?
   d. What would you like to do about your illness?

9. The family of a terminally ill patient asks a nurse if they may bathe their loved one after death, in keeping with their cultural traditions. Which response is best?
   a. "You should concentrate on the time you have with him before he dies."
   b. "Your cultural traditions are important and will be supported by our staff."
   c. "Our staff will make sure he is clean and bathed."
   d. "That won't be necessary, as the funeral home takes care of bathing the patient."

unit FOUR

UNDERSTANDING THE IMMUNE SYSTEM

CHECKLIST FOR LEARNING SUCCESS

Review of Anatomy and Physiology

- ❏ Immune:
  - ❏ Antigens
  - ❏ Lymphocytes
  - ❏ Antibodies
  - ❏ Mechanisms of immunity
  - ❏ Types of immunity
  - ❏ Aging effects

Major Disorders

- ❏ Immune:
  - ❏ Allergic rhinitis
  - ❏ Atopic dermatitis
  - ❏ Anaphylaxis
  - ❏ Urticaria
  - ❏ Angioedema
  - ❏ Hemolytic transfusion reaction
  - ❏ Serum sickness
  - ❏ Contact dermatitis
  - ❏ Transplant rejection
  - ❏ Pernicious anemia
  - ❏ Idiopathic autoimmune hemolytic anemia
  - ❏ Hashimoto's thyroiditis
  - ❏ Ankylosing spondylitis
  - ❏ Lupus erythematosus
  - ❏ Hypogammaglobulinemia
  - ❏ Human immunodeficiency virus (HIV)
  - ❏ Acquired immune deficiency syndrome (AIDS)

Nursing Assessment

- ❏ Medical history
- ❏ Physical assessment

Diagnostic Tests

- ❏ Blood studies
- ❏ Radiographic tests
- ❏ Biopsies
- ❏ Skin tests
- ❏ Gene testing

Interventions

- ❏ Immunotherapy
- ❏ Surgical management
- ❏ New therapies

Common Medications

- ❏ Antihistamines
- ❏ Antiretrovirals
- ❏ Corticosteroids
- ❏ Epinephrine
- ❏ Fusion inhibitors
- ❏ Immunosuppressives
- ❏ Immunoglobulin
- ❏ Integrase inhibitors
- ❏ Nonnucleoside analogue reverse transcriptase inhibitors
- ❏ Nucleoside analogue reverse transcriptase inhibitors
- ❏ Nucleotide analogue reverse transcriptase inhibitors
- ❏ Protease inhibitors
- ❏ Ribonucleotide reductase inhibitors
- ❏ Rho (D) immune globulin (RhoGAM)
- ❏ Thyroxine
- ❏ Vitamin B_{12}

Immune System Function, Assessment, and Therapeutic Measures

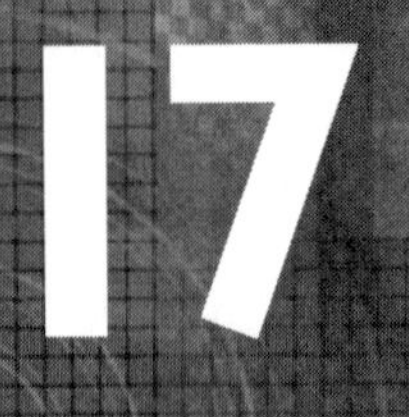

STRUCTURES OF THE IMMUNE SYSTEM

Label the following structures.

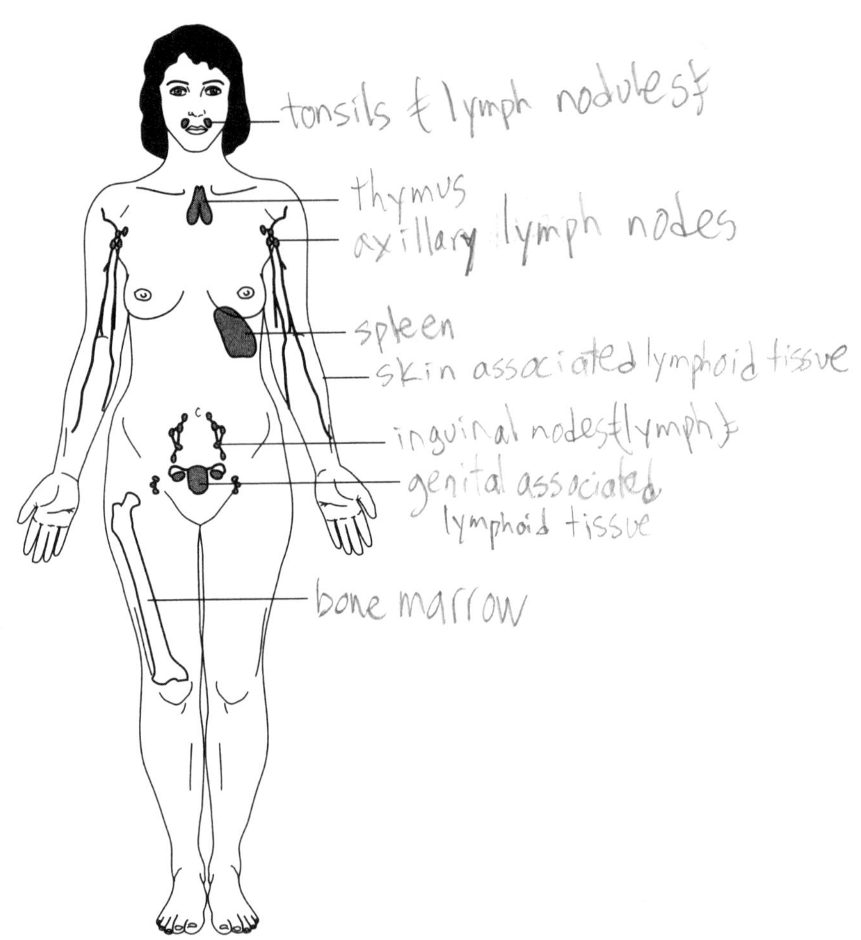

IMMUNE SYSTEM CELLS

Match each cell of the immune system with the correct description.

1. __D__ Memory cells
2. __G__ Helper T cells
3. __E__ Cytotoxic T cells
4. __B__ Plasma cells
5. __C__ Suppressor T cells
6. __A__ Macrophages
7. __F__ B cells

A. Phagocytize pathogens labeled with antibodies
B. Produce antibodies
C. Limit the immune response once the pathogen has been destroyed
D. Initiate a rapid immune response if the pathogen reenters the body
E. Destroy cells directly by lysing their membranes
F. May become plasma cells or memory cells
G. Participate in antigen recognition and activate B cells

ANTIBODIES   *IgG, IgA, IgM, IgD, IgE*

Name the proper class of antibodies for each of these functions.

Location:

1. Found on mucous membranes: __IgA__   • External secretions (eg, tears, saliva)

2. Provides long-term immunity: __IgG__   • Blood, extra-cellular fluid (ECF), lymph

3. Form the receptors on B cells: __IgD__   • B cells

4. Important in allergic reactions: __IgE__   • Mast cells or basophils
   Mast cells release histamine

5. Cross the placenta to fetal circulation: __IgG__   • Blood, ECF, lymph

6. Found in breast milk: __IgA__   • External secretions

7. The first antibody produced in an infection: __IgM__   • Blood, lymph

VOCABULARY

Fill in the blank.

1. __Antigens__ are chemical markers that identify cells or molecules.
2. __Immunity__ is the ability to destroy pathogens or other foreign material and to prevent further cases of certain infectious diseases.
3. __NK__ cells, __T-cells__, and __B-cells__ are the three types of lymphocytes.

   NK = natural killer
   T = thymus-derived
   B = bone marrow-derived

4. __T cells__ mature in the thymus gland.
5. Antibodies are also called __immunoglobulins or gamma globulins__
6. __Cell mediated__ is the type of immunity that involves only T cells.
7. __Naturally acquired active immunity__ is the type of immunity in which a person has recovered from a disease and now has antibodies and memory cells specific for that pathogen.
8. The immunoglobulin __IgG__ crosses the placenta and provides long-term immunity following recovery from an illness.
9. Lymph node enlargement with tenderness is usually indicative of __inflammation__
10. The __neutrophils__ of a white blood cell differential are increased in bacterial infections.

IMMUNE SYSTEM

Match the word with the definition.

1. ___G___ Allergy shots
2. ___D___ Tests for antibodies to human immunodeficiency virus (HIV), used as a screening test
3. ___E___ Important in allergic reactions and attaches to mast cells
4. ___A___ Swelling around the eyes
5. ___B___ A test done to confirm a diagnosis, determine a prognosis, or evaluate effectiveness of treatment
6. ___H___ Found in secretions of all mucous membranes
7. ___C___ Itching
8. ___F___ An abnormal protein found in plasma during an acute inflammatory process

A. Periorbital edema
B. Biopsies
C. Pruritus
D. Enzyme-linked immunosorbent assay *ELISA*
E. IgE
F. C-reactive protein
G. Immunotherapy
H. IgA

NURSING ASSESSMENT— SUBJECTIVE (HISTORY)

Find the 12 errors and correct the information.

Demographic data

The patient's age, gender, race, and ethnic background are important. Systemic lupus erythematosus affects men eight [*women*] times more frequently than women [*men*]. The patient's place of birth gives insight to ethnic ties. Where the patient has lived and does live may shed light on the current illness. The patient's occupation, such as that of a coal miner, may contribute to gastrointestinal [*respiratory*] symptoms. Rare [*Common*] signs and symptoms found with immune system disorders include fever, fatigue, joint pain, swollen glands, weight gain [*loss*], and skin rash.

History

Food, medication, and environmental allergies should include those that the patient experiences and those present in the family history. With a family history, a previous exposure to a substance is required [*not*] before a severe reaction occurs. Conditions such as allergic rhinitis, systemic lupus erythematosus, ankylosing spondylitis, and asthma are thought to be either familial or have a congenital genetic predisposition. If the patient's thymus gland has been removed (thymectomy), B-cell production may be altered. Corticosteroids and immunosuppressants enhance the immune response. The patient's lifestyle may place the patient at low [*high*] risk for contracting HIV. The patient's diet and usage of vitamins give insight into the depletion reserve of the immune system. Stress (environmental, physical, and psychological) can enhance [*depress*] immune system function.

CRITICAL THINKING

Read the case study and answer the following questions.

David Case, age 29, is visiting the physician because he has been extremely fatigued for several months and now has swollen lymph nodes in his neck. On palpation, the area feels enlarged, nontender, hard, and fixed.

1. What categories of data collection should the nurse obtain? ____________________

2. What might the palpation findings indicate? *Normal lymph nodes aren't palpable. Nodes that are nontender, hard, fixed, & enlarged frequently are assoc. c̄ cancer.*

3. What categories of data collection would be important to explore in detail? *If cancer is suspected: recent wt loss, occuptnl expsre, high-risk lifestyle behaviors, sexl patterns, med hx, fam hx.*

① Demographic data + age, gender, race, & ethnic background, place of birth, place of residence, occupation - past/present; pt history & blood transfusions, high-risk behaviors, allergies - drug, food, environmental; surgeries; medical hx's - past, current; physical: appearance, cardiovascular, skin, mucous membranes, respiratory, GI, renal, musculoskeletal, nervous.

REVIEW QUESTIONS

Choose the best answer.

1. A baby is born temporarily immune to the diseases to which the mother is immune. The nurse understands that this is an example of which of the following types of immunity?
   a. Naturally acquired passive immunity
   b. Artificially acquired passive immunity
   c. Naturally acquired active immunity
   d. Artificially acquired active immunity

2. Immunity to a disease after recovery is possible because the first exposure to the pathogen has stimulated the formation of which of the following?
   a. Antigens
   b. Memory cells
   c. Complement
   d. Natural killer cells

3. Which of the following immunoglobulins is first produced during an acute infection?
   a. IgG
   b. IgM
   c. IgE
   d. IgD

4. Which of the following is the function of macrophages and neutrophils?
   a. Phagocytosis
   b. Antibody production
   c. Complement fixation
   d. Suppression of autoimmunity

5. The activation of B cells in humoral immunity is assisted by which of the following?
   a. Cytotoxic T cells
   b. Helper T cells
   c. Suppressor T cells
   d. Neutrophils

6. Which of the following are chemical markers that identify cells or molecules?
   a. Antibodies
   b. Antigens
   c. T cells
   d. B lymphocytes

7. The thymus gland role with the immune system is which of the following?
   a. Maturates B cells
   b. Maturates red blood cells
   c. Maturates platelets
   d. Maturates T cells

8. Which of the following types of cells is the immune system's shutoff mechanism?
   a. Plasma cells
   b. Helper T cells
   c. Suppressor T cells
   d. B lymphocytes

9. Which of the following is the humoral immune response?
   a. B cells phagocytize the foreign antigen.
   b. T cells are stimulated by B cells and turn into plasma cells, which produce antibodies or memory cells.
   c. B cells are stimulated by T helper cells or macrophages and turn into plasma cells, which produce antibodies or memory cells.
   d. T cells produce antibodies.

10. A mother brings her children into the clinic and they are diagnosed with chickenpox. The mother had chickenpox as a child and is not concerned with contracting the disease when caring for her children. What type of immunity does this mother have?
    a. Active natural immunity
    b. Passive natural immunity
    c. Passive artificial immunity
    d. Active artificial immunity

11. Autoimmunity is defined as a phenomenon involving which of the following?
    a. Production of endotoxins that destroy B lymphocytes
    b. Inability to differentiate self from nonself
    c. Overproduction of reagin antibody
    d. Depression of the immune response

12. Antibodies are made of which of the following types of substances?
    a. Fat
    b. Sugar
    c. Protein
    d. Carbohydrate

VOCABULARY

Match the term with its definition.

1. ___J___ An anaphylactic-type reaction
2. ___K___ The type of antibodies that attach to mast cells
3. ___H___ Elimination of the offending environmental stimuli
4. ___M___ Very dry, pruritic, edematous skin
5. ___C___ Sudden, severe reaction characterized by smooth muscle spasms and capillary permeability changes
6. ___I___ Urticaria
7. ___P___ A form of lupus that affects only the skin
8. ___N___ Types of drugs used to prevent transplant rejection
9. ___B___ Painless subcutaneous and dermal erythemic eruptions with diffuse edema
10. ___D___ Requires lifelong vitamin B_{12} bec. body ∅ intrinsic factor
11. ___F___ Red blood cell (RBC) fragments seen with microscope
12. ___G___ Infant may be asymptomatic until 6 months old
13. ___O___ Antimalarial and immunosuppressent drugs may be used in treatment
14. ___A___ Causes may include heat, cold, pressure, and stress
15. ___E___ Patient education includes a diet low in iodine and high in bulk, protein, and carbohydrates
16. ___L___ Patient education includes frequent movement and the use of a hard mattress and no pillow when sleeping

A. Urticaria
B. Angioedema
C. Anaphylaxis
D. Pernicious anemia
E. Hashimoto's thyroiditis
F. Idiopathic autoimmune hemolytic anemia
G. Hypogammaglobulinemia
H. Allergic rhinitis
I. Hives
J. Type I hypersensitivity reaction
K. IgE
L. Ankylosing spondylitis
M. Atopic dermatitis
N. Immunosuppressive
O. Systemic lupus erythematosus
P. Discoid lupus erythematosus

IMMUNE DISORDERS

Fill in the blank.

1. The way hypersensitivity reactions are classified include ___I___, ___II___, ___III___, and ___IV___.
2. When allergic rhinitis occurs seasonally, it is called __hay fever__.
3. Complications of allergic rhinitis are __sinusitis__, __nasal polyps__, __asthma__, and __chronic bronchitis__.
4. __Infection__ is a complication of atopic dermatitis.
5. The first drug of choice for anaphylaxis is __IV epinephrine, dopamine__.
6. Urticaria is commonly called __hives__.
7. Angioedema differs from urticaria in that angioedema __is less pruitic__, __has more diffuse edema__, and __may last longer__.
8. The __direct coombs' test__ is used to diagnose a hemolytic transfusion reaction.
9. __Shock__ and __renal failure__ are two complications that can occur with a hemolytic transfusion reaction.
10. Today, serum sickness tends to occur when __penicillin__ and __sulfamide__ are administered to patients.
11. __Bisulfites__ and __MSG__ are two food additives that can trigger an anaphylactic reaction.
12. __Poison ivy/oak__ is the most common cause of contact dermatitis.
13. Patients with pernicious anemia are unable to absorb __Vit B_{12}__.
14. __Erythrocytapheresis__ is a process whereby abnormal RBCs are removed and replaced with normal RBCs.
15. Ankylosing spondylitis is a chronic progressive inflammatory disease of the __sacroiliac__, __costovertebral__ and __large peripheral__ joints.

IMMUNE WORD SEARCH

Figure out what words the clues represent. Then find the words in the grid. Words can go horizontally, vertically, and diagonally in all eight directions.

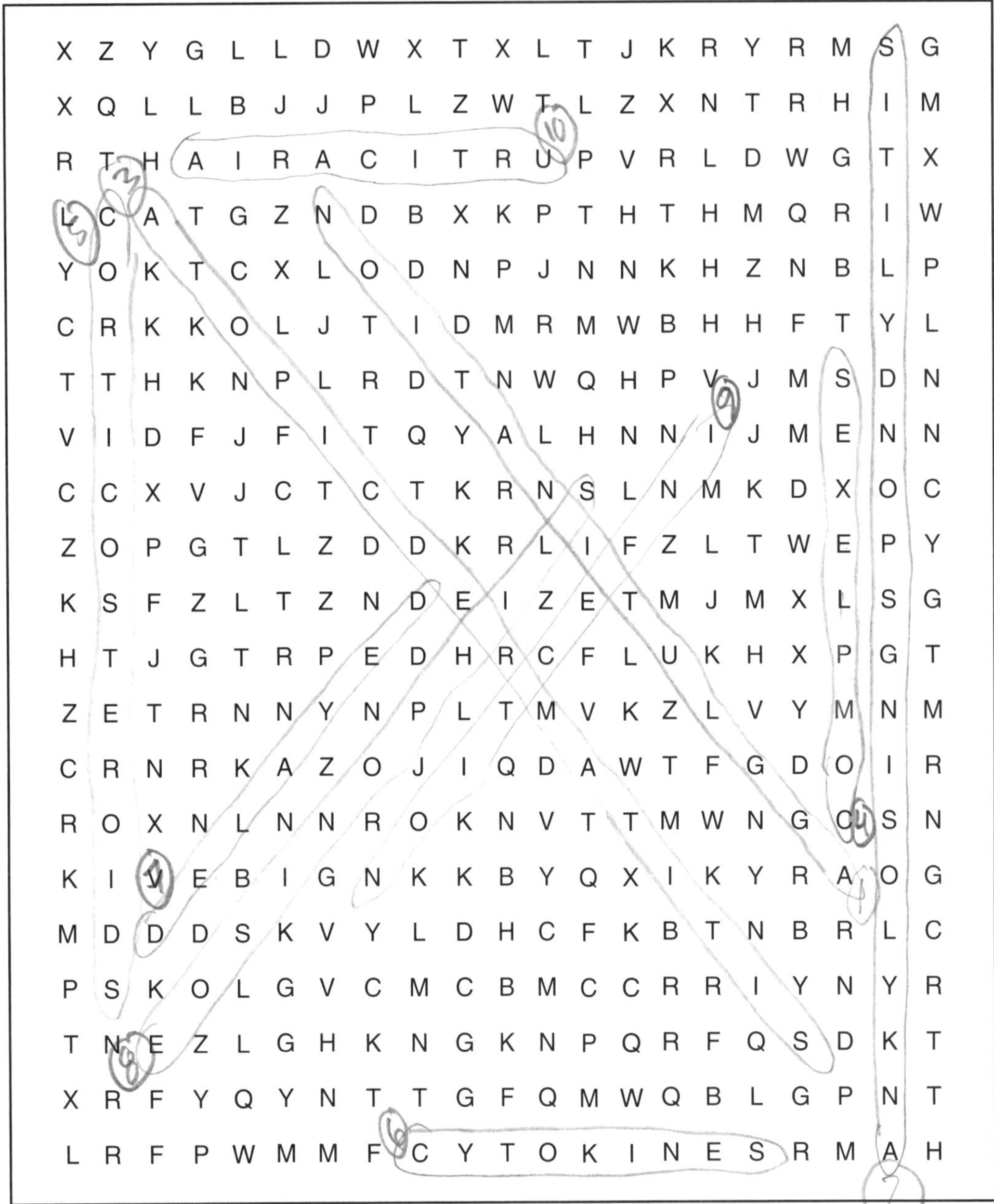

CLUES:
- When antigens clump.
- A nursing intervention for this disorder is a very firm mattress and no pillows when sleeping.
- A Type I hypersensitivity that eventually leads to a thickening of the dermis with less sweat production in these areas.
- These are formed in Type III hypersensitivity reactions, which then occlude blood vessels.
- These medications that are frequently used with immune system disorders should never be suddenly discontinued.
- Agents of the immune system that act to modify and enhance the immune and inflammatory responses.
- Type IV hypersensitivity reactions tend to be this—not immediate.
- These particular lymphocytes elevate in an allergic reaction as seen with Type I hypersensitivities.
- The main complication for a patient with hypogammaglobulinemia.
- Another term for hives.

IMMUNE PUZZLE

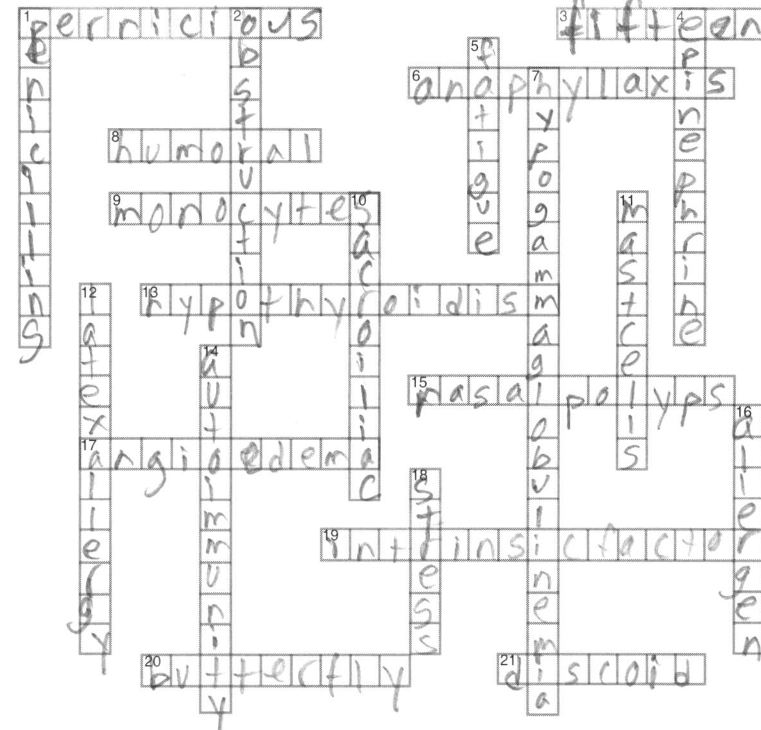

Across

1. A type of anemia that will develop in patients with autoimmune gastritis.
3. The number of minutes that a nurse should stay with a patient at the beginning of a blood transfusion.
6. This is a very serious type I hypersensitivity reaction.
8. An antibody-mediated response produced by B lymphocytes.
9. These phagocytic leukocytes are stationary.
13. Hashimoto's thyroiditis begins with this.
15. These are a complication of repeated episodes of allergic rhinitis.
17. Similar to urticaria although tends to be less pruritic, lasts longer, and involves deeper tissue.
19. The substance that is required in order for vitamin B_{12} to be absorbed in the small intestine.
20. This facial rash will occur in about 60% to 80% of systemic lupus erythematosus (SLE) patients.
21. This form of lupus erythematosus affects only the skin.

Down

1. Nowadays serum sickness tends to occur after administration of sulfonamides and these drugs.
2. A respiratory assessment finding that is considered an emergency in a patient with angioedema.
4. A drug of choice during an anaphylactic reaction.
5. This can overwhelmingly affect the activities of daily living (ADLs) of a patient with SLE.
7. This disorder is due to defective functioning B cells.
10. One group of joints that is affected in ankylosing spondylitis.
11. IgE antibodies attach to these cells in a type I hypersensitivity reaction.
12. Currently a significant type of contact dermatitis.
14. Ankylosing spondylitis is attributed to this.
16. A foreign protein or cell capable of causing an immune response.
18. An SLE flare trigger.

WORDS FOR IMMUNE PUZZLE

Allergen	Fifteen	Nasal polyps
Anaphylaxis	Humoral	Obstruction
Angioedema	Hypogammaglobulinemia	Penicillins
Autoimmunity	Hypothyroidism	Pernicious
Butterfly	Intrinsic factor	Sacroiliac
Discoid	Latex allergy	Steroids _(not used)_
Epinephrine	Mast cells	Stress
Fatigue	Monocytes	

Choose the best answer unless directed otherwise.

1. A patient has allergic rhinitis. In planning care for the patient, the nurse understands that if the patient does not remain compliant with the treatment regimen, the patient is at risk for developing which of the following?
   a. Sinusitis
   b. Anaphylaxis
   c. Lymphadenopathy
   d. Angioedema

2. A patient reports on admission being "very sick" after taking erythromycin in the past. The patient is to receive erythromycin now. Which of the following actions should the nurse take regarding giving the antibiotic?
   a. Give the antibiotic.
   b. Give half of the dose.
   c. Do not give the antibiotic.
   d. Discontinue the antibiotic.

3. A patient is being given penicillin via intravenous piggyback and develops an anaphylactic reaction. Which of the following should be the nurse's first action?
   a. Call the doctor.
   b. Call for help.
   c. Maintain the antibiotic.
   d. Turn off the antibiotic.

4. As the nurse collects data on a patient, which of the following is a symptom that may be found that the patient with anaphylaxis may be experiencing?
   a. Dermatitis
   b. Delirium
   c. Sinusitis
   d. Wheezing

5. Which of the following is the medication of choice for anaphylaxis that the nurse should anticipate would be ordered?
   a. Epinephrine
   b. Theophylline (Theo-Dur)
   c. Digoxin (Lanoxin)
   d. Furosemide (Lasix)

6. A patient is admitted with a 2-month history of fatigue, shortness of breath, pallor, and dizziness. The patient is diagnosed with idiopathic autoimmune hemolytic anemia. On reviewing the laboratory results, the nurse notes which of the following that confirms this diagnosis?
   a. RBC fragments
   b. Macrocytic, normochromic RBCs
   c. Microcytic, hypochromic RBCs
   d. Hemoglobin molecules

7. A patient, age 45, had a portion of stomach removed. The patient must take vitamin B_{12}. The nurse should include in the patient's teaching plan that if the patient does not take the vitamin B_{12}, which one of the following will develop?
   a. Iron deficiency anemia
   b. Pernicious anemia
   c. Sickle cell anemia
   d. Acquired hemolytic anemia

8. A patient is diagnosed with Hashimoto's thyroiditis and asks what causes it. The nurse would respond that the destruction of the thyroid in this condition is due to which of the following?
   a. Antigen-antibody complexes
   b. Autoantibodies
   c. Viral infection
   d. Bacterial infection

9. Which of the following is a disease process characterized by a chronic progressive inflammation of the
sacroiliac and costovertebral joints and adjacent soft
tissue?
   a. Rheumatoid arthritis
   b. Kyphosis
   c. Scoliosis
   d. Ankylosing spondylitis

Multiple response item. Select all that apply.
10. A patient who was walking in the woods disturbed a
beehive, was stung, and was taken to the emergency
department immediately due to allergies to bee stings.
Which of the following symptoms would the nurse
expect to see upon admission of this patient?
    a. Pallor around the sting bites
    b. Numbness and tingling in the extremities
    c. Respiratory stridor
    d. Retinal hemorrhage
    e. Tachycardia
    f. Dyspnea

11. A 45-year-old patient has a long-standing history of
allergies to pollen. Which of the following actions
indicates that the patient does not understand how to
control this disease?
    a. Staying indoors on dry, windy days
    b. Driving in the car with the windows open
    c. Refusing to walk outside in the spring
    d. Working in the garden on sunny days

12. The nurse would evaluate that the patient understands
what triggers allergic rhinitis by which of the following patient responses?
    a. "Injected medications"
    b. "Topical creams and ointments"
    c. "Ingested food and medications"
    d. "Airborne pollens and molds"

13. The nurse understands that an anaphylactic reaction is
considered which of the following types of hypersensitivity reactions?
    a. Type I
    b. Type II
    c. Type III
    d. Type IV

14. As the nurse cares for a patient with angioedema, the
nurse understands that angioedema differs from
urticaria in that angioedema is characterized by which
of the following?
    a. Angioedema is more pruritic.
    b. Angioedema has a deeper and more widespread
       edema.
    c. Angioedema has small, fluid-filled vesicles that
       crust.
    d. Angioedema lasts a shorter time.

19 Nursing Care of Patients with HIV Disease and AIDS

VOCABULARY

Fill in the blanks.

1. _____________ is the final phase of a chronic, progressive immune function disorder caused by the human immunodeficiency virus (HIV).   *[AIDS]*

2. The _____________ is an important part of the human immune system and helps defend the body against very primitive invaders such as fungi, yeast, and other viruses.   *[CD4+ T-lymphocyte cell]*

3. _____________ is a diagnostic test done to detect antibodies to HIV antigen on test plates.   *[enzyme-linked immunosorbent assay]*

4. _____________ are a primary complication of HIV infection and invade the body because of an impaired immune system.   *[opportunistic infxns]*

5. _____________ occurs in some patients with the acquired immune deficiency syndrome (AIDS) and is characterized by the occurrence of an involuntary baseline body weight loss of more than 10% and weakness or fever for more than 30 days or chronic diarrhea of two loose stools daily for more than 30 days.   *[Wasting Syndrome]*

6. _____________ measures the amount of HIV RNA in plasma and is extremely important for determining prognosis and monitoring the response to antiretroviral therapy.   *[viral load testing]*

DIAGNOSTIC TESTS

Describe the procedure for each of the following diagnostic tests.

1. Enzyme-linked immunosorbent assay (ELISA) test
   detects antibodies in pt's blood to HIV antigen on test plate

2. Viral load *measures amt of HIV RNA in plasma. Extremely important for determining PROGNOSIS & monitoring response to antiretroviral therapy.*

3. CD4+ cell count *In HIV/AIDS, # of cells drop but CD8+ (toxic) cell levels don't. A low ratio of CD4+ cells to CD8+ cells is seen as HIV/AIDS progresses. Recommended @ 3 mos. intervals.*

HIV

Fill in the blanks.

1. HIV is transmitted through *infected blood*, *semen*, *vagnl scrtns*, and *breast milk*.

2. HIV may stay latent for *8-12 [many]* years.

3. Fatigue, headache, fever, and generalized lymphadenopathy may be seen during the _____________ *[early]* stages of HIV infection.

4. _____________ are increasingly becoming infected with HIV.   *[women]*

HIV AND AIDS

Indicate whether the following are true or false, and correct false statements.

1. If a health-care worker is stuck with a needle from a patient with AIDS, exposure to the virus may occur even if gloves were worn. __T__

2. HIV is caused by AIDS. __F__ *AIDS → HIV*

3. Individuals who are not men who have sex with men or who are intravenous drug users probably do ~~not~~ need to worry about contracting HIV and developing AIDS. __F__

4. If the nurse suctions a patient with a fresh tracheostomy who is diagnosed with HIV and blood-tinged sputum gets in the nurse's eyes, the nurse may contract the virus. __T__

5. Once a person is infected with HIV, the diagnosis can be made using laboratory tests within 1 to 2 days. __F__ *after 2 wks*

6. A patient with AIDS should always be put into isolation for the protection of health-care workers. __F__ *not needed unless ordered for special reason*

CRITICAL THINKING

Answer the following questions.

1. Jack Swope, age 26, has been diagnosed HIV positive. He asks, "Do I have AIDS and am I going to die?" What should you say to him? *Pt is told he has HIV but does not have AIDS at this time. I tx, HIV is considered a chronic condition that may not develop into AIDS for many years. If it develops, there currently is no cure but it is treatable.*

2. When is the patient with HIV considered to have AIDS? *end-stage CD4+ T-cell count of >200/mL &/or presence of 1 of 25 conditions, usually an opportunistic infxn or cancer*

3. Jack now is diagnosed with AIDS with a CD4+ count of 200. At this time, he is asymptomatic. He is started on a combination of trimethoprim and sulfamethoxazole (Bactrim, Septra). Why? *To prevent pneumocystis carnii pneumonia (PCP) & toxoplasmosis opportunistic infxns from developing.*

4. (a) Jack is 6 feet tall and weighs 135 lb. He is malnourished. Why? *candidiasis, meds, periph. & central nrvs system disease, taste & smell. This, along c discomfort, anorexia, fatigue predispose pt to mal nourishment.*

   (b) What can you do as a nurse to improve Jack's nutrition? *medicated swish & swallows, topical anesthetic sprays, & flavor enhancers may promote an increased food intake.*

5. Six months after being diagnosed with AIDS, Jack develops dementia. Why? *It occurs from encephalopathy c/b direct infxn of brain tissue by HIV.*

6. How can a nurse contract HIV from a patient? *Bodily secretions of infected person coming into contact c recipient's blood thru a break in the skin.*

7. How should the home health nurse teach family members of a patient with AIDS to clean the patient's home? *1:10 dilution of household bleach prep'd in 24 hrs of use, clean: toilet seats, bathroom fixtures; inside of fridge to avoid mold growth; wash clothing seperately that is soiled c blood, urine, feces, or semen. Dishes are washed normal in hot soapy H2O & rinsed thoroughly after use.*

REVIEW QUESTIONS

Choose the best answer unless directed otherwise.

Multiple response item. Select all that apply.

1. In planning an educational session for a patient with HIV, the nurse would include which of the following as a method of transmission for HIV?
   a. Saliva
   b. Tears
   c. Breast milk
   d. Semen
   e. Blood

2. Which of the following would the nurse evaluate as laboratory data that support the occurrence of AIDS?
   a. 900 CD4+ cells
   b. 700 CD4+ cells
   c. 500 CD4+ cells
   d. 200 CD4+ cells

3. Which of the following diets would the nurse include in the plan of care for a person with AIDS?
   a. A high-protein, high-calorie diet divided into six small meals
   b. A low-fat, soft diet divided into eight small meals
   c. A high-carbohydrate, fat-restricted diet divided into four meals
   d. A high-fat, high-calorie diet divided into three meals

4. Which of the following is an appropriate nursing intervention to prevent infection in patients with AIDS?
   a. Prohibiting patients who are severely immunodeficient from having any visitors
   b. Prohibiting visitors with a cough
   c. Wearing protective gear such as gown, mask, gloves, and goggles when entering the room
   d. Ensuring protective barrier isolation precautions are in place

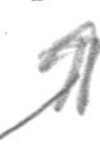

5. A patient who is being tested for HIV asks what tests are used. The nurse would be correct in stating that the tests used to confirm HIV infection are which of the following?
   a. CD4$^+$ cell count and thymus function
   b. B-cell and T-cell count
   c. ELISA and Western blot
   d. CD4$^+$, viral load, and ELISA

6. The nurse is caring for a patient with HIV who has diarrhea. Which of the following would be most therapeutic to teach the patient to avoid in the diet to reduce diarrhea?
   a. Potassium-rich food
   b. Raw fruits and vegetables
   c. Liquid nutritional supplements
   d. Frozen products

7. The nurse is teaching a patient newly diagnosed with AIDS about complications of the disease. Which of the following is the most common opportunistic infection in AIDS?
   a. *Pneumocystis carinii* pneumonia.
   b. Candidiasis
   c. Toxoplasmosis
   d. *Mycoplasma pneumoniae*

8. The nurse is taking vital signs of a pregnant woman during her first prenatal visit. The patient asks the nurse if she has to have an HIV test. Which of the following is the nurse's best response?
   a. "Yes, all pregnant women must have the test."
   b. "If you do not have multiple sex partners or inject drugs, it is not necessary."
   c. "Governmental guidelines require an HIV test for all pregnant woman."
   d. "After voluntary pretest counseling, you decide whether HIV testing should be done."

9. The nurse is caring for a patient with HIV. Which of the following foods would the nurse teach the patient is safe to eat to reduce the risk of infection?
   a. Raw fruits
   b. Cooked vegetables
   c. Raw vegetables
   d. Caesar dressing

10. When caring for a patient with AIDS, which of the following nursing actions would be most appropriate for infection control?
   a. Wear gloves at all times.
   b. Wear gloves for blood/body fluid contact.
   c. Wear gown and mask at all times.
   d. Wear a mask during patient contact times.

UNDERSTANDING THE CARDIOVASCULAR SYSTEM

CHECKLIST FOR LEARNING SUCCESS

Review of Anatomy and Physiology	Major Disorders	Nursing Assessment	Diagnostic Tests	Common Interventions
❏ Cardiovascular:	❏ Cardiovascular:	❏ Medical history	❏ Noninvasive	❏ Exercise
❏ Structures	❏ Hypertension	❏ Medications	❏ Electrocardiogram ambulatory	❏ Smoking cessation
❏ Function	❏ Inflammatory	❏ Family history	❏ Exercise tolerance testing	❏ Diet
❏ Aging effects	❏ Infectious	❏ Health promotion	❏ Echocardiogram	❏ Lifestyle and cardiac care
	❏ Occlusive	❏ Vital signs	❏ Tilt table test	❏ Antiembolism devices
	❏ Valvular	❏ Physical assessment	❏ Radioisotope imaging	❏ Cardioversion/defibrillation
	❏ Dysrhythmias		❏ Blood studies	❏ Pacemakers
	❏ Heart failure		❏ Cardiac enzymes	❏ Angioplasty
			❏ Cardiac troponin	❏ Valvuloplasty
			❏ Lipids	❏ Surgery
			❏ Invasive	❏ Cardiac rehabilitation
			❏ Angiography	
			❏ Cardiac catheterization	

Cardiovascular System Function, Assessment, and Therapeutic Measures

STRUCTURES OF THE CARDIOVASCULAR SYSTEM

Label the following structures.

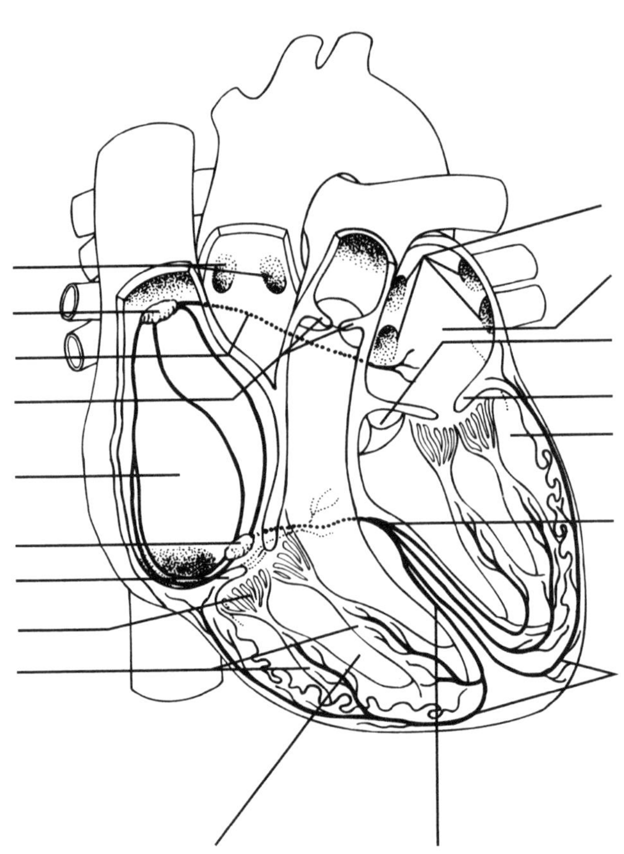

CARDIAC BLOOD FLOW

Number the following in proper sequence with respect to the flow of blood through the heart and to and from the lungs and body. Begin with the caval veins.

A. _________ Superior and inferior caval veins

B. _________ Left ventricle

C. _________ Right atrium

D. _________ Right ventricle

E. _________ Body

F. _________ Lungs

G. _________ Pulmonary artery

H. _________ Pulmonary veins

I. _________ Aorta

J. _________ Left atrium

K. _________ Mitral valve

L. _________ Aortic valve

M. _________ Tricuspid valve

N. _________ Pulmonic valve

AGING AND THE CARDIOVASCULAR SYSTEM

Find the 11 errors and insert the correct information.

It is believed that the "aging" of blood vessels, especially arteries, begins in adulthood. Average resting blood pressure tends to decrease with age and may contribute to stroke or right-sided heart failure. The thicker walled veins, especially those of the legs, may also weaken and stretch, making their valves incompetent.

With age, the heart lining becomes less efficient, and there is an increase in both maximum cardiac output and heart rate. The health of the myocardium depends on the lungs' blood supply. Hypertension causes the right ventricle to work harder, so it may atrophy. The heart valves may become thinner from fibrosis, leading to heart murmurs. Dysrhythmias become more common in the elderly as the cells of the conduction pathway become more efficient.

CARDIOVASCULAR SYSTEM

Fill in the blanks.

1. The function of the _____________ _____________ is to carry oxygen and nutrients to the tissues and remove waste products.

2. The _____________ function is to pump blood.

3. The peripheral _____________ is composed of arteries, veins, _____________ and lymph vessels.

4. With aging, the walls of blood vessels _____________.

5. The heart sound _____________ occurs at the beginning of systole when the atrioventricular valves close, and the sound *dupp* occurs at the start of _____________ when the semilunar valves close.

6. Palpation of pulse quality is recorded as _____________ 0; weak, thready 1+; _____________ 2+; bounding 3+.

7. Tests to assess _____________ function may include x-ray examination, electrocardiogram (ECG), stress test, echocardiogram, thallium scan, dipyridamole thallium scan, multiple gated acquisition (MUGA), serum troponin I, creatine kinase–myoglobin (CK-MB), lactate dehydrogenase (LDH), myoglobin, cardiac _____________, and angiography.

8. Six Ps characterize _____________ vascular disease: _____________, pulselessness, pallor, _____________, paresthesia, and paralysis.

9. Tests to assess peripheral _____________ disease are plethysmography, Doppler ultrasound, pressure measurement, stress testing, _____________, and arteriography.

ACUTE CARDIOVASCULAR NURSING ASSESSMENT

Identify a word that is obtained during a history that matches the given assessment statement.

1. _____________ Assessed before medication administration, test dyes

2. _____________ Modifiable risk factor for cardiovascular disorders that is a habit

3. _____________ Location: chest, calf; radiation: arms, jaw neck

4. _____________ Sign resulting from right-sided heart failure

5. _____________ Lung sounds with left-sided heart failure

6. _____________ Symptom of dysrhythmias

7. _____________ Effect of decreased cardiac output

8. _____________ Classic symptom of acute heart failure

CRITICAL THINKING

Make a cognitive map for a patient who is to undergo a cardiac catheterization. A cognitive map helps you visualize the patient's needs. Think of possible categories of needs of this patient and then complete activities and needs under each category. Some categories have been given to get you started, but you may think of others to include. You can get even more detailed and create subcategories for each activity or need. A cognitive map has no defined ending point.

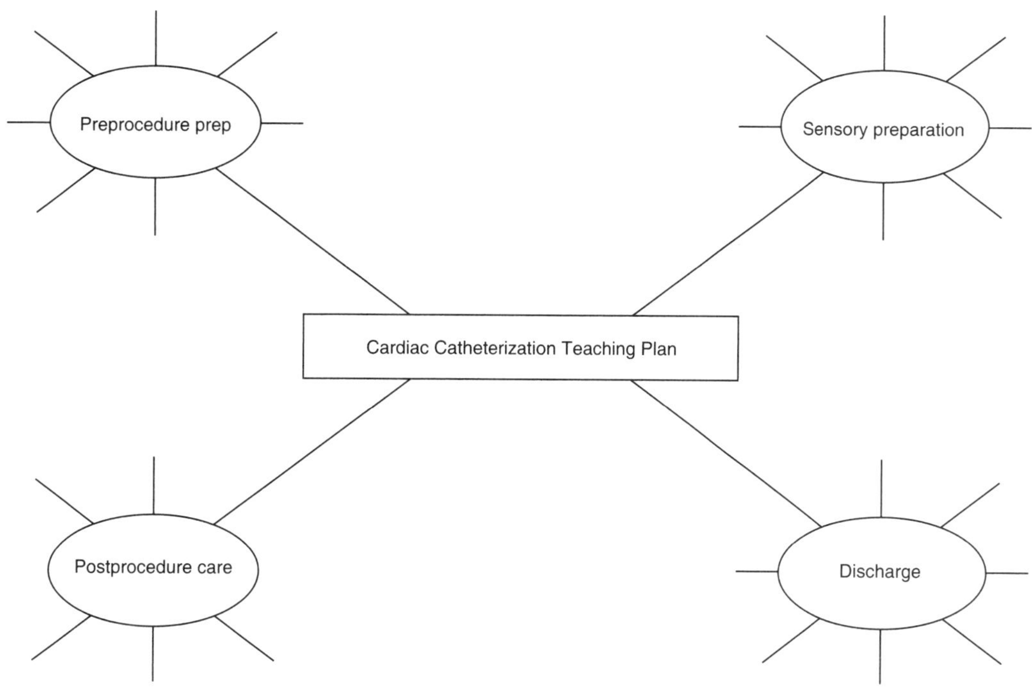

REVIEW QUESTIONS

Choose the best answer unless directed otherwise.

1. Each normal heartbeat is initiated by which of the following?
   a. Sinoatrial node in the wall of the right atrium
   b. Bundle of His in the interventricular septum
   c. Cardiac center in the medulla
   d. Sympathetic nerves from the spinal cord

2. During one cardiac cycle, which of the following occurs?
   a. Ventricles contract first, followed by the atria
   b. Atria contract first, followed by the ventricles
   c. Atria and ventricles contract simultaneously
   d. Ventricles contract twice for every contraction of the atria

3. Which of the following detects changes in blood pressure?
   a. Pressoreceptors in the medulla
   b. Blood vessels in the medulla
   c. Pressoreceptors in the carotid and aortic sinuses
   d. Coronary vessels in the myocardium

4. Epinephrine increases blood pressure because it does which of the following?
   a. Increases water resorption by the kidneys
   b. Causes vasodilation in the skin and viscera
   c. Decreases heart rate and force of contraction
   d. Increases heart rate and force of cardiac contraction

5. When blood pressure decreases, the kidneys help raise it by secreting which of the following?
   a. Renin
   b. Epinephrine
   c. Aldosterone
   d. Erythropoietin

6. Which of the following prevents the backflow of blood in veins?
   a. Precapillary sphincters
   b. Middle layer
   c. Smooth muscle layer
   d. Valves

7. A patient has had a bilateral mastectomy, so the nurse obtains blood pressure readings from the patient's legs. Which of the following does the nurse understand is the usual difference between blood pressure readings in the leg and the arm?
   a. 10 mm Hg higher
   b. 10 mm Hg lower
   c. 15 mm Hg higher
   d. 15 mm Hg lower

8. The nurse obtains a lower blood pressure on a patient's left arm than the right arm. As a result, which of the following extremities should the nurse use for ongoing blood pressure measurement?
   a. Left arm
   b. Right arm
   c. Right leg
   d. Either arm

9. The nurse is checking a patient's blood pressure for orthostatic hypotension. The nurse understands that normally when the patient stands, the blood pressure drops by which of the following amounts?
   a. Up to 15 mm Hg
   b. Up to 20 mm Hg
   c. Up to 25 mm Hg
   d. Up to 30 mm Hg

10. While the nurse checks the patient's blood pressure for orthostatic hypotension, the patient's heart rate increases. The nurse understands that normally when the patient stands, the heart rate does which of the following?
    a. Drops up to 10 beats per minute
    b. Drops up to 20 beats per minute
    c. Increases up to 20 beats per minute
    d. Increases up to 30 beats per minute

11. The nurse is examining a patient's legs for data collection and notes that there is bilateral decreased hair distribution, thick, brittle nails, and shiny, taut, dry skin. The nurse understands that this can indicate which of the following?
    a. Increased arterial blood flow
    b. Decreased arterial blood flow
    c. Increased venous blood flow
    d. Decreased venous blood flow

12. The nurse is explaining to a patient that for a thallium stress test dipyridamole (Persantine), a coronary vasodilator, will be given. Which of the following purposes will the nurse explain as the reason that this medication is being given?
    a. To decrease blood flow to cardiac cells
    b. To increase blood flow that occurs with exercise
    c. To prevent a clot from forming during the test
    d. To reduce systemic vascular resistance

Multiple response item. Select all that apply.
13. For which of the following dysrhythmias will the nurse anticipate a patient's need for a permanent pacemaker?
    a. Ventricular fibrillation
    b. First-degree heart block
    c. Atrial fibrillation
    d. Third-degree heart block
    e. Symptomatic bradycardia

Nursing Care of Patients with Hypertension

VOCABULARY

Match the word with its definition.

1. _______ Atherosclerosis
2. _______ Peripheral vascular resistance
3. _______ Normotensive
4. _______ Isolated systolic hypertension
5. _______ Hypertension
6. _______ Diastolic blood pressure
7. _______ Cardiac output
8. _______ Systolic blood pressure
9. _______ Secondary hypertension
10. _______ Primary hypertension
11. _______ Plaque

A. Most common form of arteriosclerosis, in which fats are deposited on arterial walls
B. Amount of blood the heart pumps out each minute
C. Amount of pressure exerted on the wall of the arteries when the ventricles are at rest; the bottom number in a blood pressure reading
D. Abnormally elevated blood pressure
E. Systolic pressure is 140 mm Hg or more, but the diastolic pressure is less than 90 mm Hg
F. Normal blood pressure
G. Opposition to blood flow through the vessels
H. Deposit of fatty material in the artery
I. Abnormally elevated blood pressure, the cause of which is unknown; also called essential hypertension
J. High blood pressure that is a symptom of a specific cause, such as a kidney abnormality
K. Maximal pressure exerted on the arteries during contraction of the left ventricle of the heart; top number of a blood pressure reading

DIURETICS

Select the letter that identifies the type of each diuretic.

1. _______ Spironolactone (Aldactone)
2. _______ Bumetanide (Bumex)
3. _______ Chlorothiazide (Diuril)
4. _______ Triamterene (Dyrenium)
5. _______ Furosemide (Lasix)
6. _______ Amiloride (Midamor)
7. _______ Metolazone (Zaroxolyn)
8. _______ Hydrochlorothiazide (HydroDIURIL, HCTZ)
9. _______ Torsemide (Demadex)

A. Thiazide or thiazidelike
B. Loop
C. Potassium-sparing

HYPERTENSION RISK FACTORS

Indicate whether the statement is true or false.

1. _______ Constant stress can cause hypertension.

2. _______ There is a link between a high-fat diet, obesity, and hypertension.

3. _______ High calcium, potassium, and magnesium levels are important risk factors for the development of hypertension.

4. _______ People who are not active on a regular basis are at an increased risk of developing hypertension.

5. _______ A diet high in salt is also high in vitamins and minerals.

STAGES OF HYPERTENSION AND RECOMMENDATIONS FOR FOLLOW-UP

Indicate whether the statement is true or false, and correct the false statements.

1. _______ The recommended follow-up for a systolic blood pressure of 120 to 139 is 2 years.

2. _______ The recommended follow-up for a systolic blood pressure of less than 120 is 2 years.

3. _______ The recommended follow-up for a systolic blood pressure more than 180 is now.

4. _______ The recommended follow-up for a systolic blood pressure of 160 to 179 is 2 months.

5. _______ The recommended follow-up for a systolic blood pressure of 140 to 159 is 2 months.

6. _______ The recommended follow-up for a diastolic blood pressure of 90 to 99 is 1 month.

7. _______ The recommended follow-up for a diastolic blood pressure of more than 110 is now.

8. _______ The recommended follow-up for a diastolic blood pressure of 100 to 109 is 2 months.

9. _______ The recommended follow-up for a diastolic blood pressure less than 80 is 2 years.

10. _______ The recommended follow-up for a diastolic blood pressure of 80 to 89 is 1 year.

CRITICAL THINKING

Read the case study and answer the questions.

Mrs. Laura Martin, age 42, is seen in the hypertension clinic for a follow-up visit for hypertension. Her blood pressure is 160/92 mm Hg and she is diagnosed with hypertension. The physician encourages lifestyle modification and prescribes an angiotensin-converting enzyme inhibitor.

1. What additional information should the nurse collect to develop a teaching plan for lifestyle modifications and the medication? _______________________________

____

2. Develop a teaching plan for Mrs. Martin's needs based on the data collected (see Answers for feedback).

____

____

3. What interventions will help Mrs. Martin reach her goal for controlling her hypertension? _______________

____

4. How will you know when Mrs. Martin has reached her goals? _______________________________

____

Choose the best answer unless directed otherwise.

Multiple response item. Select all that apply.
1. The nurse is developing a teaching plan for a patient. Which of the following is a modifiable risk factor for the development of hypertension?
   a. Race
   b. High cholesterol
   c. Cigarette smoking
   d. Sedentary lifestyle
   e. Age

2. If the systolic blood pressure is elevated and the diastolic blood pressure is normal, the nurse recognizes that a patient is most likely to have which type of hypertension?
   a. Primary
   b. Secondary
   c. Isolated systolic
   d. Hypertensive emergency

3. The patient asks the nurse, "What is hypertension?" Which of the following is the best response to explain hypertension?
   a. "It is measured as the heart pumps blood into the arteries."
   b. "It is higher than normal on two separate occasions."
   c. "It is regulated by stress, activity, and emotions."
   d. "It is determined by peripheral vascular resistance."

4. Which of the following is information the nurse would be correct in giving the patient about smoking and its effect on blood pressure?
   a. It is associated with stages 1 and 2 hypertension.
   b. It does not affect blood pressure regulation.
   c. It vasodilates the peripheral blood vessels.
   d. It causes sustained blood pressure elevations.

5. Which of the following medications should the nurse explain may cause headache as a side effect?
   a. Furosemide (Lasix)
   b. Atenolol (Tenormin)
   c. Clonidine (Catapres)
   d. Adalat (Procardia)

6. The nurse understands that a patient with blood pressure readings of 164/102 and 176/100 on two separate occasions would be classified in which hypertension category?
   a. Prehypertension
   b. Stage 1
   c. Stage 2

7. A patient has been prescribed bumetanide (Bumex) every morning for control of hypertension. Which of the following statements indicates correct knowledge of the treatment regimen?
   a. "I can travel to Florida and sunbathe all day."
   b. "Now I can eat whatever I want, whenever I want."
   c. "I'll take my medication in the morning, every morning."
   d. "I won't need medication once my pressure goes down."

8. Which common side effect of metolazone (Zaroxolyn) should the nurse instruct a patient to report to the health-care provider?
   a. Numb hands
   b. Muscle weakness
   c. Gastrointestinal distress
   d. Nightmares

9. The nurse understands that which of the following best describes the action of enalapril maleate (Vasotec)?
   a. It decreases levels of angiotensin II.
   b. It adjusts the extracellular volume.
   c. It dilates the arterioles and veins.
   d. It decreases cardiac output.

10. The nurse understands that which of the following is a side effect most likely to be reported by patients receiving enalapril maleate (Vasotec)?
    a. Acne
    b. Diarrhea
    c. Cough
    d. Heartburn

11. The nurse understands that which of the following best describes the action of propranolol (Inderal)?
    a. It increases heart rate.
    b. It decreases cardiac output.
    c. It decreases fluid volume.
    d. It increases cardiac contractility.

12. What instruction should the nurse give to the patient taking propranolol (Inderal) for hypertension?
    a. Have potassium level checked.
    b. Report any changes in appetite.
    c. Do not stop medication abruptly.
    d. Resume usual daily activities.

13. Which of the following nursing diagnoses is the focus of care for a patient with hypertension?
    a. Activity intolerance
    b. Ineffective airway clearance
    c. Impaired physical mobility
    d. Deficient knowledge

14. Which of the following statements, if made by a patient with hypertension, indicates to the nurse a need for more teaching?
    a. "High blood pressure may affect the kidneys and eyes."
    b. "Most people with hypertension watch their diet."
    c. "Medication will no longer be needed when I feel better."
    d. "Many people do not know when their blood pressure is high."

15. A patient teaching plan should include which of the following lifestyle modifications to help control hypertension?
    a. Regular aerobic exercise
    b. Low-tar cigarettes
    c. Three alcoholic beverages per day
    d. Daily multivitamin supplements

Nursing Care of Patients with Inflammatory and Infectious Cardiovascular Disorders

VOCABULARY

Fill in the blank with the word that is formed by the word building.

1. _____________ choreia—dance
2. _____________ peri—around + kardia—heart + itis—inflammation
3. _____________ myo—muscle + kardia—heart + itis—inflammation
4. _____________ petecchia—skin spot
5. _____________ peri—around + kardia—heart + kentesis—puncture
6. _____________ kardia—heart + tamponade—plug
7. _____________ kardia—heart + myo—muscle + pathy—disease
8. _____________ kardia—heart + mega—large
9. _____________ my—muscle + ectomy—cutting out
10. _____________ thromb—lump (clot) + phleb—vein + itis—inflammation

INFLAMMATORY AND INFECTIOUS CARDIOVASCULAR DISORDERS

Match the word with its definition.

1. _______ Solid, liquid, gaseous masses of undissolved matter traveling with the current in a blood or lymphatic vessel
2. _______ Gram-positive bacteria whose group A causes disease
3. _______ Inflammation of the heart lining caused by microorganisms
4. _______ Standardized test for reporting prothrombin to prevent variability in testing results and provide uniformity in monitoring therapeutic levels for coagulation
5. _______ Severe damage to the heart from rheumatic fever

A. Infective endocarditis
B. Emboli
C. International normalized ratio
D. Rheumatic heart disease
E. Beta-hemolytic streptococci

RHEUMATIC FEVER AND RHEUMATIC HEART DISEASE

Find the seven errors and insert the correct information.

Rheumatic fever causes a streptococcal infection such as a sore throat. Rheumatic fever signs and symptoms include polyarthritis, subcutaneous nodules, cholera with rapid, controlled movements, carditis, fever, arthralgia, and pneumonia. A throat culture diagnoses rheumatic fever. Rheumatic carditis can be a complication of rheumatic fever. The heart valves and their structures can be scarred and damaged. Rheumatic fever can be prevented by detecting and treating streptococcal infections promptly with aspirin. The signs and symptoms of a pharynx streptococcal infection include sudden sore throat, low-grade fever, chills, throat redness with exudate, sinus or ear infection, and lymph node enlargement. Nursing care focuses on relieving the patient's pain and anxiety, maintaining normal cardiac function, and educating the patient about rheumatic heart disease.

THROMBOPHLEBITIS

Complete the rationale and evaluation of the nursing care plan for a patient with thrombophlebitis.

NURSING DIAGNOSIS
Acute Pain Related to Inflammation of Vein

Interventions	Rationale	Evaluation
Assess pain using rating scale such as 0 to 10.		
Provide analgesics and non-steroidal anti-inflammatory drugs (NSAIDs) as ordered.		
Apply warm, moist soaks.		
Maintain bedrest with leg elevation above heart level.		

NURSING DIAGNOSIS
Deficient Knowledge Related to Lack of Knowledge About Disorder and Treatment

Interventions	Rationale	Evaluation
Explain condition, symptoms, and complications.		
Explain medications, therapies ordered, monthly lab test monitoring, and need for Medic Alert identification.		
Teach patient not to massage extremity.		

DIAGNOSTIC TESTS FOR INFECTIVE ENDOCARDITIS

Match the test with its finding that is indicative of infective endocarditis.

Test	**Finding**
1. ______ White blood cell count with differential	A. Abnormal heart and valve function
2. ______ Blood cultures	B. Dysrhythmias
3. ______ Erythrocyte sedimentation rate	C. Elevated
4. ______ Rheumatoid factor	D. Heart failure
5. ______ Electrocardiogram	E. Identifies causative organism
6. ______ Chest x-ray examination	F. Positive
7. ______ Echocardiogram	G. Slight elevation
8. ______ Cardiac catheterization	H. Vegetations on heart valves

CRITICAL THINKING

Read the case study and answer the questions.

Mr. Evans, age 68, is admitted to the hospital for heart failure resulting from hypertrophic cardiomyopathy. He has dyspnea, fatigue, and angina. His lung sounds reveal crackles.

1. What is the pathophysiology of hypertrophic cardiomyopathy? __________________

____

2. What occurs in hypertrophic cardiomyopathy to ventricular size and ventricular filling with blood?

____

____

3. What diagnostic test will show hypertrophic cardiomyopathy and left-sided heart failure?

____

____

4. Why is digoxin contraindicated for Mr. Evans? ____________________________

____

5. Why should Mr. Evans be taught to avoid (a) dehydration and (b) exertion?

____

____

6. Why is it important for the family to learn cardiopulmonary resuscitation (CPR)?

____

____

REVIEW QUESTIONS

Choose the best answer unless directed otherwise.

1. A patient visits the doctor for a severe sore throat and fever. As the nurse plans the patient's care, the nurse understands that it is important that which of the following diagnostic tests is obtained to help prevent cardiac complications?
   a. Chest x-ray examination
   b. Throat culture
   c. White blood cell count
   d. Erythrocyte sedimentation rate

2. Which of the following does the nurse understand usually precedes rheumatic fever?
   a. A viral infection
   b. A fungal infection
   c. A staphylococcal infection
   d. A beta-hemolytic streptococcal infection

3. A patient with a history of endocarditis is undergoing a bowel resection. The nurse explains that the prophylactic antibiotics prevent which of the following?
   a. Endocarditis
   b. Peritonitis
   c. Vegetative emboli
   d. Inflammation

4. A patient has a positive Homans' sign. Which of the following does the nurse understand explains why ambulation and performing the Homans' sign is now contraindicated?
   a. They can cause calf swelling.
   b. They can cause patient pain.
   c. They can cause an emboli.
   d. They may cause a clot to form.

5. A patient develops a postoperative deep vein thrombosis and is started on intravenous heparin. Which of the following laboratory tests is monitored during the heparin therapy?
   a. Plasma fibrinogen
   b. Prothrombin time (PT)
   c. Partial thromboplastin time (PTT)
   d. International normalized ratio (INR)

6. The nurse is caring for a patient on warfarin (Coumadin) with an elevated INR level. Which of the following would be ordered as the antidote for warfarin?
   a. Vitamin K
   b. Vitamin B_{12}
   c. Calcium chloride
   d. Protamine sulfate

7. Which of the following is a desired outcome for the nursing diagnosis of acute pain for a patient with acute thrombophlebitis?
   a. States anxiety is decreased.
   b. States pain is satisfactorily relieved.
   c. Is able to participate in desired activities.
   d. Reports ability to ambulate without pain.

8. The nurse is reviewing the patient's daily PT and INR levels. The PT level is 26 (normal = 9 to 12 seconds). Which of the following actions should the nurse take?
   a. Give the next dose of warfarin when it is ordered to be given.
   b. Inform physician before the next dose of warfarin is given.
   c. Stop the heparin infusion.
   d. Continue monitoring heparin infusion.

Multiple response item. Select all that apply.
9. A patient, who had a hysterectomy 2 days ago, reports tenderness in her left calf. The nursing assessment reveals the following: left calf 17.5″, right calf 14″, left thigh 32″, right thigh 28″, and a shiny, warm, and reddened left leg. Which of the following interventions should be given priority in the patient's plan of care?
   a. Maintain bedrest.
   b. Encourage ambulation tid.
   c. Apply bilateral antiembolism stockings.
   d. Encourage bilateral leg exercises.
   e. Apply right antiembolism stocking.
   f. Apply warm moist heat as ordered.

10. The nurse is caring for a patient receiving warfarin therapy. Which of the following findings is essential to report to the physician?
    a. Bleeding time 3 (normal = 2 to 5 seconds)
    b. INR 4 (normal = 2 to 3 seconds)
    c. PTT 29 (normal = 30 to 45 seconds)
    d. PT 20 (normal = 9 to 12 seconds)

11. A patient has end-stage dilated cardiomyopathy. He comes to the emergency department with dyspnea. He says he went to bed and awoke with a feeling of suffocation. He says it was frightening. Which of the following responses by the nurse is most appropriate?
    a. "You must have been dreaming."
    b. "Reclining decreases the heart's ability to pump blood."
    c. "Sleeping increases heart rate, which increases the body's need for oxygen."
    d. "Reclining increases fluid returning to the heart, which builds up fluid in the lungs."

12. The nurse is caring for a patient, age 68, who is receiving digoxin (Lanoxin) 0.125 mg qd for cardiac myopathy. Which of the following assessments of the patient would indicate that he is experiencing a side effect of digoxin that requires follow-up?
    a. Skin flushing
    b. Anorexia
    c. Hypertension
    d. Constipation

13. The physician writes a "now" order for codeine 45 mg intramuscular (IM) for a patient with thrombophlebitis. The nurse has on hand codeine 60 mg/2 mL. Which of the following doses should be given?
    a. 1.45 mL
    b. 1.50 mL
    c. 1.75 mL
    d. 2.15 mL

14. A patient, age 46, is admitted for observation following an auto accident. He hit the steering wheel and has a chest contusion. Which of the following creates a pericardial friction rub?
    a. Inflamed cardiac tricuspid and mitral valves
    b. Decreased cardiac output
    c. Increased pulmonary pressures
    d. Rubbing of pericardial and epicardial layers

15. Which of the following is the most common symptom of pericarditis?
    a. Dyspnea
    b. Intermittent claudication
    c. Chest pain
    d. Calf pain

Nursing Care of Patients with Occlusive Cardiovascular Disorders

VOCABULARY

Match the word with its definition.

1. ______ Arteriosclerosis
2. ______ Atherosclerosis
3. ______ Stenosis
4. ______ Ischemia
5. ______ Skin breakdown as a result of chronic venous insufficiency
6. ______ High-density lipoprotein
7. ______ Collateral circulation
8. ______ Percutaneous transluminal coronary angioplasty
9. ______ Chest pain caused by decreased blood supply to the heart
10. ______ Chest pain that usually subsides with rest
11. ______ Chest pain that increases in frequency and is not relieved by rest
12. ______ Tortuous and bulging veins, usually in lower extremity
13. ______ Disease causing venospasms when exposed to cold
14. ______ A bulging or dilation of an artery
15. ______ Death of a portion of the myocardium
16. ______ Laboratory value that determines degree of damage to the heart
17. ______ A moving clot
18. ______ A stationary clot
19. ______ Intermittent claudication
20. ______ Obstructed blood flow in the coronary arteries

A. Varicose veins
B. Procedure that compresses plaque against wall of artery
C. Unstable angina
D. Hardening of arteries
E. Angina pectoris
F. Coronary artery disease
G. Stable angina
H. Raynaud's disease
I. Plaque buildup within arterial wall
J. Lack of blood supply
K. Aneurysm
L. Vessels grow to compensate for blocked blood flow
M. Narrowing of a vessel
N. Myocardial infarction
O. Embolism
P. "Good" cholesterol
Q. Thrombus
R. Venous stasis ulcer
S. Troponin I
T. Exertional calf pain that ceases with rest

ATHEROSCLEROSIS

Answer the following questions.

1. What is the pathophysiology of atherosclerosis?

____

____

____

2. What are modifiable risk factors that contribute to atherosclerosis?

____

____

____

3. Develop a teaching plan for one of the modifiable risk factors for atherosclerosis.

____

____

____

MYOCARDIAL INFARCTION

Find the 23 errors and insert the correct information.

Myocardial infarction (MI) is the death of a portion of the pericardial sac caused by blockage or spasm of a coronary artery. When the patient has an MI, the affected part of the muscle becomes damaged and no longer functions properly. Ischemic injury takes a few minutes before complete necrosis and infarction take place. The ischemic process affects the subendocardial layer, which is the least sensitive to hypoxia. Myocardial contractility is depressed, so the body attempts to compensate by triggering the parasympathetic nervous system. This causes a decrease in myocardial oxygen demand. After necrosis, the contractility function of the muscle is temporarily lost. If treatment is initiated after several signs of an MI, the area of damage can be minimized. If prolonged ischemia occurs, the size of the infarction can be small.

The area that is affected by an MI depends on which coronary artery is involved. The left anterior descending (LAD) branch of the left main coronary artery is the area that feeds the lateral wall. The right coronary artery (RCA) feeds the anterior wall and parts of the atrioventricular node and the sinoatrial node. An occlusion of the RCA leads to an inferior MI and abnormalities of impulse conduction and formation. The left circumflex coronary artery feeds the inferior wall and part of the posterior wall of the heart.

Pain is the least common complaint. The pain does not radiate. The patient usually believes that an MI is occurring. Other symptoms may include restlessness, a feeling of impending doom, nausea, diaphoresis, and cold, clammy, ashen skin. The only symptom that might be present in the elderly patient is vomiting.

The three strong indicators of an MI are patient history, abnormal electrocardiographic (ECG) reading, and high triglyceride levels.

Initially, patients are kept on bedrest to increase myocardial oxygen demand. Patients are medicated promptly when complaining of chest pain. Meperidine (Demerol) is the most widely used narcotic for several reasons. It helps decrease anxiety, increases respirations, and has a vasoconstrictive effect on coronary arteries. Oxygen is given usually at 1 L/hr via nasal cannula. Nitroglycerin sublingual, topical, or by intravenous drip can also be administered. Thrombolytic therapy is a frequent option for preventing a clot that can occlude a coronary artery.

A nursing care plan should include factors that may contribute to decreased cardiac workload. Changes in diet, stress reduction, regular exercise program, cessation of smoking, and following a medication schedule require extensive patient and family teaching.

PHARMACOLOGICAL TREATMENT

Match the medication to the appropriate description.

1. _______ A calcium channel blocker
2. _______ Beta blocker
3. _______ Drug of choice for anginal attacks
4. _______ Does not dissolve existing clots
5. _______ Drug used to lower cholesterol
6. _______ Decreases platelet aggregation
7. _______ Long-acting nitrate
8. _______ Thrombolytic therapy agent
9. _______ Decreases blood viscosity

A. Nitroglycerin

B. Cholestyramine (Questran)

C. Propranolol (Inderal)

D. Nifedipine (Procardia)

E. Streptokinase

F. Dipyridamole (Persantine)

G. Heparin

H. Pentoxifylline (Trental)

I. Isosorbide dinitrate (Isordil)

CRITICAL THINKING

Read the following case study and answer the questions.

Mr. Edwards is a 43-year-old man with a history of peripheral vascular disease and hypertension. He smokes two packs of cigarettes per day. He complains of calf pain during minimal exercise that decreases with rest.

1. Which of the following nursing diagnoses would be the most appropriate relating to Mr. Edwards' symptoms?

    A. Ineffective tissue perfusion related to compromised circulation
    B. Fatigue related to pain on exertion
    C. Impaired mobility relating to stress associated with pain
    D. Self-care deficit related to pain and muscle spasms

2. Explain what happens when intermittent claudication occurs. ______________________________________
____
____

3. Why does rest decrease the pain? ________________
____
____

4. Describe how smoking contributes to decreased circulation. ___________________________________
____
____

REVIEW QUESTIONS

Choose the best answer unless directed otherwise.

1. A patient who has been scheduled for a stress ECG asks why this ECG is needed. Which of the following is the nurse's best response?
    a. It can predict whether the patient may soon have a heart attack.
    b. It verifies how much more physically fit the patient needs to become.
    c. It determines the patient's potential target heart rate.
    d. It shows how the heart performs during exercise.

2. During a stress ECG, a patient reports chest pain and the test is stopped. When the patient is asked to undergo a heart catheterization, the patient appears very apprehensive and worried. Which of the following is the most appropriate action for the nurse to take to reduce the patient's anxiety?
    a. Explain how coronary artery disease is treated.
    b. Avoid discussing the heart catheterization until the patient has relaxed.
    c. Explain how well others have done after having this procedure.
    d. Listen to the patient express feelings about the situation.

3. Before a cardiac catheterization and coronary arteriogram, it is essential that the nurse ask a patient if he or she is allergic to which of the following?
    a. Eggs
    b. Codeine
    c. Iodine
    d. Penicillin

4. Which of the following statements by a patient demonstrates to the nurse that the patient understands when to replace nitroglycerin tablets?
    a. Pills no longer tingle when used.
    b. Pills disintegrate when touched.
    c. Pills smell like vinegar.
    d. Pills become discolored.

5. After hospitalization for a myocardial infarction, a patient is placed on a low-sodium diet. In discussing foods allowed on this diet, the nurse should tell the patient that this list includes which of the following?
    a. Hot dogs
    b. Fresh vegetables
    c. Milk and cheese
    d. Canned soups

6. A patient, hospitalized with an MI, suddenly begins to have severe respiratory distress with frothy sputum. These signs indicate that the patient probably has developed which of the following?
    a. Pneumonia
    b. Cardiac tamponade
    c. Pulmonary edema
    d. Pneumothorax

7. As the nurse assesses a patient for decreased circulation in the lower extremities, which of the following findings would indicate adequate circulation?
    a. Loss of hair on the extremity
    b. Capillary refill less than 3 seconds
    c. Diminished pulses in the extremity
    d. Thickened nails of the extremity

8. The percentage of calories from fat in the diet should be limited to no more than which of the following to help prevent atherosclerosis?
   a. 10%
   b. 25%
   c. 30%
   d. 45%

9. The nurse understands that pain associated with coronary artery disease occurs from which of the following?
   a. Lack of nutrients to the heart
   b. Interrupted electrical activity to the areas of the heart
   c. Lack of sufficient oxygen to the myocardium
   d. Overexertion of heart muscle due to the workload

Multiple response item. Select all that apply.
10. Which of the following does the nurse correctly include in a teaching plan as modifiable risk factors for coronary artery disease?
    a. Hypertension
    b. Race
    c. Age
    d. Gender
    e. Smoking
    f. Diabetes

11. Which of the following should the nurse correctly include in a teaching plan as a saturated fat?
    a. Cottonseed oil
    b. Coconut oil
    c. Safflower oil
    d. Sunflower oil

Multiple response item. Select all that apply.
12. The nurse is collecting data on a patient. Which of the following clinical manifestations would the nurse expect to find with acute venous insufficiency?
    a. Full superficial veins
    b. An aching, cramping type of pain
    c. Initial absence of edema
    d. Cool and cyanotic skin
    e. Positive Homans' sign

13. The nurse understands that which of the following is the most characteristic symptom of Buerger's disease?
    a. Numbness
    b. Pain
    c. Cramping
    d. Swelling

14. A patient has been diagnosed with Raynaud's disease and asks the nurse what occurs with this disease. Which of the following is the most appropriate response by the nurse?
    a. "Arterial vessel occlusion is caused by many clots that develop in the heart and are carried to the bloodstream."
    b. "Arteriolar vasoconstriction occurs, most often on the fingertips with symptoms of coldness, pain, and pale skin."
    c. "Peripheral vasospasm occurs in the lower limbs as a result of valve damage from long-standing venous stasis."
    d. "Thrombosis related to prolonged vasoconstriction caused by overexposure to the cold occurs."

Nursing Care of Patients with Cardiac Valvular Disorders

24

VOCABULARY

Fill in the blank with the word that is formed by the word building.

1. _______________ annulus—ring + plasty—formed
2. _______________ commissura—joining together + tome—incision
3. _______________ in—not + sufficiens—sufficient
4. _______________ re—again + gurgitare—to flood
5. _______________ stenos—narrow
6. _______________ valvula—leaf of a folding door + plasty—formed

MITRAL VALVE PROLAPSE

Find the eight errors and insert the correct information.

During ventricular diastole, when pressures in the left ventricle rise, the leaflets of the mitral valve normally remain open. In mitral valve prolapse (MVP), however, the leaflets bulge backward into the left ventricle during systole. Often there are functional problems seen with MVP. However, if the leaflets do not fit together, mitral stenosis can occur with varying degrees of severity.

MVP tends to be hereditary, and the cause is known. Infections that damage the mitral valve may be a contributing factor. It is the most common form of valvular heart disease and typically occurs in men age 20 to 55. Most patients with MVP have symptoms. Symptoms that may occur include chest pain, dysrhythmias, palpitations, dizziness, and syncope. No treatment is needed unless symptoms are present. Stimulants and caffeine should be avoided to prevent symptoms. Information on endocarditis prevention is essential.

VALVULAR DISORDERS

Indicate whether the statement is true or false, and correct false statements.

1. _______ Stenosis is widening of the opening of a heart valve.

2. _______ Stenosis inhibits the forward flow of blood.

3. _______ Regurgitation, or insufficiency, is failure of the valve to close completely.

4. _______ Regurgitation inhibits backflow of blood.

5. _______ Rheumatic heart disease and congenital defects are primary causes of valvular disease.

6. _______ The primary valves affected by disease are the tricuspid and pulmonic valves.

7. _______ Compensatory mechanisms in valvular disease are dilation to handle the increased blood volume and hypertrophy to increase the strength of contractions.

8. _______ Symptoms of valvular disease often occur early and reflect decreased cardiac output and pulmonary congestion: fatigue, dyspnea, orthopnea, cough.

9. _______ In severe valvular disease, heart failure occurs, and symptoms reflect the backup of blood from the failing chamber.

10. _______ In acute valve disorders, symptoms of shock are seen.

11. _______ Valve disease diagnosis is made with electrocardiogram (ECG), chest x-ray examination, echocardiogram, and cardiac catheterization.

12. _______ Valvuloplasty uses a balloon to separate the valve leaflets.

13. _______ Commissurotomy narrows the valve opening.

14. _______ Annuloplasty surgically repairs the valve.

15. _______ Patient teaching for valvular disorder includes understanding the importance of prophylactic antibiotics before all invasive procedures.

CRITICAL THINKING

Read the case study and answer the questions.

Mrs. Murphy, age 72, has aortic stenosis and is scheduled for an aortic valve replacement. She reports fatigue and dyspnea with exertion.

1. What may be the cause of Mrs. Murphy's aortic stenosis? ____

2. When obtaining Mrs. Murphy's medical history, what should the nurse ask that is relevant to the cause of aortic stenosis? ____

3. How does the heart compensate for aortic stenosis? ______________________________________

4. What should the nurse anticipate may occur in severe aortic stenosis? ____________________________

5. Why is angina a common symptom of aortic stenosis? ______________________________________

6. What medication might the nurse expect to be ordered preoperatively? _________________________

7. Why does Mrs. Murphy's chest x-ray examination show an enlarged heart? ____

8. Why is aortic stenosis treated with valvular replacement? __________________________________

REVIEW QUESTIONS

Choose the best answer unless directed otherwise.

1. Which of the following does the nurse understand occurs in aortic stenosis?
   a. Aortic valve does not close tightly.
   b. Emptying of blood from left ventricle is impaired.
   c. Blood backflows into the left atrium.
   d. Emptying of the left atrium is impaired.

2. The nurse understands that which of the following occurs in mitral regurgitation?
   a. Backflow of blood into the left atrium
   b. Backflow of blood into the right atrium
   c. Impaired emptying of the right ventricle
   d. Impaired emptying of the left ventricle

3. Which of the following compensatory mechanisms does the nurse understand occurs with ventricular valve disorders?
   a. Decreased atrial kick
   b. Atrial hypertrophy
   c. Ventricular hypertrophy
   d. Systolic hypertension

4. Which of the following does the nurse understand causes fatigue in patients with chronic aortic stenosis?
   a. Atrial fibrillation
   b. Left ventricular failure
   c. Decreased pulmonary blood flow
   d. Increased coronary artery blood flow

Multiple response item. Select all that apply.

5. Which of the following medications does the nurse anticipate that the patient will be given to prevent complications associated with decreased cardiac output?
   a. Furosemide (Lasix)
   b. Cephalexin (Keflex)
   c. Penicillin (Bicillin)
   d. Warfarin (Coumadin)
   e. Potassium (K-Dur)

6. Which of the following diagnostic tests does the nurse understand measures the pressures in the cardiac chambers?
   a. ECG
   b. Exercise stress test
   c. Echocardiogram
   d. Cardiac catheterization

7. Which of the following should the nurse include in the plan of care as a patient outcome for deficient knowledge related to mitral stenosis?
   a. Clear breath sounds, no edema or weight gain
   b. Normal changes in vital signs with less fatigue during self-care
   c. Verbalizes knowledge of disorder
   d. States fear is reduced

8. The nurse is caring for a patient, age 70, who has a nursing diagnosis of deficient knowledge related to furosemide administration. Which of the following interventions is essential to include when planning a teaching session to promote successful learning?
   a. Assess patient's learning priorities.
   b. Tell patient what he needs to learn first about furosemide.
   c. Assess patient's dietary intake of potassium.
   d. Give patient a written test at the end of the teaching session.

9. A patient, age 65, is being discharged after a mechanical valve replacement for aortic stenosis. Which of the following should be taught regarding the warfarin therapy?
   a. Wear Medic Alert identification.
   b. Increase intake of green leafy vegetables.
   c. Keep yearly blood test appointments.
   d. Use a straight razor when shaving.

10. The nurse is teaching a patient with heart failure how to avoid activity that results in Valsalva's maneuver. Which of the following statements by the patient indicates to the nurse that the teaching has been effective?
    a. "I will breathe normally when moving."
    b. "I will use a straw to drink oral fluids."
    c. "I will take fewer but deeper breaths."
    d. "I will clench my teeth when moving."

11. The nurse is planning care for a patient with chronic mitral regurgitation. Which of the following is the nurse correct in assessing to determine the cause of dyspnea and cough in patients with chronic mitral regurgitation?
    a. Cardiac rhythm
    b. Heart tones
    c. Peripheral edema
    d. Lung sounds

25 Nursing Care of Patients with Cardiac Dysrhythmias

VOCABULARY

Match the words and definitions.

1. _______ Amplitude
2. _______ Atrial depolarization
3. _______ Atrial systole
4. _______ Bigeminy
5. _______ Cardioversion
6. _______ Complete heart block
7. _______ Contractility
8. _______ Decompensation
9. _______ Defibrillate
10. _______ Inherent
11. _______ Ischemia
12. _______ Isoelectric line
13. _______ Multifocal
14. _______ Quadrigeminy
15. _______ Right bundle branch block
16. _______ Trigeminy
17. _______ Unifocal
18. _______ Ventricular diastole
19. _______ Ventricular escape rhythm
20. _______ Ventricular repolarization
21. _______ Ventricular systole

A. Beat occurring every fourth complex, as in premature ventricular contractions (PVCs)

B. Belonging to anything naturally

C. Coming or originating from one site

D. Condition in which there is a complete dissociation between atrial and ventricular systoles

E. Contraction of the atria

F. Contraction of the two ventricles

G. Defect in heart conduction system in which right bundle does not conduct impulses normally

H. Elective procedure in which synchronized shock of 25 to 50 joules is delivered to restore normal sinus rhythm

I. Electrical activation of the atria

J. Electrical tracing is at zero and is neither positive nor negative

K. Failure of the heart to maintain adequate circulation

L. Force with which left ventricular ejection occurs

M. Local and temporary deficiency of blood supply resulting from obstruction of the circulation to another part

N. Occurring every third beat, as in PVCs

O. Occurs every second beat, as in PVCs

P. Originating from many foci or sites

Q. Period of relaxation of the ventricle

R. Reestablishment of the polarized state of the muscle after contraction

S. Size or fullness of voltage

T. Naturally occurring rhythm of the ventricles when the rest of the conduction system fails

U. Use of electrical device to apply countershocks to the heart through electrodes placed on the chest wall to stop fibrillation

COMPONENTS OF A CARDIAC CYCLE

Label the components of a cardiac cycle.

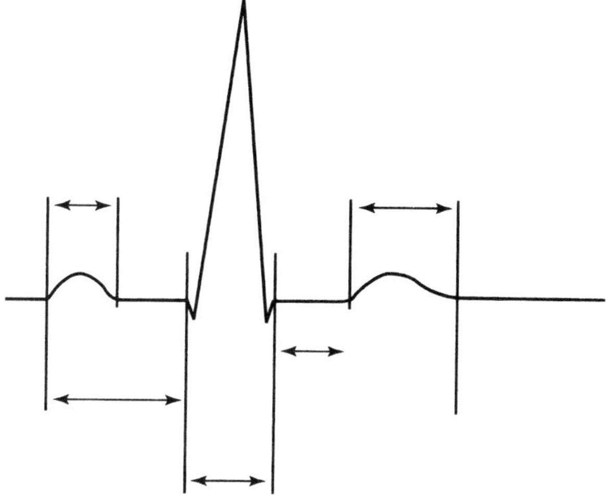

HEART RATE

Count the heart rate using the 6-second method.

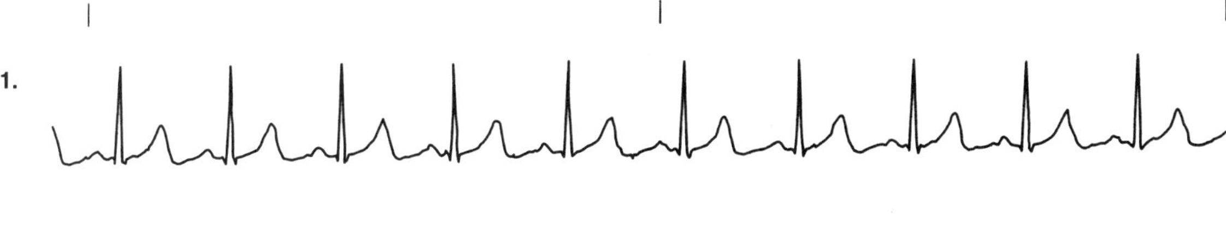

1.

Heart rate = _______________________

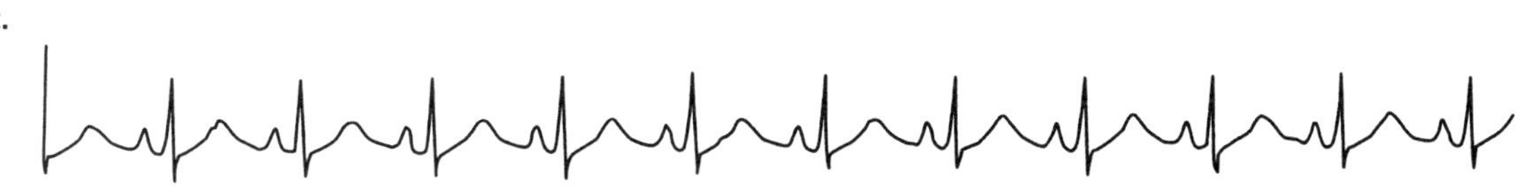

2.

Heart rate = _______________________

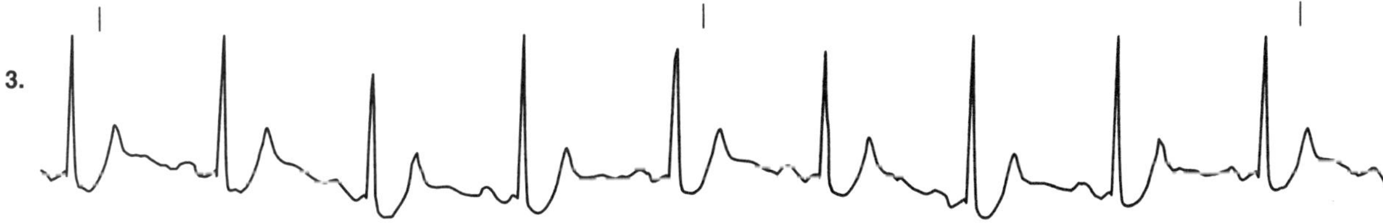

3.

Heart rate = _______________________

CARDIAC CONDUCTION

Match the words and definitions.

1. _______ Sinoatrial node
2. _______ Atrioventricular node
3. _______ Normal sinus rhythm
4. _______ Right atrium
5. _______ Right ventricle
6. _______ Left atrium
7. _______ Left ventricle
8. _______ Bradycardia
9. _______ Tachycardia
10. _______ Q wave
11. _______ P wave
12. _______ R wave
13. _______ S wave
14. _______ T wave
15. _______ U wave
16. _______ Premature
17. _______ Sinus tachycardia
18. _______ Sinus bradycardia
19. _______ Premature atrial contraction
20. _______ Atrial fibrillation
21. _______ Premature ventricular contraction
22. _______ Ventricular tachycardia
23. _______ Ventricular fibrillation
24. _______ Asystole

A. Rate less than 60
B. No QRS complexes seen—straight line
C. An early beat
D. An early beat that has a P wave and a normal QRS complex
E. Where an impulse originates
F. A chaotic pattern—no visible cardiac cycles
G. No identifiable P waves with a normal QRS complex; irregularly, irregular
H. Wave that precedes a QRS complex
I. Where an impulse is delayed before going to the Purkinje fibers
J. An early beat with no P wave and a wide, bizarre QRS complex
K. Successive beats of three or more wide, bizarre QRS complexes
L. Rhythm with normal P waves, QRS, T waves with a heart rate of 60 to 100 beats per minute
M. The first negative deflection of a QRS complex
N. A small wave seen after the T wave
O. The first positive deflection on a QRS complex
P. Rhythm with normal P waves, QRS, T waves with a heart rate of less than 60 beats per minute
Q. The chamber of the heart that pumps the blood to the rest of the body
R. Chamber that receives blood returning to the heart
S. Rhythm with normal P waves, QRS, T waves with a heart rate of more than 100 beats per minute
T. The wave that follows the QRS complex
U. The chamber that receives blood from the pulmonary veins
V. The downward deflection after the R wave
W. Heart rate of more than 100 beats per minute
X. Chamber that propels blood into the pulmonary artery

ELECTROCARDIOGRAM INTERPRETATION

Analyze the electrocardiogram (ECG) rhythms using the five-step interpretation process.

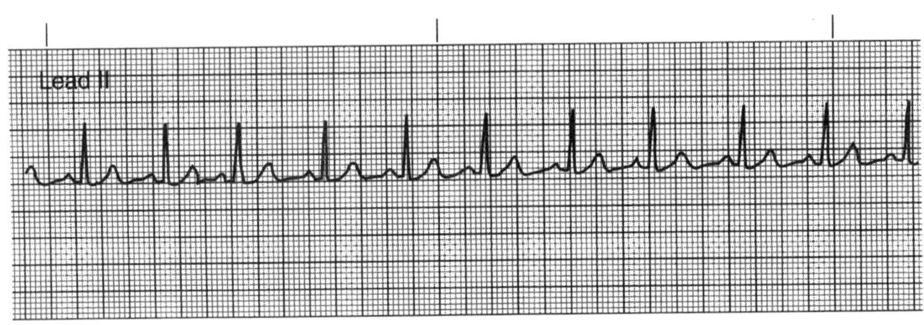

A.

1. Rhythm: ____

2. Heart rate: ____

3. P waves: ____

4. PR interval: ____

5. QRS interval: ____

6. ECG interpretation: ____

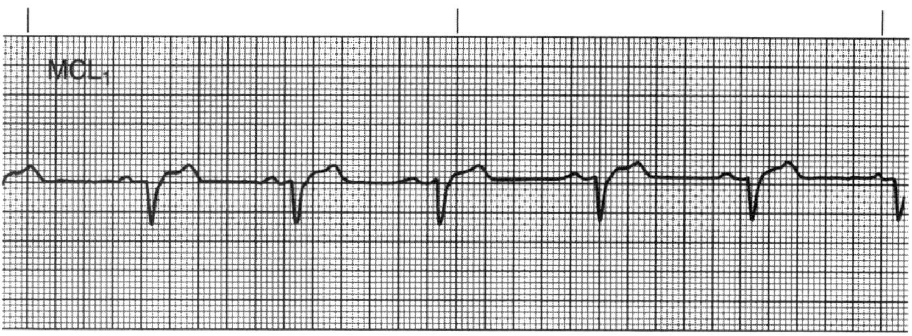

B.

1. Rhythm: ____

2. Heart rate: ____

3. P waves: ____

4. PR interval: ____

5. QRS interval: ____

6. ECG interpretation: ____

CRITICAL THINKING

Read the case study and answer the questions.

Mrs. Samuels is admitted to the hospital for chest pain. Tests are run, and her ECG shows bigeminal PVCs of more than 6 per minute that are close to her T wave. Her potassium level is 3 mEq/L. She is short of breath on exertion. Her blood pressure is 104/56, her pulse is 72, and her respirations are 16.

1. What should the nurse do first? _______________________________________

2. What actions should the nurse take regarding the dysrhythmia? _______________

3. What might some of the causes be for this dysrhythmia? ___________________

4. What additional symptoms might the nurse anticipate? ____________________

5. What type of orders should the nurse expect from the doctor? ______________

REVIEW QUESTIONS

Choose the best answer unless directed otherwise.

1. The nurse understands that which of the following defines a cardiac cycle?
   a. Circulation of the blood through the body
   b. Circulation of the blood through the heart
   c. Depolarization and repolarization of heart chambers
   d. Pumping action of the heart

2. When a life-threatening dysrhythmia is seen on a cardiac monitor, which of the following is the nurse's first appropriate action?
   a. Notify the physician immediately.
   b. Assess the patient.
   c. Administer the appropriate medication for the noted dysrhythmia.
   d. Obtain vital signs.

3. The heart receives blood returning from the body through which of the following?
   a. Pulmonary vein
   b. Aorta
   c. Vena cavae
   d. Right coronary artery

4. Which of the following separates the right side of the heart from the left?
   a. Valve
   b. Pericardium
   c. Chamber
   d. Septum

5. Which of the following chambers of the heart is largest and has the thickest myocardium?
   a. Left ventricle
   b. Right ventricle
   c. Right atrium
   d. Left atrium

6. Which of the following waveforms represents the resting state of the ventricle on the ECG?
   a. U wave
   b. QRS complex
   c. P wave
   d. T wave

7. Which of the following is the inherent rate for the atrioventricular node?
   a. 20 to 40 beats per minute
   b. 40 to 60 beats per minute
   c. 60 to 100 beats per minute
   d. More than 100 beats per minute

8. The nurse understands that rhythms arising from the primary pacing node of the heart are referred to as which of the following?
   a. Escape beats
   b. Bundle branch blocks
   c. Sinus rhythms
   d. Ectopic rhythms

9. The nurse is teaching a patient about digoxin. Which of the following would the nurse be correct in including in the teaching plan as the action of digoxin?
   a. Decreases ectopic beats.
   b. Increases force of contractions.
   c. Increases heart rate.
   d. Raises blood pressure.

10. The nurse is providing care to a patient with atrial fibrillation. Which of the following is a possible serious complication of atrial fibrillation for which the nurse should be alert?
    a. Formation of a thrombus
    b. Swelling of hands and feet
    c. Cardiac tamponade
    d. Coronary occlusion

Multiple response item. Select all that apply.
11. Which of the following treatments is appropriate for a patient with atrial fibrillation?
    a. Lidocaine (Xylocaine)
    b. Nitroglycerin
    c. Isoproterenol (Isuprel)
    d. Digoxin (Lanoxin)
    e. Cardioversion

12. The nurse is caring for a patient who has had a run of three or more PVCs together. The nurse should document this as which of the following?
    a. Ventricular tachycardia
    b. Bigeminy
    c. Trigeminy
    d. Multifocal PVCs

13. The nurse is caring for a patient in ventricular tachycardia who is hemodynamically stable; which of the following is the first choice of treatment?
    a. Cardioversion
    b. Pacemaker
    c. Defibrillation
    d. Antiarrhythmic intravenous medication

14. The nurse is caring for a patient whose ECG monitor shows a total absence of electrical impulse. The nurse does not detect a pulse. The nurse documents this as which of the following rhythms?
    a. Agonal
    b. Ventricular standstill
    c. Asystole
    d. Sinus arrest

15. A patient with a cardiac disorder is having increased PVCs and feels "anxious." After assessment and vital signs, what is the next action for the nurse to take?
    a. Order an ECG and cardiac enzymes.
    b. Call the physician.
    c. Elevate the head of the bed and start oxygen at 2 L/min.
    d. Put the bed in Trendelenburg's position.

Nursing Care of Patients with Heart Failure

VOCABULARY

Fill in the blank with the appropriate word found in the word list.

Afterload

Cor pulmonale

Hepatomegaly

Orthopnea

Paroxysmal nocturnal dyspnea

Peripheral vascular resistance

Preload

Pulmonary edema (acute heart failure)

Splenomegaly

1. _Pulmonary edema_ is the acute inability of the heart to pump enough blood to meet the body's oxygen and nutrient needs.

2. _Cor pulmonale_ occurs when the right side of the heart fails because of an increased workload caused by pulmonary disease.

3. Organ enlargement that may occur with right-sided heart failure is known as _hepatomegaly_ and _splenomegaly_.

4. The goal of treatment for heart failure is to improve the heart's pumping ability and decrease the heart's workload by reducing _periph vasc resistance_.

5. _Paroxysmal noct. dyspnea_ causes supine patients to awaken suddenly with a feeling of suffocation.

6. The end-diastole stretch in the ventricles produced by ventricular volume is _preload_.

7. The tension in the ventricular wall during systole necessary to overcome vascular resistance is _afterload_.

8. _Orthopnea_ is dyspnea that occurs when the patient lies down.

FLUID ACCUMULATION PATTERNS

Label the backward accumulation of fluid and shade areas of fluid congestion.

The heart pumps blood in a closed circuit. If one side of the heart fails to adequately pump blood forward, it pools and backs up from the failing chamber. On the drawing, use arrows to mark the path of the backward accumulation of fluid from the side of the heart that is failing. Shade in areas where fluid congestion occurs.

To increase your understanding of where the backward accumulation of fluid occurs from a certain side of the heart, use blue shading to illustrate the side with deoxygenated blood accumulation. Use red shading for the side with oxygenated blood accumulation.

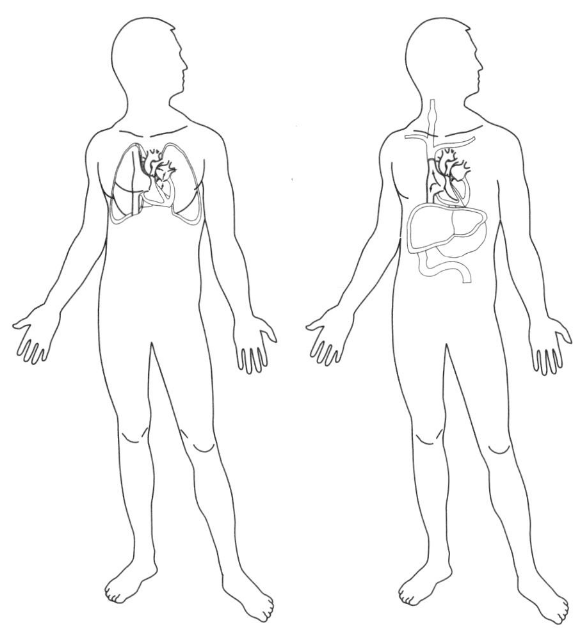

SIGNS AND SYMPTOMS OF HEART FAILURE

In heart failure, certain signs and symptoms occur based on the side of the heart that is failing as a pump.

Match the following sign or symptom to the failing side of the heart that is causing it.

1. ___*L*___ Dry cough
2. ___*R*___ Peripheral edema
3. ___*L*___ Crackles
4. ___*R*___ Hepatomegaly
5. ___*R*___ Jugular vein distention
6. ___*L*___ Dyspnea
7. ___*R*___ Splenomegaly
8. ___*L*___ Orthopnea

L. Left-sided heart failure

R. Right-sided heart failure

CRITICAL THINKING

Read the following case study and answer the questions.

Mr. Donner, age 72, is admitted to the cardiac unit for increasing dyspnea on exertion and fatigue.

Subjective Data
History of heart failure for 2 years
Unable to walk one block without increasing dyspnea
Sleeps at 60-degree angle in reclining chair
Increasing fatigue during the last 2 weeks

Objective Data
BP 140/78, P 108, R 24, T 98.8°F (37.1°C)
Jugular vein distention at 45 degrees
Has frequent dry cough
Bilateral crackles in lung bases
Nonpitting edema
Diagnostic studies
Chest x-ray examination: left and right ventricular hypertrophy, bilateral fluid in lower lung lobes

1. Explain the cause of Mr. Donner's fatigue, cough, and shortness of breath. *L-sided ♡ failure leading to backward fluid accum. in lung tissues + ↓ CO.*

2. Which of Mr. Donner's signs and symptoms are from left-sided heart failure and which are from right-sided heart failure?
   Left: *dyspnea, cough, crackles, orthopnea*
   Right: *jug. vein distention, peripheral edema*

3. Explain the purpose of each of the following therapies. How would they be beneficial in treating Mr. Donner's heart failure?
   A. Furosemide (Lasix) 40 mg PO bid: _______________
   B. Digitalis 0.125 mg PO qd: _______________
   C. 2-g sodium diet: _______________
   D. Oxygen 4 L/min: _______________

4. Mr. Donner suddenly becomes dyspneic and anxious, has moist crackles throughout his lungs, and pink frothy sputum. Explain what is happening. *He is experiencing acute ♡ failure - pulmonary edema. Fluid accumulation in lungs.*

5. Explain the purpose of each of the following therapies. How are they beneficial in treating Mr. Donner's acute heart failure? *Is severe & needs immed. tx.*
   A. High-Fowler's position: _______________
   B. Oxygen 6 L/min: _______________
   C. Furosemide (Lasix) 40 mg IVP: _______________
   D. Digitalis 0.25 mg PO: _______________
   E. Morphine 2 mg IVP: _______________

6. List two priority nursing diagnoses and goals for Mr. Donner's chronic heart failure. _______________

7. What are Mr. Donner's health learning needs to manage his chronic condition? *S/S of ♡ failure; meds: purpose of, monitoring (♡ rate, potassium), sx's; diet; energy conservation; daily wts*

REVIEW QUESTIONS

Choose the best answer unless directed otherwise.

1. A patient is admitted to a medical unit with a diagnosis of heart failure. The patient reports that she has had increasing fatigue during the past 2 weeks. Which of the following is the most likely cause of this fatigue?
   a. Dyspnea
   b. Decreased cardiac output
   c. Dry cough
   d. Orthopnea

2. A patient asks the nurse what her diagnosis of heart failure means. Which of the following is the nurse's best response?
   a. "Your heart briefly stops."
   b. "Your heart has an area of muscle that is dead."
   c. "Your heart is pumping too much blood."
   d. "Your heart is not an efficient pump."

3. A patient's chest x-ray examination indicates fluid in both lung bases. Which of the following signs or symptoms present during the nurse's assessment most reflects these x-ray examination findings?
   a. Fatigue
   b. Peripheral edema
   c. Bilateral crackles
   d. Jugular vein distention

4. To monitor the severity of a patient's heart failure, which of the following assessments is the most appropriate for the nurse to include as a daily assessment in the plan of care?
   a. Weight
   b. Calorie count
   c. Appetite
   d. Abdominal girth

5. A patient is being given digoxin (Lanoxin) to treat heart failure. Which of the following is a usual adult daily dosage of digoxin (Lanoxin)?
   a. 0.005 mg
   b. 0.025 mg
   c. 0.25 mg
   d. 2.5 mg

6. Which of the following signs indicates to the nurse that digoxin (Lanoxin) has been effective for a patient?
   a. Urine output decreases
   b. Urine output increases
   c. Heart rate higher than 95
   d. Heart rate lower than 50

7. When the nurse is reviewing a patient's daily laboratory test results, which of the following electrolyte imbalances should the nurse recognize as predisposing the patient to digoxin toxicity?
   a. Hypokalemia
   b. Hyperkalemia
   c. Hyponatremia
   d. Hypernatremia

8. For a patient who is being discharged on digoxin, the nurse should include which of the following in an explanation to the patient on the signs and symptoms of digoxin toxicity?
   a. Poor appetite
   b. Constipation
   c. Halos around lights
   d. Tachycardia

9. The patient is being discharged on furosemide (Lasix). The nurse evaluates the patient as understanding her medication teaching if she states that she will have which of the following laboratory tests monitored as ordered?
   a. "I will have my urine sodium checked."
   b. "I will have my calcium level checked."
   c. "I will have my prothrombin time checked."
   d. "I will have my potassium level checked."

Multiple response item. Select all that apply.
10. Which of the following does the nurse understand are the reasons a patient with pulmonary edema is given morphine sulfate?
    a. To reduce anxiety
    b. To relieve chest pain
    c. To strengthen heart contractions
    d. To increase blood pressure
    e. To reduce preload and afterload

11. If a patient has elevated pulmonary vascular pressures, the nurse understands that the patient is most likely to develop which of the following physiological cardiac changes?
    a. Left atrial atrophy
    b. Right atrial atrophy
    c. Left ventricular hypertrophy
    d. Right ventricular hypertrophy

12. The nurse evaluates that furosemide IV is effective in treating pulmonary edema if which of the following patient signs or symptoms is resolved?
    a. Pedal edema
    b. Jugular vein distention
    c. Pink, frothy sputum
    d. Bradycardia

13. A patient is being taught the action of digoxin, which is an inotropic agent. The nurse defines an inotropic agent as a medication that has which of the following actions?
    a. Decreases heart rate
    b. Increases heart rate
    c. Increases conduction time
    d. Strengthens heart contraction

14. For a patient receiving furosemide, the nurse evaluates the medication as being effective if which of the following effects occurs?
    a. Urine output increased
    b. Serum potassium decreased
    c. Heart rate increased
    d. Pulse pressure increased

15. When caring for an anxious patient with dyspnea, which of the following nursing actions is most helpful to include in the plan of care to relieve anxiety?
    a. Increasing activity levels
    b. Staying at patient's bedside
    c. Pulling the privacy curtain
    d. Closing the patient's door

UNDERSTANDING THE HEMATOPOIETIC AND LYMPHATIC SYSTEMS

CHECKLIST FOR LEARNING SUCCESS

Review of Anatomy and Physiology

- ❑ Blood components
- ❑ Functions of different blood cells
- ❑ Lymphatic system
- ❑ Effects of aging

Major Disorders

- ❑ Anemias
- ❑ Disseminated intravascular coagulation
- ❑ Idiopathic thrombocytopenic purpura
- ❑ Hemophilia
- ❑ Leukemias
- ❑ Multiple myeloma
- ❑ Hodgkin's disease
- ❑ Lymphoma
- ❑ Spleen disorders

Nursing Assessment

- ❑ Signs and symptoms of bleeding
- ❑ Lymph nodes
- ❑ Skin

Diagnostic Tests

- ❑ Complete blood cell count
- ❑ White blood cell differential
- ❑ Coagulation studies
- ❑ Bone marrow biopsy
- ❑ Lymphangiography
- ❑ Lymph node biopsy

Interventions

- ❑ Blood product administration
- ❑ Chemotherapy
- ❑ Thrombocytopenia precautions
- ❑ Infection precautions
- ❑ Bone marrow transplant

Common Medications

- ❑ Iron
- ❑ Colony-stimulating factors
- ❑ Chemotherapy
- ❑ Clotting factors

VOCABULARY

Fill in the blank with the appropriate word.

1. _Ecchymoses_ is a blue-black discoloration from hemorrhage under the skin.
2. _Lymphedema_ is the term used to describe swelling from blockage of lymph circulation.
3. Tiny hemorrhages into the skin creating a polka-dot appearance are called _petechiae_.
4. _Purpura_ is caused by hemorrhages into the skin, mucous membranes, or internal organs.
5. The patient with _thrombocytopenia_ has an increased risk for bleeding because of a lack of platelets.

LYMPHATIC SYSTEM

Match each part of the lymphatic system with its proper description.

1. _B_ Lymph capillaries
2. _D_ Lymph nodules MALT
3. _E_ Thoracic duct
4. _A_ Lymph nodes
5. _C_ Valves

A. Destroy pathogens in the lymph from the extremities before the lymph is returned to the blood
B. Collect tissue fluid from intercellular spaces
C. Prevent backflow of lymph in larger lymph vessels
D. Destroy pathogens that penetrate mucous membranes
E. Empties lymph from the lower body and upper left quadrant into the left subclavian vein

lymph nodules, aka MALT = mucosa-associated lymphatic tissue

Structures of the Lymphatic System
Label the following structures.

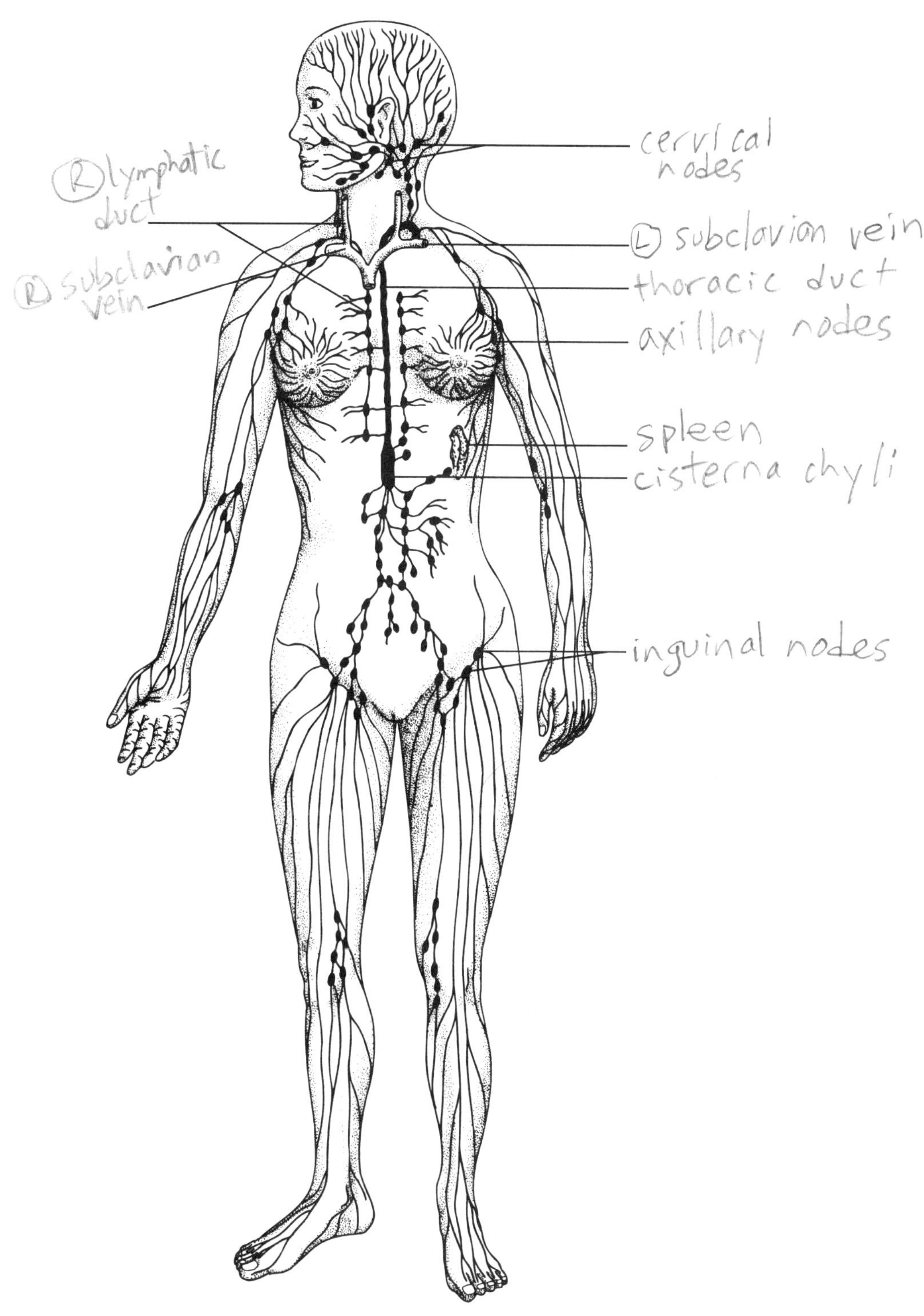

HEMATOPOIETIC SYSTEM

Match each term with its definition.

1. ____ Albumin
2. ____ Macrophages
3. ____ Calcium ions
4. ____ Intrinsic factor
5. ____ Hemoglobin
6. ____ Basophils
7. ____ Red bone marrow
8. ____ Stem cell
9. ____ Megakaryocyte
10. ____ Lymphocytes

A. May become any kind of blood cell
B. Essential for chemical clotting
C. Release histamine
D. A hematopoietic tissue
E. May become cells that produce antibodies
F. Large phagocytic cells
G. Promotes absorption of vitamin B_{12}
H. Its fragments become platelets
I. Carries oxygen in RBCs
J. Pulls tissue fluid into capillaries to maintain blood volume

CRITICAL THINKING

Read the case study and answer the questions.

Mr. Foster is receiving a unit of packed red blood cells. You assist with identification of the patient before it starts. The registered nurse then delegates monitoring of his vital signs every half hour to you.

1. Why should Mr. Foster be monitored for each of the following symptoms?
   A. Fever
   B. Back pain
   C. Respiratory distress
   D. Crackles
   E. Hives

2. Mr. Foster's respiratory rate increases from 16 to 20 breaths per minute. What do you do?

3. The physician asks that the transfusion be slowed down. How many hours can the blood hang before it must be stopped?

Choose the best answer.

1. Which of the following items are transported in blood plasma? Choose all that apply.
   a. Oxygen
   b. Nutrients
   c. Carbon dioxide
   d. Hormones

2. What is the mineral necessary for chemical clotting?
   a. Iron
   b. Sodium
   c. Potassium
   d. Calcium

3. Through which of the following does lymph return to the blood?
   a. Carotid arteries
   b. Aorta
   c. Inferior vena cava
   d. Subclavian veins

4. Which of the following is a normal hemoglobin value?
   a. 38% to 48%
   b. 12 to 18 g/100 mL
   c. 48 to 54 mg %
   d. 27 to 36 g/dL

5. Which laboratory study is monitored for the patient receiving heparin therapy?
   a. International normalized ratio (INR)
   b. Prothrombin time
   c. Partial thromboplastin time
   d. Bleeding time

6. Which blood product replaces missing clotting factors in the patient who has a bleeding disorder?
   a. Platelets
   b. Packed red blood cells
   c. Albumin
   d. Cryoprecipitate

7. A patient is on warfarin (Coumadin) therapy and has an INR of 1.6. Which action by the nurse is appropriate?
   a. Observe the patient for abnormal bleeding.
   b. Notify the physician and expect an order to increase the warfarin dose.
   c. Advise the patient to double today's dose of warfarin.
   d. Administer vitamin K per protocol.

8. Which gauge intravenous cannula should the nurse choose when preparing to initiate a blood transfusion?
   a. 18
   b. 22
   c. 24
   d. 28

9. A patient receiving a transfusion of packed red blood cells complains of chest and back pain. How do you respond?
   a. Do a complete physical assessment.
   b. Ask the patient to rate his pain on a 0 to 10 scale.
   c. Stop the transfusion or call the RN STAT depending on agency policy.
   d. Administer his analgesic, as needed (PRN).

10. The nurse is preparing to assist the physician with a bone marrow biopsy. Which of the following interventions is most important for the nurse to do before the procedure?
    a. Explain the procedure to the patient's family.
    b. Administer an analgesic to the patient.
    c. Observe the patient for bleeding.
    d. Drape the biopsy site.

Nursing Care of Patients with Hematological and Lymphatic Disorders

VOCABULARY

Label each statement true or false.

1. __F__ Anemia is a reduction in white blood cells. *[handwritten: red]*
2. __T__ Hemolysis is the destruction of red blood cells.
3. __T__ Pancytopenia is reduced numbers of all blood cells.
4. __T__ Polycythemia is the production of excess blood cells.
5. __F__ Phlebotomy is the excision of a vessel. *[handwritten: 'drawal of blood]*
6. __T__ Disseminated intravascular coagulation involves accelerated clotting throughout *[handwritten: periphrl bl. vssls]* the circulation.
7. __F__ Thrombocytopenia is an increase in platelets.
8. __F__ Hemarthrosis is bleeding into the muscles. *[handwritten: jts]*
9. __T__ Leukemia literally means "white blood."
10. __F__ Cancer of the lymph system is called lymphemia. *[handwritten: leukemia]*
11. __T__ Abnormalities in B cells and T cells can result in lymphoma.
12. __T__ Enlargement of the spleen is called splenomegaly.

CRITICAL THINKING: LEUKEMIA

Read the case study and answer the questions.

Mr. Frantzis is a 60-year-old man in the acute stage of chronic lymphocytic leukemia. He is admitted to a nursing home because he has no family to help care for him. He has had chemotherapy in the past but has decided against further treatment. You are assigned to his care today. You find him pale and weak, with no energy to get out of bed. He also complains of pain in his chest.

1. Mr. Frantzis says he is too weak to get up for breakfast. What do you do? *[handwritten: On those days when he's too tired to get up, bring him breakfast in bed. A liquid supplement that is easy to drink might be another option if ordered by doct]*

2. How do you follow up on the pain in his chest? *[handwritten: Do pain assmnt w/ WHAT'S UP? may be due to sternal or rib tndrnss from crowding of bone marrow]*

3. The nursing assistant assigned to Mr. Frantzis has a runny nose. What should you do? *[handwritten: Not all rhinorrhea is intxs; find out if LNA has a cold. If so, reassign pt's care to another LNA bec. he is @ risk of intxn]*

4. Mr. Frantzis calls you "Jennifer" when you enter his room, but that is not your name. How do you respond? *[handwritten: Clarify who "Jennifer" is – u may resemble someone. However, he may be developing confusion if the leukemia has invaded CNS,]*

5. You note bleeding from Mr. Frantzis' gums. What care can you provide? *[handwritten: Provide good mouth care after ea. meal & as required. Use soft toothbrush or swab if irritation is severe. Avoid giving him foods that are irritating, acidic, or extremely hot or cold. Remove dentures for cleaning @ HS. Inspect mouth carefully while dentures are out.]*

CRITICAL THINKING: HODGKIN'S DISEASE

Circle the errors in the following paragraph and write in the correct information.

Joe is a 28-year-old construction worker diagnosed with stage I Hodgkin's disease. He initially went to his physician because of a painful lump in his neck. He is also experiencing high fevers and weight loss. The diagnosis was confirmed in laboratory test by the presence of Reed-Steinway cells. He expresses his fears to his nurse, who tells him that Hodgkin's disease is not really cancer, and that it is often curable. Joe takes a leave from work and begins palliative radiation therapy.

SICKLE CELL ANEMIA

Fill in the signs and symptoms of sickle cell anemia.

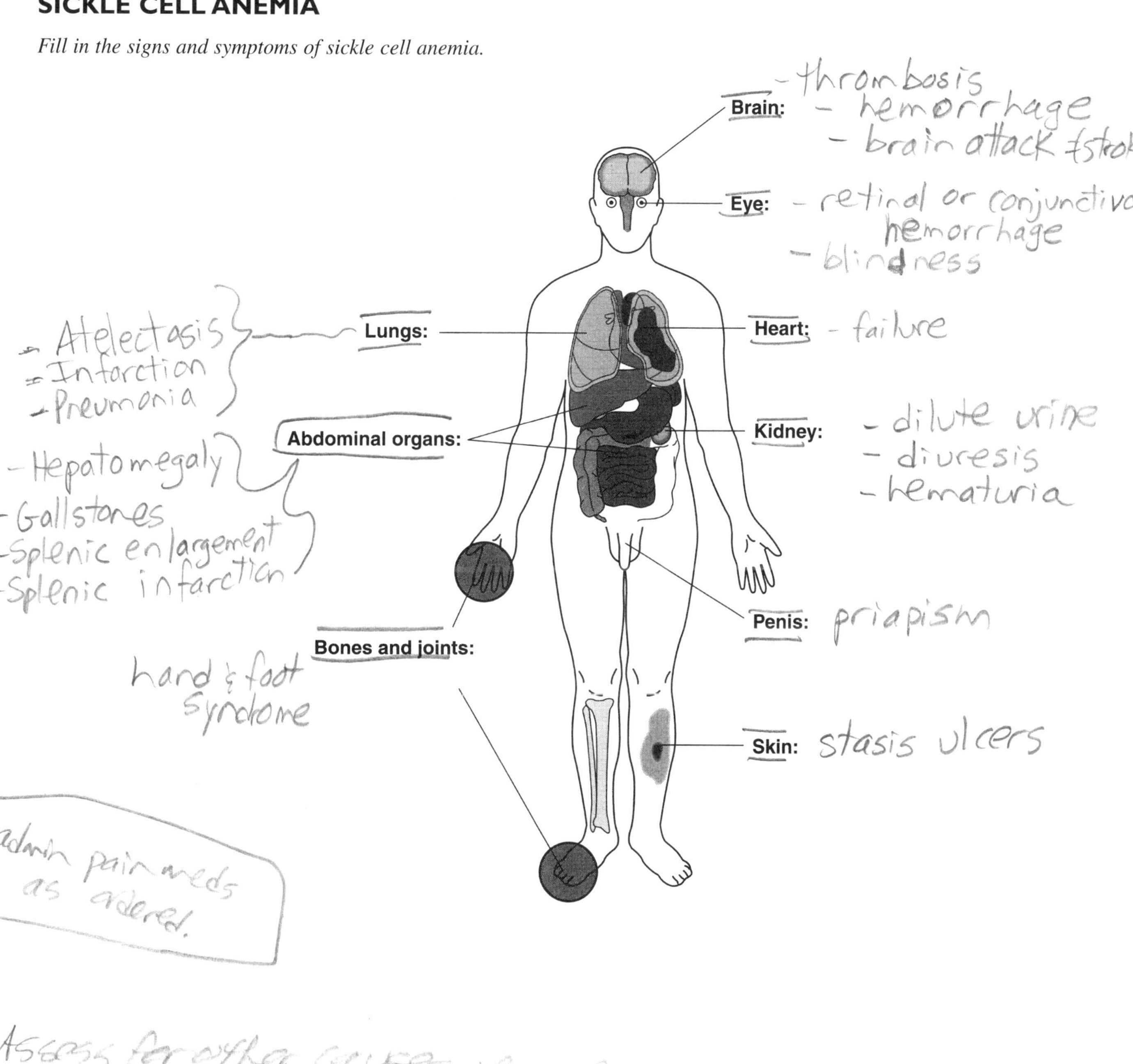

REVIEW QUESTIONS

Choose the best answer.

1. A patient has iron deficiency anemia. Which of the following foods will best help provide dietary iron?
   a. Fresh fruits
   b. Lean red meats
   c. Dairy products
   d. Breads and cereals

2. A patient admitted with gastrointestinal tract bleeding has a hemoglobin level of 6 g/dL. She asks the nurse why she feels short of breath. Which response is best?
   a. "Anemia prevents your lungs from absorbing oxygen effectively."
   b. "You do not have enough hemoglobin to carry oxygen to your tissues."
   c. "You don't have enough blood to feed your cells."
   d. "You have lost a lot of blood, and that has damaged your lungs."

3. A 50-year-old African American patient is diagnosed with anemia. Where can the nurse assess for pallor?
   a. Scalp
   b. Axillae
   c. Chest
   d. Conjunctivae

4. Which of the following is an early sign of anemia?
   a. Palpitations
   b. Glossitis
   c. Pallor
   d. Weight loss

5. A 17-year-old African American boy is admitted in sickle cell crisis. Which of the following events most likely contributed to the onset of the crisis?
   a. He started a new job last week.
   b. He walked home in a cold rain yesterday.
   c. He had seafood for dinner last night.
   d. He has not exercised for a week.

6. A patient has hand-foot syndrome related to his sickle cell anemia. What findings does the nurse expect to see as the patient is assessed?
   a. Unequal growth of fingers and toes
   b. Webbing between fingers and toes
   c. Purplish discoloration of hands and feet
   d. Deformities of the wrists and ankles

7. The nurse has taught a patient with thrombocytopenia how to prevent bleeding. Which of the following is the best evidence that the teaching has been effective?
   a. The patient states that he will be careful to avoid injury.
   b. The patient can list signs and symptoms of bleeding.
   c. The patient uses an electric razor instead of his safety razor.
   d. The patient states when he should call the doctor.

8. A patient with a history of hemophilia A arrives in the emergency department complaining of a "funny feeling" in his elbow. The patient states that he thinks he is bleeding into the joint. Which response by the nurse is correct?
   a. Palpate the patient's elbow to assess for swelling.
   b. Notify the physician immediately and expect an order for factor VIII.
   c. Prepare the patient for an x-ray examination to determine whether bleeding is occurring.
   d. Apply heat to the patient's elbow and wait for the physician to examine the patient.

9. For which of the following problems should the nurse monitor in the patient with multiple myeloma?
   a. Uncontrolled bleeding
   b. Respiratory distress
   c. Liver engorgement
   d. Pathological fractures

10. Which of the following interventions can help minimize complications related to hypercalcemia?
    a. Encourage 3 to 4 L of fluid daily.
    b. Have the patient cough and deep breathe every 2 hours.
    c. Place the patient on bed rest.
    d. Apply heat to painful areas.

11. A patient with a new diagnosis of lymphoma is experiencing fatigue. Which of the following is the best way to assess her fatigue?
    a. Observe her activity level.
    b. Monitor for changes in vital signs.
    c. Monitor hemoglobin and hematocrit values.
    d. Have her rate her fatigue on a scale of 0 to 10.

12. Patients with lymphoma are at risk for infection. Which of the following activities increases this risk?
    a. Going to church
    b. Taking a walk outside
    c. Cleaning the house
    d. Watching television

13. The patient is having difficulty coping with her new diagnosis of lymphoma. Which response by the nurse is most helpful?
    a. "Don't worry. You'll be okay."
    b. "The treatments you are receiving will make you feel better very soon."
    c. "Who do you usually go to when you have a problem?"
    d. "Have you made end-of-life decisions?"

14. A patient is admitted for a splenectomy. Why is an injection of vitamin K ordered before surgery?
    a. To correct clotting problems
    b. To promote healing
    c. To prevent postoperative infection
    d. To dry secretions

15. Which of the following conditions places a patient at risk for respiratory complications following his splenectomy?
    a. A low platelet count
    b. An incision near the diaphragm
    c. Early ambulation
    d. Early discharge

16. Patients are at risk for overwhelming postsplenectomy infection (OPSI) following splenectomy. Which of the following symptoms alerts the nurse to this possibility?
    a. Bruising around the operative site
    b. Irritability
    c. Pain
    d. Fever

17. What discharge teaching is most important to help the patient who has had a splenectomy prevent infection?
    a. Avoid showering for 1 week.
    b. Sleep in a semi-Fowler's position.
    c. Receive vaccines against infection.
    d. Stay on antibiotics for life.

unit SEVEN

UNDERSTANDING THE RESPIRATORY SYSTEM

CHECKLIST FOR LEARNING SUCCESS

Chis 29-31

Review of Anatomy and Physiology and Aging Changes
- ❑ Lungs and bronchial tree
- ❑ Mechanisms of breathing
- ❑ Acid-base balance
- ❑ Aging changes

Major Disorders
- ❑ Upper respiratory infections
- ❑ Influenza
- ❑ Cancer of larynx
- ❑ Pneumonia
- ❑ Tuberculosis
- ❑ Pleural effusion
- ❑ COPD
- ❑ Chronic bronchitis
- ❑ Asthma
- ❑ Emphysema
- ❑ Cystic fibrosis
- ❑ Pulmonary embolism
- ❑ Pneumothorax
- ❑ Respiratory failure
- ❑ Lung cancer

Nursing Assessment
- ❑ Adventitious lung sounds
- ❑ Dyspnea
- ❑ Activity tolerance

Diagnostic Tests
- ❑ Red blood cell count
- ❑ White blood cell count
- ❑ Sputum culture and sensitivity (C&S)
- ❑ Oximetry
- ❑ Arterial blood gases
- ❑ Chest x-ray
- ❑ Pulmonary function studies
- ❑ Bronchoscopy

Interventions
- ❑ Breathing exercises
- ❑ Cough and deep breathe (C&DB)
- ❑ Smoking cessation
- ❑ Oxygen therapy
- ❑ Nebulized mist treatments
- ❑ Metered-dose inhalers
- ❑ Chest physiotherapy
- ❑ Incentive spirometry (IS)
- ❑ Chest tubes
- ❑ Tracheostomy
- ❑ Mechanical ventilation
- ❑ Noninvasive positive pressure ventilation (NIPPV)
- ❑ Thoracic surgery

Respiratory System Function, Assessment, and Therapeutic Measures

VOCABULARY

Complete the sentences with words provided below.

Adventitious   Barrel chest   Dyspnea   Thoracentesis   Tracheostomy
Apnea   Crepitus   Respiratory excursion   Tidaling   Tracheotomy

1. A patient with a low oxygen saturation may develop _________.
2. _________ may develop if air leaks into tissues from a chest tube site.
3. A _________ may be necessary for severe pleural effusion.
4. The patient with air trapping may develop a _________.
5. The nurse can measure respiratory _________ to check chest expansion.
6. Crackles are an example of a/an _________ sound.
7. A patient who is choking may need an emergency _________.
8. The _________ in the water-seal chamber shows that a chest tube is intact.
9. _________ is the absence of respirations.
10. A patient is taught to remove the inner cannula of a _________ tube every 8 hours for cleaning.

ANATOMY

Number the following structures in the order in which air flows through them.

_________ Nose   _________ Nasal cavities   _________ Trachea
_________ Larynx   _________ Oropharynx   _________ Secondary bronchi
_________ Primary bronchi   _________ Bronchioles   _________ Alveoli
_________ Laryngopharynx   _________ Nasopharynx

VENTILATION

Number the events of breathing in proper sequence beginning with the medulla.

_______ The medulla generates motor impulses.

___4___ The chest cavity is enlarged in all directions.

___3___ The diaphragm and external intercostal muscles contract.

___6___ Intrapulmonic pressure decreases.

___2___ Motor impulses travel along the phrenic and intercostal nerves.

___5___ The chest wall expands the parietal pleura, which expands the visceral pleura, which in turn expands the lungs.

___7___ Air enters the lungs until intrapulmonic pressure equals atmospheric pressure.

ADVENTITIOUS LUNG SOUNDS

Match the adventitious lung sound to its description.

1. ___E___ Coarse crackles
2. ___A___ Fine crackles
3. ___F___ Wheezes
4. ___D___ Stridor
5. ___C___ Pleural friction rub
6. ___B___ Diminished

A. Velcro being torn apart
B. Faint lung sounds
C. Leather rubbing together
D. Loud crowing noise
E. Moist bubbling
F. High-pitched violins

CHEST DRAINAGE

Label the three chambers of the chest drainage system and explain the function of each.

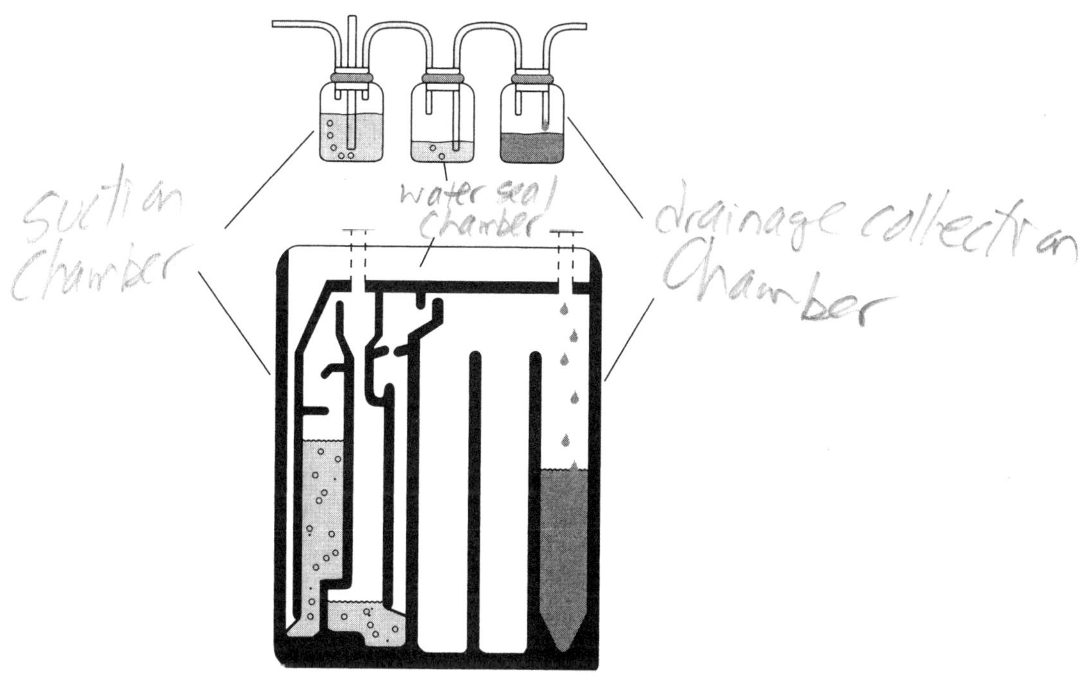

THE RESPIRATORY SYSTEM

Label the parts.

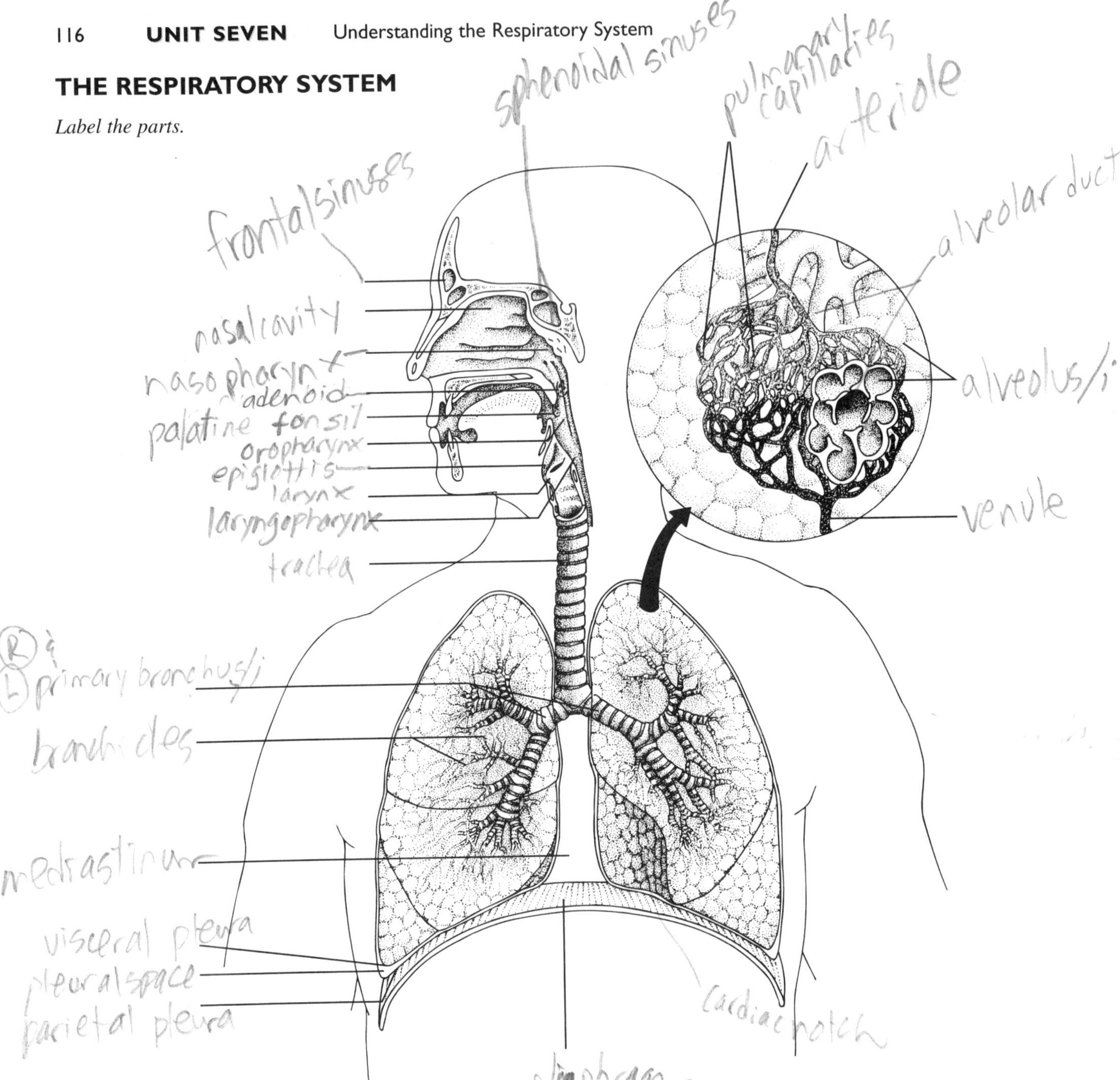

CRITICAL THINKING

Read the case study and answer the questions.

Bill, a licensed practical nurse (LPN), is collecting admission data on Mr. Howe, who has been admitted for dyspnea and weight loss. While questioning Mr. Howe, Bill learns that he has had progressive weight loss over the past several months and that he has a productive cough. He also complains of waking up at night "wringing wet," and his wife has to change the bed sheets.

1. What additional questions should Bill ask about Mr. Howe's cough? _WHAT'S UP?_

2. What disorder is suggested by Mr. Howe's symptoms? _______________________________

3. What diagnostic tests do you expect to see ordered? _______________________________

4. Mr. Howe is scheduled for a bronchoscopy. What preprocedure care should Bill provide? Postprocedure? _______________________________

REVIEW QUESTIONS

Choose the best answer.

1. Which of the following structures covers the larynx during swallowing?
   a. Hyoid cartilage
   b. Vocal cords
   c. Soft palate
   d. Epiglottis

2. Where are the respiratory centers located in the brain?
   a. Cerebral cortex and cerebellum
   b. Medulla and pons
   c. Hypothalamus and cerebral cortex
   d. Hypothalamus and temporal lobes

3. What is the purpose of the serous fluid between the pleural membranes?
   a. Enhance exchange of gases
   b. Facilitate coughing
   c. Destroy pathogens
   d. Prevent friction

4. Within the alveoli, surface tension is decreased and inflation is possible because of the presence of which substance?
   a. Tissue fluid
   b. Surfactant
   c. Pulmonary blood
   d. Mucus

5. What is the function of the nasal mucosa?
   a. Assist with gas exchange
   b. Sweep mucus and pathogens to the trachea
   c. Warm and moisten the incoming air
   d. Increase the oxygen content of the air

6. Deteriorating cilia in the respiratory tract predispose the elderly to which of the following problems?
   a. Chronic hypoxia
   b. Pulmonary hypertension
   c. Respiratory infection
   d. Decreased ventilation

7. Which of the following adventitious lung sounds is a violinlike sound?
   a. Crackles
   b. Wheezes
   c. Friction rub
   d. Crepitus

8. An LPN checks the oxygen saturation on a patient with chronic lung disease. The result is 79%. The patient has removed her oxygen cannula, and it is lying on the bed. Which of the following actions is appropriate next?
   a. Call the registered nurse stat.
   b. Put the oxygen cannula back on the patient.
   c. Do a nebulized mist treatment.
   d. No action necessary; this is a normal saturation.

9. The purpose of pursed-lip breathing is to promote which of the following?
   a. Carbon dioxide excretion
   b. Carbon dioxide retention
   c. Oxygen excretion
   d. Oxygen retention

10. Which position will help increase oxygen saturation in the patient with lung disease?
    a. Prone
    b. Supine with head on pillow
    c. Trendelenburg
    d. Side lying with good lung dependent

11. What care should the nurse provide for the patient with a transtracheal catheter?
    a. Assist with cleaning the catheter two to three times a day.
    b. Provide supplemental oxygen via mask at all times.
    c. Help remove the catheter at night for sleeping.
    d. Assist to connect the catheter to a humidification source.

12. What is the purpose of chest physiotherapy?
    a. It helps the patient strengthen chest muscles.
    b. It humidifies thick respiratory secretions.
    c. It promotes lung expansion.
    d. It helps the patient expectorate secretions.

13. The nurse notes that the suction-control chamber on a chest-drainage system is bubbling vigorously. Which intervention is appropriate?
    a. Check the system for leaks.
    b. Replace the drainage system with a new one.
    c. Reduce the level of wall suction.
    d. Increase the water level in the suction control chamber.

30

Nursing Care of Patients with Upper Respiratory Tract Disorders

VOCABULARY

Unscramble the letters of the following words to fill in the blanks in the statements below.

hiitsrin   aadihpysg
pixessait   daxueet
laiohnpstry   cayetorlemeng

1. The patient who has had his or her larynx removed is called a *laryngectamee*
2. A nosebleed is called *epistaxis*.
3. *Exudate* is the term used to describe drainage or pus.
4. A "nose job" is called *rhinoplasty*
5. Difficulty swallowing is called *dysphagia*.
6. *Rhinitis* is the correct term for a runny nose.

CRITICAL THINKING: NASAL SURGERY

Read the case study and answer the questions that follow.

Mr. Jones has a submucous resection done for a deviated nasal septum.

1. Following surgery, you note that Mr. Jones is swallowing repeatedly while he sleeps. What do you do?
   Assess for bleeding — wake Mr. Jones to examine. VS checked for signs of blood loss. Make sure he's in semi-Fowler's position to prevent aspiration & swelling

2. Before discharge you explain to Mr. Jones that he should not do anything that can increase bleeding, such as sneezing, coughing, or straining to have a bowel movement. He says, "How can I avoid doing those things? It sounds impossible." How do you respond?
   Get Rx for antihistamine, cough suppressant. Drink plenty of fluids, take in ample fiber, use laxatives to keep stools soft.

3. Mr. Jones asks if he can use aspirin for pain. What do you say?
   No — because it can cause bleeding. Check doc re: acetaminophen & other similar meds (ibuprofen) can as well.

CRITICAL THINKING: INFLUENZA

Read the case study and answer the questions that follow.

Your son comes down with influenza. He is feverish, tired, and has a sore throat and headache. The physician did a throat culture and told you it is viral. She told you to put your son to bed and give him fluids and acetaminophen.

1. Why didn't the physician order antibiotics? *antibiox kill bacteria, not virus. Discretion must be used t antibiox - overuse can cause resistent bacteria strains*

2. How will fluids help? *thin mucus, secretions which facilitates lungs' cough production & expels*

3. When should you give the acetaminophen? *Fever may be benificial if not too high. ask doc what temp to give acetaminophen or other evidence of discomfort*

4. Your daughter develops the same symptoms. Is it necessary to take her to the physician? *Flu is contagious, so it is reasonable to provide same care as son reqired to do if symptoms are same. Call doc to discuss - probably unnecessary to go see doc unless other sxs present. Don't share rx's if any given.*

5. Your elderly grandmother was visiting when your son first developed symptoms. She is now calling to say she has gotten the flu, and her chest hurts. She asks what she should do. What should you tell her? *Older adults are more vulnerable - she could more easily develop pneumonia. She ought to go to dr's to be evaluated. If t in 48 hours of exposure, she could take tamiflu.*

REVIEW QUESTIONS

Choose the best answer.

1. A patient visits her nurse practitioner (NP) after she has had a cold for a week and is now experiencing a severe headache and fever. Her NP diagnoses a sinus infection. Which of the following additional symptoms is the patient likely to exhibit?
   a. Facial tenderness
   b. Chest pain
   c. Photophobia
   d. Ear drainage

2. In addition to antibiotics, which of the following recommendations can the nurse make to increase comfort in a patient experiencing sinusitis? Choose all answers that are correct.
   a. Coughing and deep breathing
   b. Sinus irrigation
   c. Hot moist packs
   d. Room humidifier
   e. Percussion and postural drainage
   f. Semi-Fowler's position

3. When evaluating the effectiveness of nursing interventions for sinusitis discomfort, which of the following does the nurse assess?
   a. White blood cell count
   b. Amount and color of sinus drainage
   c. Capillary refill
   d. Comfort level

4. A 58-year-old man is diagnosed with cancer of the larynx. Which of the following are early symptoms of this cancer?
   a. Anemia and fatigue
   b. Crackles and stridor
   c. A noticeable lump in the neck
   d. Dysphagia or hoarseness

5. Place the following four nursing actions for the new laryngectomee in correct order of priority.
   3 a. Assist with ambulation.
   4 b. Set up a visit from a well-adjusted laryngectomee.
   1 c. Maintain a patent airway.
   2 d. Control postoperative pain.

6. Which of the following communication methods is not an option for a patient following laryngectomy surgery?
   a. Placing a finger over the stoma
   b. Using a special valve that diverts air into the esophagus
   c. Using a picture board
   d. Learning esophageal speech

7. A narcotic analgesic is ordered for postoperative pain. Why are narcotics given in low doses to the laryngectomy patient?
   a. They depress the respiratory rate and cough reflex.
   b. They increase respiratory tract secretions.
   c. They have a tendency to cause stomal edema.
   d. They can cause addiction.

8. The nurse teaches a patient how to live with a new tracheostomy. Which of the following instructions is appropriate?
   a. "Never suction your tracheostomy; you might damage your trachea."
   b. "You should not feel bad about the tracheostomy— you should feel lucky to be alive."
   c. "Be sure to protect your tracheostomy from pollutants such as powders, hair, and chemicals."
   d. "Your tracheostomy will be cleaned each time you visit your doctor."

9. A 17-year-old student enters the emergency department with a nosebleed that won't quit. Which of the following positions is recommended for the patient with a nosebleed?
   a. Lying down with feet elevated
   b. Sitting up with neck extended
   c. Lying down with a small pillow under the head
   d. Sitting up leaning slightly forward

10. The physician orders local application of epinephrine 1:1000 solution to treat a nosebleed. The patient asks how this will help. Which of the following responses by the nurse is best?
    a. "It will raise your blood pressure, which is necessary because of blood loss."
    b. "It will dilate your bronchioles and make your breathing easier."
    c. "It will help your blood to clot to reduce bleeding."
    d. "It will constrict your vessels and slow down the bleeding."

31

Nursing Care of Patients with Lower Respiratory Tract Disorders

VOCABULARY

Complete the crossword puzzle.

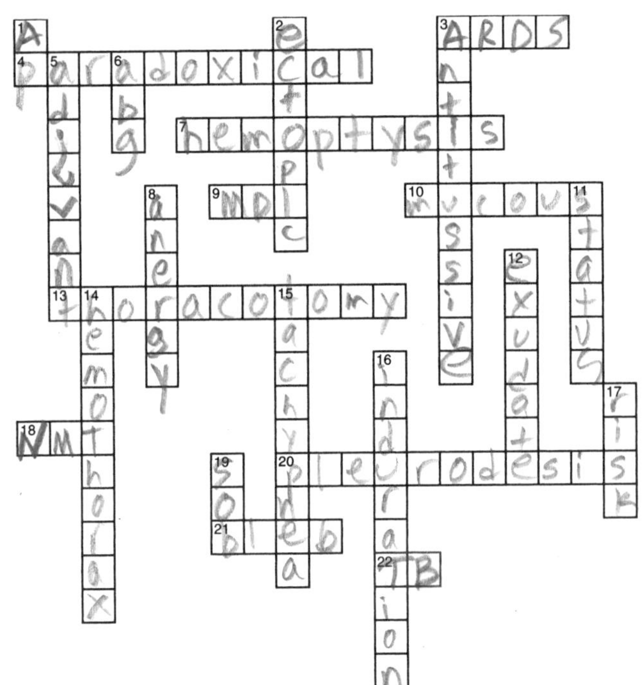

Across

3. Also called "white lung"
4. Chest collapses during inspiration during this type of respiration
7. Bloody sputum
9. Abbreviation for inhaler *metered dose inhaler*
10. Respiratory membrane secretion
13. Incision into the chest
18. Abbreviation for inhaled nebulized medication *nebulized mist tx*
20. Treatment for repeat pneumothorax
21. Blister on lung
22. Abbreviation for tuberculosis

Down

1. Abbreviation for "front to back" when referring to the chest *anteroposterior (AP)*
2. Term used to describe hormones produced by tumors *ectopic*
3. Medication that relieves coughing *antitussive*
5. Treatment in addition to standard therapy *adjuvant*
6. Abbreviation for laboratory tests done to measure respiratory status *arterial blood gases (ABG)*
8. Unable to react, as in skin testing *anergy*
11. Continuous asthma is called ___ *status* ___ asthmaticus.
12. Drainage on infected tonsils *exudate*
14. Blood in the chest *hemothorax*
15. Rapid respirations *tachypnea*
16. Firm raised area in positive tuberculosis skin test *induration*
17. Smoking is a ___ *risk* ___ factor for cancer
19. Abbreviation for short of breath *SOB (shortness of breath)*

RESPIRATORY MEDICATIONS

Match the medication with its action.

1. __B__ Prednisone
2. __D__ Albuterol (Ventolin)
3. __E__ Tiotropium (Spiriva)
4. __F__ Cromolyn sodium (Intal)
5. __A__ Guaifenesin (Humibid)
6. __C__ Zafirlukast (Accolate)
7. __G__ Codeine

A. Expectorant
B. Potent anti-inflammatory
C. Leukotriene inhibitor (reduces inflammation in asthma)
D. Beta-adrenergic bronchodilator
E. Anticholinergic bronchodilator
F. Mast cell stabilizer to prevent asthma
G. Antitussive

CRITICAL THINKING

Read the case study and answer the questions.

Edith is a 56-year-old homemaker admitted to the hospital with emphysema and acute dyspnea. She is a smoker with a 48-pack-year history.

1. What data do you collect for Edith's admission database?

2. What does a 48-pack-year history mean?

3. Explain the pathophysiology involved in emphysema. How does the disease cause dyspnea?

4. What do you expect Edith's lungs to sound like when you auscultate?

5. Why is it important for Edith to receive no more than 2 L of oxygen per minute?

6. Why might Edith be at risk for pneumothorax?

7. What position will help Edith's shortness of breath? Why?

8. How can you encourage Edith to stop smoking?

REVIEW QUESTIONS

Choose the best answer.

1. A 72-year-old chemist has left lower lobe pneumonia. His nurse checks his oxygen saturation and the result is 86%. Which of the following actions by the nurse is best?
   a. Call the physician for an order for oxygen.
   b. No action necessary; this is a normal SaO_2.
   c. Call the respiratory therapist stat for assistance.
   d. Walk the patient in the hall and recheck his O_2 saturation.

2. Which of the following explanations by the nurse will help a patient understand what to expect during a bronchoscopy?
   a. "The physician will place a small tube through your nose or mouth and into the bronchi to look at your airways."
   b. "You will breathe a radioactive substance that will show diseased areas in your lungs."
   c. "You will need to drink a thick white liquid, which will be opaque on the x-rays."
   d. "A dye will be injected to help visualize the structures of the bronchioles. Do you have any allergies?"

3. Which of the following nursing actions is appropriate when a patient returns to his or her room after a bronchoscopy?
   a. Order a meal because the patient has been nil per os (NPO) for 8 hours.
   b. Encourage fluids to flush dye from the patient's system.
   c. Monitor the patient for return to consciousness.
   d. Check for a gag reflex before allowing the patient to drink.

4. A patient asks how to avoid lung cancer. Which risk factors should the nurse relate? Choose all that apply.
   a. Living in a cold climate
   b. Smoking
   c. Exposure to passive smoke
   d. Air pollution
   e. Crowded living conditions
   f. Diet low in fruits and vegetables

5. A patient with a new diagnosis of lung cancer decides to have radiation therapy. Which of the following expectations of this treatment is most appropriate?
   a. Complete cure of the cancer
   b. Increased comfort
   c. Prevention of the need for oxygen
   d. Prevention of cancer spread

6. A newly diagnosed patient asks what asthma is. Which of the following explanations by the nurse is correct?
   a. "Your airways are inflamed and spastic."
   b. "You have fluid in your lungs that is causing shortness of breath."
   c. "Your airways are stretched and nonfunctional."
   d. "You have a low-grade infection that keeps your bronchial tree irritated."

7. Which of the following is the best explanation of emphysema for a newly diagnosed patient?
   a. "You have inflamed bronchioles, which causes a lot of secretions."
   b. "Your lungs have lost some of their elasticity, and air gets trapped."
   c. "The blood supply to your lungs is damaged, so you can't absorb oxygen."
   d. "You have large dilated sacs of sputum in your lungs."

8. A patient is treated with intravenous (IV) methylprednisolone (Solu-Medrol) for emphysema. What is the purpose of corticosteroid treatment in lung disease?
   a. Dry secretions.
   b. Treat the infection that causes an exacerbation.
   c. Improve the oxygen-carrying capacity of hemoglobin.
   d. Reduce airway inflammation.

9. How many liters per minute of oxygen should be administered to the patient with emphysema?
   a. 2 L/min
   b. 6 L/min
   c. 10 L/min
   d. 95 L/min

10. Which of the following medications can be used to quickly reduce shortness of breath in a crisis situation for a patient with end-stage respiratory disease?
    a. Oral cortisone
    b. Intramuscular meperidine (Demerol)
    c. IV morphine
    d. IV propanolol (Inderal)

11. Which of the following positions is best for a chest-drainage system when the patient is being transported by wheelchair?
    a. Hang it on the top of the wheelchair backrest.
    b. Place it on the patient's feet and ask the patient to hold it.
    c. Hang it on the same pole as the patient's IV.
    d. Place it in the patient's lap.

12. The nurse notes vigorous bubbling in the water-seal chamber of a chest-drainage system. Which of the following actions should the nurse take to correct the bubbling?
    a. Examine the entire system and tubing for air leaks.
    b. Lower the level of suction.
    c. Nothing; vigorous bubbling is expected.
    d. Ask the patient to cough forcefully.

13. How can the nurse help monitor effectiveness of therapy for the patient with a pneumothorax and a chest-drainage system?
    a. Palpate for crepitus.
    b. Auscultate lung sounds.
    c. Document color and amount of sputum.
    d. Monitor suction level.

14. Which of the following risk factors presents the greatest threat for respiratory disease?
    a. Smoking
    b. High-fat diet
    c. Exposure to radiation
    d. Alcohol consumption

UNDERSTANDING THE GASTROINTESTINAL, HEPATIC, AND PANCREATIC SYSTEMS

CHECKLIST FOR LEARNING SUCCESS

Review of Anatomy and Physiology

- ❏ Gastrointestinal:
  - ❏ Oral cavity/pharynx
  - ❏ Esophagus
  - ❏ Stomach
  - ❏ Small intestine
  - ❏ Large intestine
  - ❏ Aging
  - ❏ Liver structure and function
  - ❏ Gallbladder structure and function
  - ❏ Pancreas structure and function
  - ❏ Aging changes

Major Disorders

- ❏ Oral disorders
- ❏ Nausea/vomiting
- ❏ Eating disorders
- ❏ Oral/esophageal cancer
- ❏ Gastroesophageal reflux disease (GERD)
- ❏ Gastritis
- ❏ Peptic ulcer disease
- ❏ Gastric bleeding
- ❏ Gastric cancer
- ❏ Constipation/diarrhea
- ❏ Appendicitis
- ❏ Peritonitis
- ❏ Diverticulosis
- ❏ Inflammatory bowel disease
- ❏ Absorption disorders
- ❏ Intestinal obstructions
- ❏ Lower gastrointestinal (GI) bleeding
- ❏ Colon cancer
- ❏ Hepatitis
- ❏ Liver failure
- ❏ Pancreatitis
- ❏ Cholecystitis
- ❏ Cholelithiasis
- ❏ Cancer

Nursing Assessment

- ❏ Nursing data collection
- ❏ Medical history
- ❏ Physical assessment
- ❏ Pain
- ❏ Alcohol use history
- ❏ Medication history
- ❏ GI S&S
- ❏ Skin
- ❏ Abdomen
- ❏ Mental status

Diagnostic Tests

- ❏ Laboratory tests
- ❏ Flat plate of abdomen
- ❏ Upper GI series
- ❏ Lower GI series
- ❏ Esophagogastroduodenoscopy (EGD)
- ❏ Colonoscopy
- ❏ Gastric analysis
- ❏ Stool studies
- ❏ IgG antibody test
- ❏ ALT, AST
- ❏ Albumin
- ❏ Amylase
- ❏ Ammonia
- ❏ Bilirubin
- ❏ Prothrombin time
- ❏ Occult blood
- ❏ UGI, LGI series
- ❏ Cholecystogram
- ❏ Liver scan
- ❏ ERCP
- ❏ Liver biopsy

Interventions

- ❏ GI intubation
- ❏ Tube feedings
- ❏ Total parenteral nutrition (TPN)/peripheral parenteral nutrition (PPN)
- ❏ GI decompression
- ❏ Gastric surgeries/complications
- ❏ Nursing care after gastric surgery
- ❏ Ostomy management
- ❏ TIPS
- ❏ Tamponade
- ❏ Transplant
- ❏ Cholecystectomy
- ❏ Nutrition
- ❏ ESWL
- ❏ Pain control

Common Medications

- ❏ Antacids
- ❏ Antidiarrheals
- ❏ Antiemetics
- ❏ Bulk-forming agents
- ❏ H_2 receptor antagonists
- ❏ Laxatives
- ❏ Proton pump inhibitors
- ❏ Stool softeners
- ❏ Sulfasalazine (Azulfidine)
- ❏ Vitamin B_{12}
- ❏ Diuretics
- ❏ Analgesics
- ❏ Histamine antagonists
- ❏ Lactulose
- ❏ Neomycin

Gastrointestinal, Hepatic, and Pancreatic Systems Function, Assessment, and Therapeutic Measures

FUNCTIONS OF THE GASTROINTESTINAL SYSTEM

Fill in the blanks with the appropriate part of the gastrointestinal system.

1. The ___lower___ ___esophageal___ sphincter prevents back-up of stomach contents into the esophagus.
2. The ___ileocecal___ valve prevents back-up of fecal material from the large intestine into the small intestine.
3. The ___pyloric___ sphincter prevents back-up of duodenal contents into the stomach.
4. The absorption of most of the end products of digestion occurs in the ___small___ intestine.
5. The digestion of protein begins in the ___stomach___.
6. Water and the vitamins produced by the normal flora are absorbed in the ___large___ intestine.
7. The ___small___ intestine is the site of action of bile and pancreatic enzymes.
8. The passageway for food into the stomach from the mouth is the ___esophagus___.
9. Voluntary control of defecation is provided by the ___external___ ___anal___ sphincter.
10. The watery secretion that permits taste and swallowing is produced by the ___salivary___ glands.
11. The process of mechanical digestion is produced by the ___tongue___ and ___teeth___ in the mouth.
12. The structures in the small intestine that contain capillaries and lacteals for absorption are the ___villi___.
13. The part of the colon that contracts in the defecation reflex is the ___rectum___.

STRUCTURES OF THE GASTROINTESTINAL SYSTEM

Label the following structures.

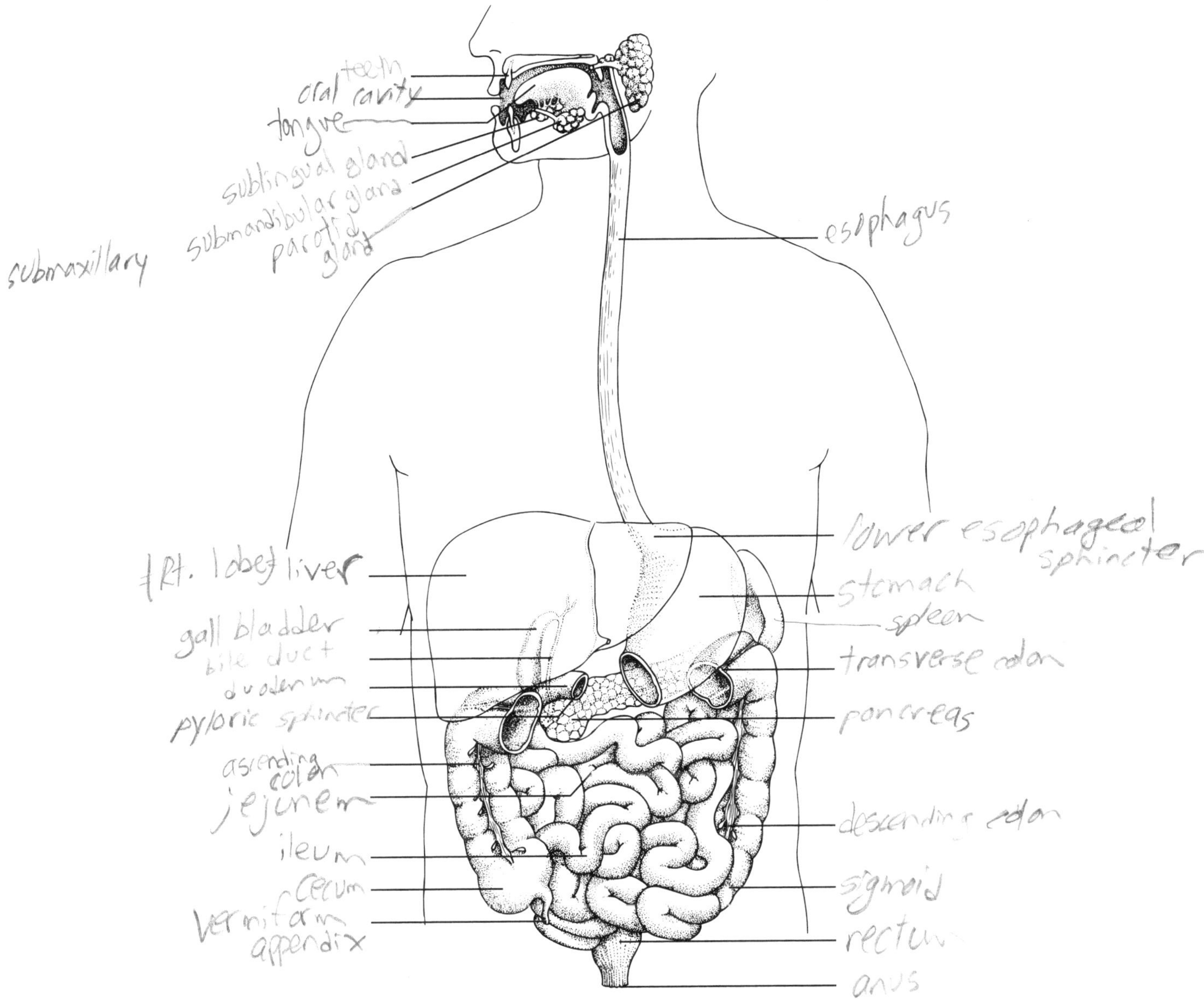

VOCABULARY

Unscramble the letters to identify the word described by the definition.

1. Flexible or rigid device consisting of a tube and optical system for observing the inside of a hollow organ or cavity. __endoscope__ donscepeo

2. Gurgling and clicking heard over the abdomen caused by air and fluid movement from peristaltic action normally occurring every 5 to 15 seconds at a rate of 5 to 35 per minute. __bowel sounds__ wlebo onudss

3. Examination of the upper portion of the rectum with an endoscope. __colonscopy__ ocnooscypo

4. Feeding via a tube placed in the stomach. __gavage__ gvaaeg

5. Immovable accumulation of feces in the bowels. __impaction__ mipcaitno

6. Resin obtained from trees to test for occult blood in feces. __guaiac__ gaiuca

7. Device consisting of a fluorescent screen that makes the shadows of objects interposed between the tube and the screen visible. __fluoroscope__ ulfroocspeo

8. Fatty stools. __steatorrhea__ estaotrhrae

9. A test performed to measure secretions of hydrochloric acid and pepsin in the stomach. __gastric analysis__ stgairc naayliss

10. Examination of the stomach and abdominal cavity by use of an endoscope. __gastroscopy__ stgarsopcoy

LABORATORY TESTS

Match the test with its definition.

1. _____ Stool for lipids
2. _____ Stool cultures
3. _____ Stool for occult blood
4. _____ Carcinoembryonic antigen (CEA)
5. _____ Stool for ova and parasites

A. Levels may indicate colorectal or other cancer.
B. Testing stool for blood that is not visible to the eye
C. Testing stool for intestinal infections caused by parasites
D. Testing stool for the presence of pathogenic organisms in the GI tract
E. Testing stool for excessive amounts of fat

BOWEL PREPARATION

Circle the eight errors in the following paragraph, and insert the correct information.

A stomach preparation is required for several procedures that visualize the lower bowel. This preparation is important for effective test results. An incomplete bowel preparation may prevent the test from being done or cause the need for it to be repeated. This can result in the patient's early discharge and cost savings. The patient usually receives a soft diet 24 hours before the test. A bowel preparation medication (liquid or pill) may be given. A cool tap-water enema or Fleet enema may be given once. Elderly or debilitated patients should be carefully assessed during the administration of multiple enemas, which can fatigue the patient and improve electrolytes. In patients with bleeding or constipation, the bowel preparation may not be ordered by the physician.

PANCREAS

Name the pancreatic enzyme with its function.

1. Digests polypeptides to short chains of amino acids
   ____
2. Digests emulsified fats to fatty acids and glycerol
   ____
3. Digests starch to maltose
   ____

CRITICAL THINKING

Read the following case study and answer the questions.

Mrs. Davis is a 41-year-old schoolteacher who is admitted to your unit with recurrent lung cancer. She is debilitated and her physician orders total parenteral nutrition (TPN) to be started.

1. Why is the TPN rate started slowly at first? _____________

2. Why are serum glucose levels monitored on Mrs. Davis during TPN administration? _____________

3. In what types of veins may TPN be administered with (a) dextrose of 12% or less; (b) dextrose greater than 12%? _____________

4. Why is it necessary to use an infusion control pump for TPN? _____________

5. The TPN is behind schedule. What action should the nurse take? _____________

6. When TPN is discontinued, why is the infusion slowly weaned off? _____________

7. When TPN is ordered to be stopped, why should the patient be fed first if it is not contraindicated? _____________

8. Identify one nursing diagnosis and outcome with interventions for the patient on TPN. _____________

REVIEW QUESTIONS

Choose the best answer.

1. Which of the following structures are connected by the ileocecal valve?
   a. Duodenum to the stomach
   b. Colon to the small intestine
   c. Stomach to the esophagus
   d. Ileum to the jejunum

2. Mechanical digestion in the stomach is accomplished by which of the following structures?
   a. Mucosa
   b. Smooth muscle layers
   c. Striated muscle layers
   d. Gastric glands

3. Gastric juice contributes to the digestion of which of the following types of nutrients?
   a. Proteins
   b. Fats
   c. Starch

4. The enzymes of the small intestine contribute to the digestion of which of the following types of nutrients?
   a. Proteins
   b. Fats
   c. Disaccharides

5. Which of the following structures carries bile and pancreatic juices to the duodenum?
   a. Pancreatic duct
   b. Cystic duct
   c. Hepatic duct
   d. Common bile duct

6. Bowel sounds heard as soft clicks and gurgles at a rate of four per minute would be documented by the nurse as which of the following types of findings?
   a. Absent
   b. Hyperactive
   c. Hypoactive
   d. Normal

7. Which of the following diagnostic procedures on stool specimens must the nurse collect using sterile technique?
   a. Stool for ova and parasites
   b. Stool for occult blood
   c. Stool culture
   d. Stool for lipids

8. Which of the following diagnostic procedures does the nurse understand does not require the patient to be nil per os (NPO)?
   a. Upper GI series (barium swallow)
   b. Flat plate of the abdomen
   c. Magnetic resonance imaging (MRI)
   d. EGD

9. Which of the following nursing diagnoses would be most appropriate to include in the patient's plan of care following a barium swallow?
   a. Risk for constipation
   b. Risk for diarrhea
   c. Risk for pain
   d. Imbalanced nutrition; more than body requirements

10. Which of the following colors would the nurse recognize as an expected finding for the patient's stools immediately after a barium swallow?
    a. Brown
    b. Black
    c. White
    d. Green

11. Which of the following does the nurse understand is the primary reason a patient is NPO until the gag reflex returns after an EGD procedure?
    a. To rest the vocal cords
    b. To prevent aspiration
    c. To keep the throat dry
    d. To prevent vomiting

12. Which of the following positions would the nurse be correct in using for nasogastric (NG) tube insertion?
    a. Trendelenburg's
    b. Prone
    c. Sims'
    d. High-Fowler's

13. A patient who has an NG tube and an intravenous (IV) line states, "I'm so embarrassed to have my family here I have tubes coming out of me everywhere." Which of the following would be an appropriate nursing diagnosis?
    a. Impaired adjustment
    b. Defensive coping
    c. Disturbed body image
    d. Anxiety

14. When inserting an NG tube, it is recommended to have the patient do which of the following to make the insertion easier?
    a. Cough
    b. Swallow
    c. Hold breath
    d. Exhale

Nursing Care of Patients with Upper Gastrointestinal Disorders

VOCABULARY

Unscramble the letters to identify a word described by the definition.

1. Most common cause of peptic ulcers; its recent discovery has revolutionized treatment and cure of most peptic ulcers. _helicobacter pylori_ lehicbocatre ypoilr
2. Loss of appetite _anorexia_ noraxeai
3. Inflammation of the stomach _gastritis_ sagrtisti
4. Small, white, painful ulcers that appear on the inner cheeks, lips, gums, tongue, palate, and pharynx _aphthous stomatitis_ hpatouhs tsoamtisti
5. Recurrent episodes of binge eating and self-induced vomiting _bulimia nervosa_ lubiami ernvsoa
6. Rapid entry of food into the jejunum causing dizziness, tachycardia, fainting, sweating, nausea, diarrhea, and abdominal cramping _dumping syndrome_ umdpnig nysdomre
7. Surgical removal of the stomach _gastrectomy_ gtrasetcmyo
8. 20% to 30% over average weight for age, sex, and height _obesity_ boesiyt
9. Condition in which the stomach may protrude above the diaphragm _hiatal hernia_ ihaatl erhian
10. Following surgical removal of part of the stomach, reanastomosis of the remaining portion to the proximal jejunum _gastrojejunostomy_ satgorjujeonsotym

GASTRITIS

Match the description with the type of gastritis associated with it.

1. _a_ Heartburn or indigestion
2. _b_ Autoimmune gastritis
3. _a_ Often caused by overeating
4. _c_ Associated with the bacteria *Helicobacter pylori*
5. _b_ Associated with difficulty in absorbing vitamin B_{12}
6. _a_ Can lead to peritonitis
7. _c_ Can be treated with antibiotics
8. _a_ Treatment includes a bland diet

A. Acute gastritis
B. Chronic gastritis type A _can lead to pern. anemia_
C. Chronic gastritis type B

PEPTIC ULCER DISEASE

Circle the seven errors in the following paragraph and write the correct information.

Most peptic ulcers are caused by stress. Peptic ulcers are commonly found in the sigmoid colon. Symptoms of peptic ulcers include burning and a gnawing pain in the chest. With a duodenal ulcer, there is pain and discomfort with a full stomach, which may be relieved by avoiding food. Peptic ulcers cannot be cured. Medication treatment for most peptic ulcers should include anticoagulants as indicated.

GASTRECTOMY

Label the structures as they appear following various types of gastric surgery.

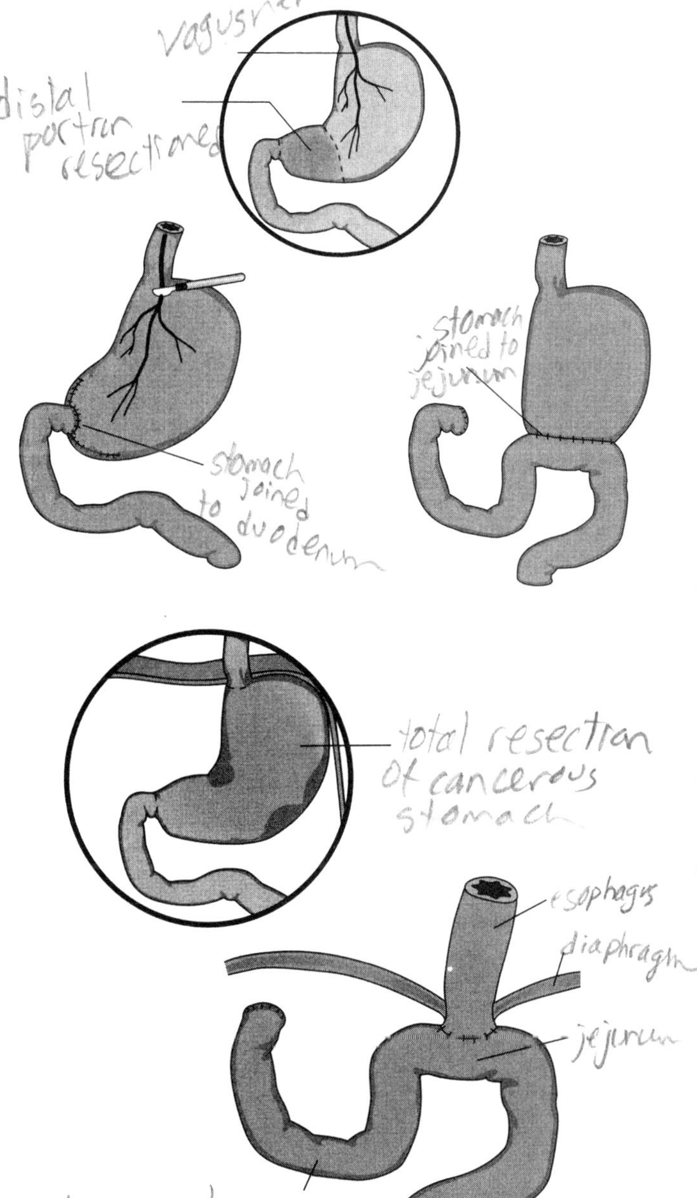

CRITICAL THINKING

Read the following case study and answer the questions.

Mrs. Sheffield has just returned from surgery. She had a Billroth I procedure. She has a nasogastric tube, a 1000-mL intravenous (IV) of lactated Ringer's solution infusing at 100 mL/h, and a Foley catheter. She is nil per os (NPO). Her vital signs are stable: blood pressure 118/90, pulse 80, respirations 16, and temperature 98°F (36.6°C). Her abdominal dressing is clean, dry, and intact. She is drowsy but easily aroused. After getting Mrs. Sheffield settled in the bed, you connect her nasogastric tube to intermittent low wall suction as ordered by her physician and add another blanket to warm her. Mrs. Sheffield requests something for pain. You administer morphine 5 mg intramuscularly and allow her to rest. An hour later, the nurse's aid tells you that Mrs. Sheffield is vomiting bright red blood. You go to her room and find her lying on her side propped up on one arm vomiting into an emesis basin. Her nasogastric suction catheter contains 250 mL of bright red drainage. Her dressing remains clean and dry. She is diaphoretic and complaining of nausea.

1. What is your first response? _______________________

____

2. What is your next action? ________________________

____

3. Vital signs are now blood pressure 86/60, pulse 96, respirations 24, and temperature 97.6°F (36.4°C). What is your assessment of the new data, and what is your next step? _____________________________________

____

____

4. As you lightly palpate her abdomen, it feels slightly distended, and you suspect that she may be bleeding into her peritoneum. What is your next step?

____

____

5. What do you need to tell the physician? _____________

____

6. The physician orders a hematocrit and hemoglobin, electrolytes, and oxygen at 2 L via nasal cannula. The physician also tells you to get Mrs. Sheffield ready to return to surgery. What is your priority nursing action?

____

____

REVIEW QUESTIONS

Choose the best answer unless directed otherwise.

1. A patient has a duodenal peptic ulcer and is taking cimetidine (Tagamet). Which of the following side effects related to cimetidine should be included in the teaching plan?
   a. Confusion
   b. Hypertension
   c. Blurred vision
   d. Dry mouth

2. A patient is admitted with chronic gastritis type B. Which of the following signs and symptoms is the nurse likely to find on assessment?
   a. Anorexia
   b. Dysphagia
   c. Diarrhea
   d. Feeling of fullness

3. Which of the following surgical procedures is the most likely treatment for a patient with gastric cancer?
   a. Gastroplasty
   b. Gastrorrhaphy
   c. Gastric stapling
   d. Gastrectomy

Multiple response item. Select all that apply.

4. An asymptomatic patient is admitted with gastric bleeding. For which of the following signs or symptoms of severe gastric bleeding should the nurse monitor?
   a. Hypertension
   b. Diaphoresis
   c. Bounding pulse
   d. Edema
   e. Hypotension

5. A patient had a gastrectomy 2 months ago. The patient comes to the clinic complaining of greasy stools and frequent bowel movements. After the patient's surgical recovery and current eating habits are assessed, which of the following types of diet would be most appropriate for the nurse to teach the patient to use?
   a. Bland diet
   b. High-carbohydrate diet
   c. Low-fat diet
   d. Pureed diet

6. A patient visits her gynecologist and reports that she is very unhappy with her weight, which is 310 lb on her 5-foot 7-inch frame. When planning her care, the nurse knows that the initial treatment for obesity includes which of the following?
   a. Gastroplasty
   b. Billroth I procedure
   c. Billroth II procedure
   d. Diet management

7. A patient has been diagnosed with a hiatal hernia. The patient complains of heartburn and occasional regurgitation. Which of the following interventions should the nurse teach the patient to reduce the symptoms?
   a. Eat small, frequent meals.
   b. Recline for 1 hour after meals.
   c. Sleep flat without a pillow.
   d. Eat a bedtime snack.

8. A patient is having an acute episode of gastric bleeding. The physician orders an IV of 1000 mL of 0.9% normal saline, a complete blood cell (CBC) count, a nasogastric tube to low-wall suction, and oxygen by nasal cannula. Which of the following orders should the nurse perform first?
   a. Administer the IV of 1000 mL of 0.9% normal saline.
   b. Draw the blood for the CBC cell.
   c. Insert the nasogastric tube.
   d. Apply oxygen by nasal cannula.

9. Which of the following does the nurse understand is a sign or symptom of oral cancer?
   a. Painless ulcer
   b. White painful ulcers
   c. Feeling of fullness
   d. Heartburn

10. Which of the following procedures does the nurse understand is done palliatively for the dysphagia that occurs in inoperable esophageal cancer?
    a. Gastrectomy
    b. Esophageal dilation
    c. Radical neck dissection
    d. Modified neck dissection

11. Which of the following statements by the patient would the nurse evaluate as indicating understanding by the patient of preventive measures for gastroesophageal reflux disease?
    a. I need to eat large meals.
    b. I will sleep without pillows.
    c. I need to lie down for 2 hours after each meal.
    d. I will identify foods that cause discomfort.

VOCABULARY

Match the vocabulary word to the correct definition.

1. ____ Appendicitis
2. ____ Colectomy
3. __b__ Colitis
4. __k__ Colostomy
5. __a__ Diverticulosis
6. __d__ Fistula
7. __h__ Hernia
8. ____ Ileostomy
9. __C__ Intussusception
10. ____ Melena
11. __g__ Peritonitis
12. __f__ Volvulus

A. Outpouchings in colon
B. Inflammation of colon
C. Telescoping of the bowel
D. Tunnel connection between bowel and another organ
E. Blood in stool
F. Twisting of bowel
G. Inflammation or infection of peritoneum
H. Bulging of abdominal contents through abdominal wall
I. Diversion of small bowel through abdominal wall
J. Removal of large bowel
K. Diversion of large bowel through abdominal wall
L. Inflamed appendix

OSTOMIES

Circle the errors in the following paragraphs and insert the correct information.

1. Michelle Braun is a 16-year-old with ulcerative colitis. She is taking cortisone and ~~amoxicillin (Amoxil)~~. She is on a ~~high~~-residue diet. She is now admitted to the hospital for a colectomy and ~~elective loop ostomy~~. You monitor her intake and output (I&O), daily weights, and electrolytes. You also monitor for signs of inflammation in her joints, skin, and other parts of her body. You teach her to ~~restrict~~ fluids following surgery to limit the number of stools she has daily.

2. James Key is a 46-year-old with a new sigmoid colostomy. Following surgery you monitor his stoma every shift for 3 days to ensure that it remains ~~gray~~ and moist. You explain that the stool will be ~~semiformed~~ and that he will have to irrigate his ostomy every 1 to 2 days to

have bowel movements. You contact the dietitian to provide a list of the high-fiber foods that he should avoid.

CRITICAL THINKING

Read the case study and answer the questions.

Mrs. Millie Hendricks is a 90-year-old resident in the nursing home where you work as an LPN. She has a history of severe osteoarthritis and no teeth or dentures, but otherwise she is quite healthy. She normally has a bowel movement every other day but has occasional constipation, which she takes care of herself by requesting a dose of milk of magnesia. Today when you take Mrs. Hendricks' medications to her, she says, "I think I need a second dose of that milk of magnesia; my bowels haven't moved in three days." You look at her medication administration record and find as needed (prn) orders for milk of magnesia, psyllium (Metamucil), Senna (Sennakot), or a tap water enema.

1. What should you do before you administer more medication? ___________________________

   ____

   ____

2. What factors most likely led to Mrs. Hendricks' constipation? _______________________

   ____

   ____

   ____

3. What will happen if Mrs. Hendricks' bowels do not move today? _______________________

   ____

   ____

   ____

4. What nondrug interventions will help Mrs. Hendricks' move her bowels? _______________

   ____

   ____

   ____

5. After Mrs. Hendricks' bowels have moved, what measures can you institute to prevent constipation next time?

   ____

   ____

   ____

   ____

REVIEW QUESTIONS

Choose the best answer unless directed otherwise.

1. A patient visits his physician with complaints of chronic diarrhea that is sometimes bloody. Ulcerative colitis is diagnosed. How should the nurse explain the patient's diagnosis to him?
   a. "You have inflamed sacs throughout your colon."
   b. "Your colon and rectum are inflamed and ulcerated."
   c. "You have ulcerations and fistulas in your small bowel."
   d. "Your colon is spastic and hypertonic."

Multiple response item. Select all that apply.
2. Which of the following laboratory studies does the nurse understand helps monitor ulcerative colitis?
   a. Aspartate aminotransferase (AST)
   b. Creatine phosphokinase (CPK) isoenzymes
   c. Amylase
   d. Complete blood count (CBC)
   e. Electrolytes
   f. Lipase

3. Which of the following diet instructions should be included in the plan of care to help a patient control ulcerative colitis symptoms?
   a. Drink milk or eat a milk product at least six times daily.
   b. Include four servings daily of whole grain breads or cereals.
   c. Limit coffee to six cups daily.
   d. Avoid fresh fruits and vegetables.

4. A patient who has ulcerative colitis is taken to the emergency department with severe rectal bleeding. Which of the following is the best option for maintaining nutritional status for this patient with ulcerative colitis who must be nil per os (NPO) for an extended period of time?
   a. Nasogastric (NG) tube feedings
   b. Percutaneous endoscopic gastrostomy (PEG) tube feedings
   c. Total parenteral nutrition (TPN)
   d. Intravenous (IV) 5% dextrose and water

5. A patient is diagnosed with acute diverticulitis. Which of the following may have placed the patient at risk for developing diverticulitis?
   a. Eating a low-fiber diet
   b. Chronic diarrhea
   c. History of nonsteroidal anti-inflammatory drug (NSAID) use
   d. Family history of colon cancer

6. Which of the following foods might a patient with diverticulitis be instructed to avoid in his plan of care?
   a. Peanuts and raspberries
   b. Apples and pears
   c. Red meat and dairy products
   d. Bran and whole grains

7. Which of the following nursing diagnoses is most appropriate to include in the plan of care for a patient with symptoms of a bowel obstruction?
   a. Risk for impaired swallowing related to NPO status
   b. Risk for urinary retention related to fluid volume depletion
   c. Risk for deficient fluid volume related to nausea and vomiting
   d. Risk for impaired coping related to prolonged hospitalization

8. Which of the following explanations by the nurse to reinforce the patient's preoperative education for a loop ostomy would be correct?
   a. "You will have a stoma in the middle of your abdomen that will constantly drain liquid stool."
   b. "You will have a looped bag system to collect stool from your stoma."
   c. "You will have a loop of bowel on your abdomen, but it will not drain stool."
   d. "You will have a loop of bowel on your abdomen that can be put back in after your bowel has healed."

9. Which of the following dietary instructions is most important to include in the plan of care to prevent complications for a patient with an ileostomy?
   a. "Drink lots of fluids to prevent dehydration."
   b. "Avoid fruits and vegetables to prevent diarrhea."
   c. "Avoid milk products to prevent gas."
   d. "Eat plenty of fiber to prevent constipation."

10. A patient is concerned about ileostomy odor. Which of the following responses by the nurse would be best?
    a. "A teaspoon of baking soda in your pouch will absorb all the odor."
    b. "The plastic your pouch is made of is odorproof. You shouldn't have to worry about odor as long as you don't have a leak."
    c. "Effluent from an ileostomy has no odor. It's colostomies that can smell bad from time to time."
    d. "Changing your pouch and face plate daily will help prevent odor."

Nursing Care of Patients with Liver, Gallbladder, and Pancreatic Disorders

VOCABULARY

Match the following terms with the appropriate description.

1. ____d____ Ascites
2. ____c____ Asterixis
3. ____j____ Cirrhosis
4. ____e____ Encephalopathy
5. ____g____ Fetor hepaticus
6. ____k____ Hepatorenal syndrome
7. ____l____ Hepatitis
8. ____a____ Jaundice
9. ____i____ Portal hypertension
10. ____b____ Pancreatectomy
11. ____h____ Steatorrhea
12. ____f____ Varices

A. Yellowing of the sclerae and skin from excess bilirubin
B. Removal of all or part of the pancreas
C. Liver flap
D. Fluid in the abdomen from decreased albumin
E. Neurological changes from excess ammonia
F. Weakened, swollen veins
G. Foul breath
H. Fatty, foul-smelling stools
I. Increased pressure in the portal circulation
J. Scarring and hardening of the liver from inflammation
K. Oliguria and sodium retention without kidney defects
L. Inflammation of the liver cells

LIVER

Fill in the crossword with terms related to the liver.

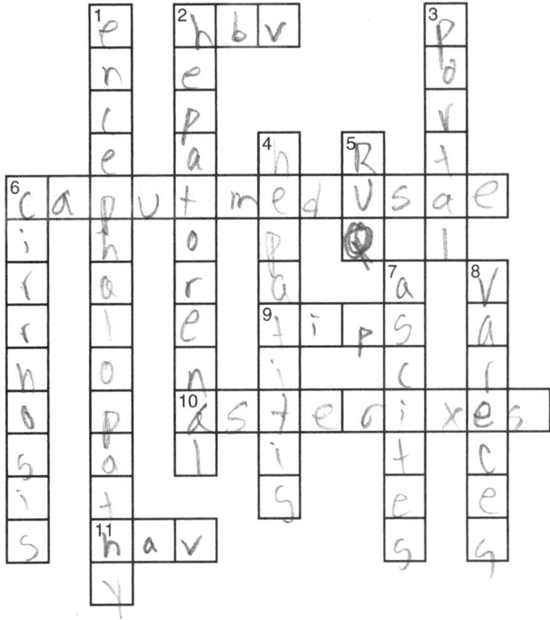

Across

2. Abbreviation for serum hepatitis
6. Visible veins around umbilicus
9. Abbreviation for liver shunt
10. Liver flap
11. Abbreviation for infectious hepatitis

Down

1. Confusion and coma are symptoms
2. This syndrome causes anuria
3. Abdomen circulation
4. Liver inflammation
5. Abbreviation for liver location
6. Chronic liver failure is Laënnec's _____________
7. Collection of fluid in peritoneal cavity
8. Dilated esophageal veins

GALLBLADDER

Match the following terms with the appropriate description.

1. ____d____ Cholecystitis
2. ____f____ Cholesterol
3. ____g____ Flatulence
4. ____e____ Murphy's sign
5. ____a____ Bilirubin
6. ____h____ Extracorporeal shock wave lithotripsy (ESWL)
7. ____i____ T-tube
8. ____j____ Laparoscopic cholecystectomy
9. ____b____ Chenodeoxycholic acid
10. ____c____ Choledochoscopy

A. Pigment from the breakdown of red blood cells
B. Dissolves cholesterol gallstones
C. Use of an endoscope to explore the common bile duct
D. Inflammation of the gallbladder
E. Inability to take a deep breath when fingers are pressed under liver margin
F. Composition of gallstones
G. Intestinal gas expelled via the rectum
H. A procedure that shatters gallstones using sound waves
I. A surgical drain used to ensure that bile freely drains from the gallbladder after surgery
J. Removal of the gallbladder through a small abdominal incision

PANCREAS

In the space on the left, write N or A to indicate whether the assessment finding is normal or abnormal. If the finding is abnormal, indicate the possible (liver-, gallbladder-, or pancreas-related) cause for the finding in the space on the right.

1. Serum glucose >150 mg% ___A___ *panc* __________
2. Serum amylase >500 IU/L ___A___________
3. Serum lipase = 15 U/L ___N___________
4. Pleural effusion ___A___________
5. Blood pressure and pulse 15% from patient's baseline
   ___N___________
6. Serum albumin <3.2 g/dL __________
7. Positive Cullen's sign __________
8. Urinary output <30 mL/hr __________
9. Positive Chvostek's sign __________
10. Foul-smelling, fatty stools __________

CRITICAL THINKING

Read the case study and answer the questions.

Ms. Betty Smith has been diagnosed with hepatic encephalopathy secondary to Laënnec's cirrhosis or chronic liver failure. During the admission process, you note the following findings: abdomen grossly distended, yellow sclerae and skin, multiple bruises, and 2+ pitting edema of the lower extremities. You also note that Ms. Smith is irritable and has difficulty answering questions, and appears to doze off frequently during the interview. You observe that Ms. Smith scratches her arms and legs frequently. Her laboratory data indicate that her serum bilirubin, ammonia, and prothrombin time are elevated and that her serum albumin, total protein, and potassium are below normal.

1. What data support the diagnosis of Laënnec's cirrhosis?
   ____
   ____
   ____

2. What data suggest that Ms. Smith has hepatic encephalopathy? What other evidence might you observe? ____
   ____
   ____

3. Why is Ms. Smith exhibiting 2+ pitting edema and abdominal distention? ____
   ____
   ____

4. What medical treatments can you expect the physician to order for the hepatic encephalopathy? __________________
   ____

Two days after Ms. Smith was admitted, you see bright red blood in Ms. Smith's emesis. Ms. Smith also complains of feeling cold, and her pulse is 115 and thready. You call for help and place Ms. Smith in a semi-Fowler's position.

5. What further treatment can you anticipate for Ms. Smith? ____
   ____

6. For what complications related to placement of a Senstaken-Blakemore tube should you watch?
   ____
   ____

7. What observations should you make to detect bleeding from lack of clotting factors? __________________________
   ____

8. What nursing measures can you provide to help Ms. Smith maintain her fluid balance? __________________
   ____

9. What should you teach Ms. Smith about taking acetaminophen (Tylenol)? Why? __________________
   ____

REVIEW QUESTIONS

Choose the best answer unless directed otherwise.

1. A patient with ascites is placed on a low-sodium diet. The nurse knows that diet teaching has been successful if the patient selects which of the following meals?
   a. Cottage cheese and peaches with tomato juice
   b. Frankfurter on a bun with pickle relish and skim milk
   c. Baked chicken, white rice, and apple juice
   d. Turkey and lettuce sandwich on whole wheat bread with tomato soup

2. Which of the following nursing interventions related to esophageal tamponade with a Senstaken-Blakemore tube is *inappropriate*?
   a. Keeping a pair of scissors at the bedside
   b. Having oral suction available
   c. Maintaining traction on the tube, if ordered
   d. Deflating the gastric balloon periodically

3. Which of the following instructions should be given to the patient with portal hypertension?
   a. Cough and deep breathe every 2 hours.
   b. Avoid straining to have a bowel movement.
   c. Increase fluid intake.
   d. Expect urine to be tea colored.

4. Which of the following precautions will protect the nurse who is caring for the patient with hepatitis B?
   a. Reverse isolation
   b. Standard precautions
   c. Respiratory precautions
   d. Enteric precautions

5. Fulminant liver failure is most often caused by which of the following?
   a. Antibiotic use
   b. Vitamin use
   c. Alcohol use
   d. Hepatitis B virus (HBV)

6. A patient with chronic liver failure has asterixis and fetor hepaticus and is confused. The nurse recognizes these as symptoms of which complication?
   a. Hepatic encephalopathy
   b. Hepatorenal syndrome
   c. Portal hypertension
   d. Ascites

7. After treatment of esophageal varices by tamponade, the nurse must closely and carefully observe the patient because bleeding recurs in up to _______ % of patients.
   a. 20
   b. 60
   c. 80
   d. 100

Multiple response item. Select all that apply.
8. Which of the following are risk factors for gallbladder disease?
   a. Male
   b. Obese
   c. Multiple pregnancies
   d. Age 40 or older
   e. Fasting

9. The nurse can expect which of the following pain medications to be ordered for the patient with biliary colic?
   a. Codeine
   b. Morphine
   c. Apomorphine
   d. Meperidine

10. Which of the following is a nonsurgical intervention for the management of biliary colic?
    a. Encouraging a high-fat diet
    b. Administering vitamin K
    c. Administering chenodeoxycholic acid (Chenodiol)
    d. Administering probantheline (Pro-Banthine)

11. Patients with a history of pancreatic disease commonly have a history of which of the following?
    a. High-protein diet
    b. Very-low-fat diet
    c. Excessive alcohol consumption
    d. Excessive intake of vitamin C

12. Patients with acute pancreatitis frequently describe their pain as
    a. Dull, boring, beginning in the mid epigastrium and radiating to the back
    b. Knifelike, centered in the left lower quadrant
    c. Burning, focused over the left flank and radiating to the shoulder
    d. Sharp, severe pain that begins in the right upper quadrant

unit NINE

UNDERSTANDING THE URINARY SYSTEM

CHECKLIST FOR LEARNING SUCCESS

Review of Renal/Urinary Anatomy and Physiology	Major Renal/ Urinary Disorders	Nursing Assessment	Diagnostic Tests	Interventions	Common Medications
❑ Kidneys	❑ Incontinence	❑ Medical history	❑ Urinalysis	❑ Urinary catheters	❑ Diuretics
❑ Urine	❑ Urinary retention	❑ Medications	❑ Urine culture	❑ Lithotripsy	❑ Kayexalate (sodium
❑ Elimination of urine	❑ Urinary tract infections	❑ Vital signs	❑ Blood urea nitrogen	❑ Hemodialysis	polystyrene sulfonate)
❑ Aging effects	❑ Urological obstructions	❑ Physical assessment	❑ Creatinine	❑ Peritoneal dialysis	❑ Phosphate binders
	❑ Tumors	❑ Intake and output	❑ Creatinine clearance	❑ Continuous renal	
	❑ Polycystic kidney disease	❑ Daily weights	❑ Kidneys-ureter-bladder	replacement therapy	
	❑ Chronic renal diseases		❑ Intravenous pyelogram	❑ Urinary diversion	
	❑ Acute/chronic renal failure		❑ Cystoscopy and pyelogram		
	❑ Kidney transplantation				

VOCABULARY

Match the term for an abnormality of the urine or urination with the correct description.

1. __C__ Hematuria
2. __A__ Dysuria
3. __D__ Nocturia
4. __B__ Oliguria
5. __H__ Enuresis
6. __F__ Anuria
7. __E__ Polyuria
8. __G__ Pyuria

A. Painful urination
B. Decreased urine output (<400 mL per 24 hours)
C. Blood in the urine
D. Voiding during the night
E. Excessive urination (>2000 mL per 24 hours)
F. Absence of urination
G. Presence of pus in the urine
H. Bedwetting

ANATOMY

Label the parts of the kidney and nephron.

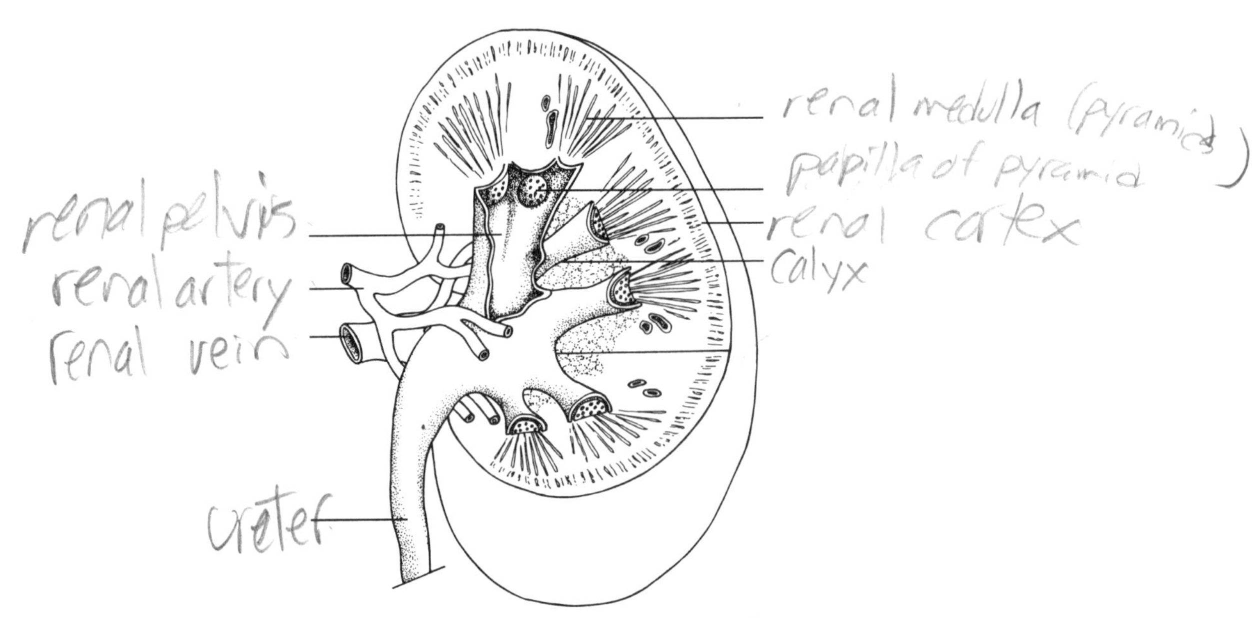

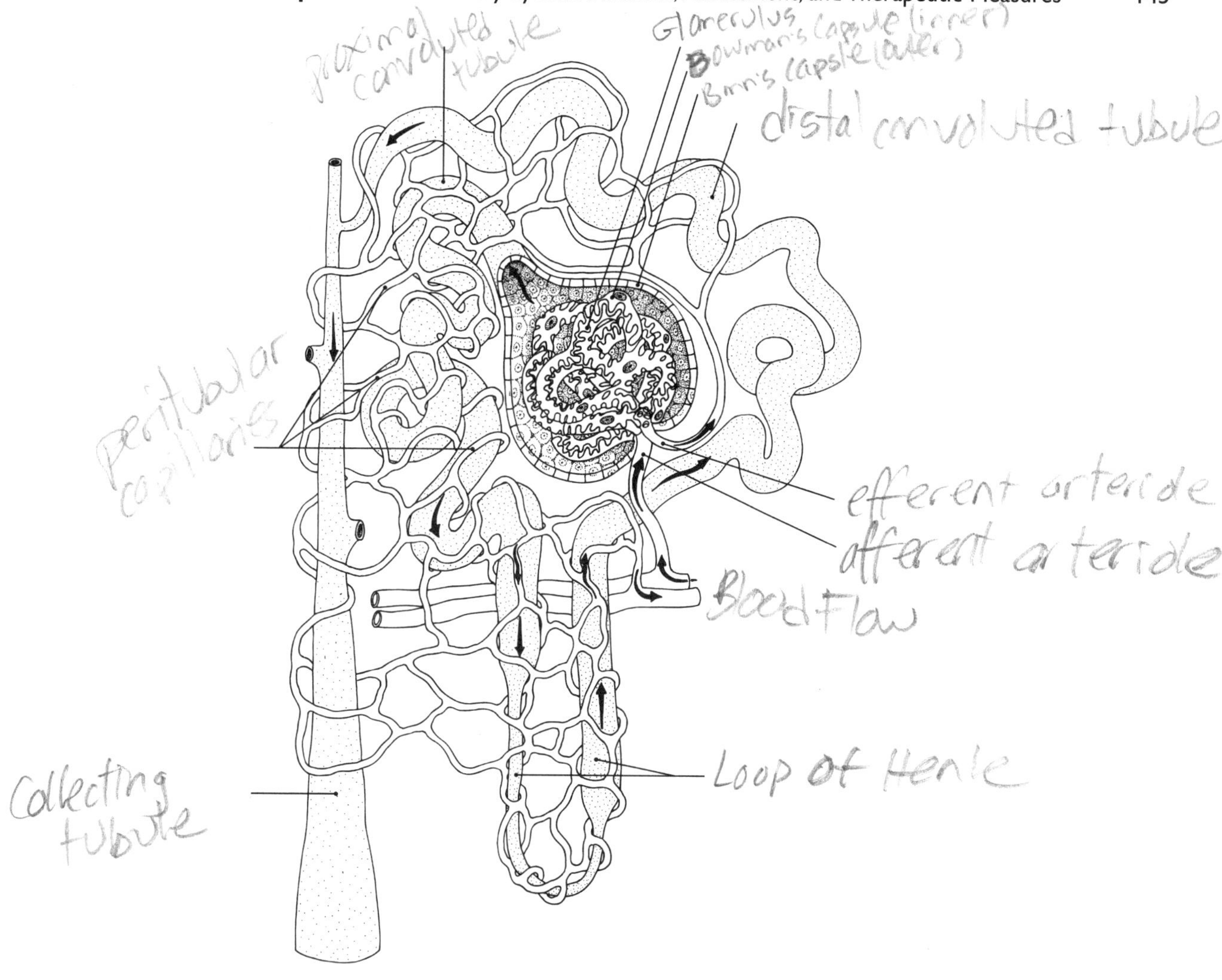

SAMPLE URINALYSIS RESULTS

Review the urinalysis results of the following three patients and determine the most likely cause of the abnormal results.

	Patient A	Patient B	Patient C
Color	Yellow	Dark amber	Yellow-green
Character	Cloudy	Concentrated	Clear
Glucose	Negative	Negative	Negative
Bilirubin	Negative	Negative	2+
Ketones	Small	Negative	Negative
Specific gravity (1.010–1.025)	1.024	1.035	1.025
Hemoglobin	Small	Negative	Negative
pH (5.0–9.0)	6.0	5.2	5.5
Protein	100	Negative	Negative
Urobilinogen (0.2–1.0)	0.2	0.2	0.2
Nitrite	Positive	Negative	Negative
Urine microscopic casts	White blood cell, Red blood cell	Negative	Negative
White blood cells (0–4 HPF)	400	4	1
Red blood cells (0–4 HPF)	90	2	2
	Patient A	**Patient B**	**Patient C**
Crystals	Negative	2	Negative
Amorphous	Negative	Negative	Negative
Epithelial cells (negative)	3	Negative	2
Bacteria (negative)	4+	Negative	Negative
Yeast (negative)	Negative	Negative	Negative

Patient A: _infection c diarrhea, vomiting, anorexia   UTI_

Patient B: _dehydration, deficient fluid volume_

Patient C: _liver dysfunction_

RENAL DIAGNOSTIC TESTS

Indicate whether each statement is true or false.

1. ___F___ An x-ray of the renal structures after injection of a radiopaque dye into the venous system is called a renal ultrasound.

2. ___F___ A diagnostic test in which sound waves are used to outline the structure of the kidney is an intravenous pyelogram.

3. ___F___ A urine sample that is cultured to determine the kind of bacteria it contains is called a creatinine clearance urine test. *culture*

4. ___T___ A diagnostic test in which the inside of the bladder is visualized is called a cystoscopy.

5. ___F___ The radiopaque dye used when doing diagnostic tests of the renal system is harmless.
possibility of allergic RXN → Nephrotoxicity can occur!

CRITICAL THINKING

Read the case studies and answer the following questions.

Mrs. Bohke is a 54-year-old female patient admitted to the hospital with a diagnosis of pneumonia. During her stay, she tells you she has trouble getting to the bathroom on time and often dribbles before she can get to the bathroom.
Some people can become continent by going to bathroom, fluids intake & setting up regular toileting schedule.

1. What type of urinary incontinence does she have?
stress incontinence

2. What teaching could be done to help her decrease her incontinence? *Kegels. Also, should be referred to urologist*

Mrs. Simmon is a 79-year-old woman with a fractured hip and a previous cerebrovascular accident (CVA). She has poor vision but is alert mentally. You find her lying in bed in a puddle of urine, crying. She explains that she was unable to find her call light. You find it lying on the floor out of her reach.

3. What kind of incontinence did Mrs. Simmon experience? *functional incontinence*

4. What actions should the nurse take to ensure that this does not happen again? *secure call light - she can feel, pin it to gown. Having roommate who could turn or call light for her.*

5. When caring for a patient with incontinence, is it helpful to decrease fluid intake? Why or why not? *NO! Because complications that result significantly outweigh any benefit of "not needing to go".*

REVIEW QUESTIONS

Choose the best answer unless otherwise directed.

1. Which of the following is secreted when the blood level of oxygen decreases?
   a. Erythropoietin *(circled)*
   b. Renin
   c. Angiotensin II
   d. Vitamin D

2. Urea is a nitrogenous waste product from the metabolism of which of the following?
   a. Nucleic acids
   b. Amino acids *(circled)*
   c. Muscle tissue
   d. Carbohydrates

3. The kidneys are located behind which of the following structures?
   a. Spinal column
   b. Diaphragm
   c. Peritoneum *(circled)*
   d. Inferior vena cava

4. The renal pyramids make up which kidney structure?
   a. Renal cortex
   b. Renal medulla *(circled)*
   c. Renal pelvis
   d. Renal fascia

5. The process of tubular resorption takes place in which of the following parts of the kidney?
   a. From the glomerulus to Bowman's capsule
   b. From the afferent arteriole to the efferent arteriole
   c. From the peritubular capillaries to the glomerulus
   d. From the renal tubule to the peritubular capillaries *(circled)*

6. When collecting a urine specimen on a newly admitted patient, the nurse should take which of the following actions?
   a. Direct the patient to wash perineum before collecting the urine specimen. *(circled)*
   b. Have the patient void, throw that urine away, and then collect another specimen at least 2 hours later.
   c. Obtain the first voided urine of the day.
   d. Direct the patient to drink at least three glasses of water.

7. A patient's urinalysis results show the following findings: urine dark amber, bacteria–small amount, nitrite negative, specific gravity 1.035. Which of the following is the best explanation for these results?
   a. Dehydration
   b. Urinary tract infection
   c. Contamination of the specimen from bacteria on the perineum
   d. Contamination from menstruation

Multiple response item. Select all that apply.

8. Which of the following diagnostic test results would the nurse evaluate as being related to renal failure?
   a. Hematocrit 39% (38% to 47%)
   b. Potassium 4.0 mEq/L (3.6 to 5.0 mEq/L)
   c. Uric acid 2 ng/dL (2.5 to 5.5 ng/dL)
   d. Creatinine 3 mg/dL (0.6 to 1.5 mg/dL)
   e. BUN 35 mg/dL (8 to 20 mg/dL)

9. A patient is scheduled for an intravenous pyelogram. When giving care, the nurse should recognize that restriction of which of the following is part of the preparation for an intravenous pyelogram?
   a. Salt intake
   b. Fluid intake
   c. Use of tobacco
   d. Physical activities

10. The patient is scheduled for a cystoscopy with basket extraction. Which of the following is the most important nursing care after this kind of surgery?
   a. Measuring urine output
   b. Monitoring daily weights
   c. Observing for symptoms of acute renal failure
   d. Limiting fluid intake

11. A patient, age 48, has urge incontinence. When assessing the patient, the nurse would expect to find which of the following symptoms?
   a. Patient unable to reach the bathroom in time and ends up urinating in underwear
   b. Patient incontinent of small amounts of urine when coughs, sneezes, or bears down
   c. Patient incontinent of urine when has many responsibilities and becomes overloaded
   d. Patient incontinent because unable to tell when needs to urinate and unable to control urination

12. Which of the following actions should the nurse take to prevent development of a urinary tract infection in a patient who has a urinary catheter inserted?
   a. Limit fluid intake to 2000 mL per 24 hours to decrease the flow of urine, which can result in increased contamination.
   b. Wash the perineum with an antibacterial soap three times per 24 hours.
   c. Keep catheter securely taped to the patient, preventing back-and-forth motion of the catheter.
   d. Empty the urinary catheter bag only when needed to prevent contamination of the exit spout.

13. Which of the following actions should the nurse take for a patient who has total urinary incontinence?
   a. Give patient cranberry juice to keep the urine acidic.
   b. Ensure that patient has ready access to the urinal.
   c. Teach patient how to do Kegel's exercises to increase perineal tone.
   d. Apply an adult incontinence brief to catch urine and change when necessary.

Nursing Care of Patients with Disorders of the Urinary System

VOCABULARY

Fill in the blank with the correct term.

1. _Urethritis_ is inflammation of the urethra.
2. _Cystitis_ is inflammation of the bladder.
3. _Pyelonephritis_ is inflammation of the kidney.
4. Surgical repair of the urethra is called _urethroplasty_.
5. Kidney stones are also called _renal calculi_.
6. _Nephrolithotomy_ is surgical incision into the kidney to remove a stone.
7. Unrelieved obstruction of the urinary tract can lead to _hydronephrosis_.
8. A _nephrostomy_ tube may be inserted directly into the kidney pelvis to drain urine.
9. Surgical removal of a kidney is called a _nephrectomy_.
10. Thickening and hardening of the renal blood vessels is called _nephrosclerosis_.

URINARY TRACT INFECTIONS

Answer the following questions.

1. What is the usual cause of urinary tract infections (UTIs) in women? _Contamination from shorter urethra, close proximity of urethra/meatus to rectum, infrequent urination_

2. What is the usual cause of UTIs in men? _enlarged prostate "prostatic hypertrophy"_

3. What advice regarding fluids should be given to patients who are susceptible to UTIs? _↑ intake, but avoid irritants such as alcohol, caffeine, chocolate. Drink cranberry juice daily_

4. What is the single most important thing a patient with a history of UTIs should be taught? _Never delay tx! Get referral to specialist, may lead to serious complications. Get urine C&S_

5. Compare cystitis (bladder infection) versus pyelonephritis (kidney infection) by filling out the following chart.

	Cystitis	Pyelonephritis
Symptoms	foul smelling urine, dysuria, frequency, urgency, cloudy urine	fever & chills, fatigue, urgency, frequency, dysuria, flank pain
Urinalysis results	↑ WBC's, + leukocyte esterase, bacteria (+), RBC's, nitrite +	same as, but + casts, ↑ "much sicker" & shows sx of systemic disease, blood cultures may be obtained
Prognosis	good c tx, can become chronic c repeat infections	Prog = good if full antibiox course taken, but complix occur if bacteria invade bloodstream, renal failure can result

URINARY TRACT OBSTRUCTIONS

Answer the following questions.

1. What is the most common symptom of cancer of the bladder? _painless hematuria because cancer tissue readily bleeds_

2. What is the most common risk factor for cancer of the bladder? _smoking_

3. What is the most common symptom of cancer of the kidney? _hematuria_

4. What does the urine look like when a patient has an ileal conduit? _cloudy due to mucus still being produced from ileum (part of sm intestine) which still secretes_

5. What nursing care should be provided for a patient with an ileal conduit? _Appliance kept on all times that either holds urine or drains. Necessary to use appliance, needs Δing, necessary to use a week_

6. What is the most important care that should be given a patient with a kidney stone? _Strain all urine. Pain mgt!_

7. What teaching should be done for the patient to prevent further stone formation if the stone is composed of calcium oxalate? Uric acid? _avoid purines = sardines, organ meats, avoid too much Ca (milk) or oxalate, cola, beer, keep urine acidic_

CRITICAL THINKING

Read the case study and answer the questions.

Mrs. Zins is a 47-year-old woman who has had type 1 diabetes mellitus for over 20 years. Recently she has begun having incidents of hypoglycemia, she is edematous, and her blood pressure has elevated. She is admitted to the hospital for diagnosis and treatment of probable renal failure.

Subjective Data

States that she has been exhausted lately and her skin is itchy.

States that she has been very irritable and her husband says she is hard to live with.

Objective Data

BP 194/104, P 98, R 22, T 98.4°F (36.9°C)

Jugular vein distention present at 45 degrees

3+ pitting edema of feet and ankles, generalized edema throughout body, including periorbital edema

Weight gain of 20 pounds in 2 months

Skin very dry, flaky

Diagnostic Tests

Fasting blood sugar 56 mg/100 L

Serum sodium 145 mEq/L

Serum creatinine 5.4 mg/100 L

Serum potassium 5.9 mEq/L

Uric acid 8.2 ng/dL

Hemoglobin (Hgb) 7.2 g/100 mL, Hematocrit (Hct) 22%

1. Mrs. Zins has been having incidents of hypoglycemia. Why is this happening? _bec. she's developing renal failure. Kidneys help degrade insulin & excrete it from body. As kidneys fail, smaller amounts of insulin are needed bec. it isn't removed from the body._

2. With Mrs. Zins present blood sugar of 56, what kind of juice should the nurse give her? _cranberry or another low potassium juice. OJ is not OK - too high in K+. Her K is high enough_

3. How does diabetes cause chronic renal failure? _causes arthersclerotic Δ's in kidney vessels. Also, thickens glomerulus. Predis-poses to pyelonephritis = damage to kidney, see back, *_

4. Is there anything Mrs. Zins could have done to decrease the possibility of developing renal failure? _Yes — good dbts mgt, keep BS WNL — can ↓ dbtc complexns including RF_

5. Identify two nursing diagnoses that would be appropriate for Mrs. Zins based on her assessment. _FVE = edema, wt gain, juglr distxn. Fatigue = reports exhaustxn, hgb = 7.2_

6. What diagnostic test was most indicative of renal failure for Mrs. Zins? _Serum creatinine of 5.4 mg_

7. Why is Mrs. Zins anemic? _Bec. kidneys have ↓'d or stopped producing erythropoietin, which stimulates marrow to make RBC's. GI bleed is possible_

8. What would be the three most important nursing assessments for Mrs. Zins related to her chronic renal failure? _daily wts, I's O's fluid restrxn if rx'd & monitor lab values of electrolytes_

9. What kind of diet will Mrs. Zins most likely receive? _probly a defined diabetic diet of low so, low potassium, ↓ protein, & fluid restrxn AND if phosphorus levels are elevated, low phosphorus too, bec. that is common in RF. VERY difficult to follow — most restrictive diet._

* Also dbtc pt can develop neurogenic bladder which predisposes pt to both infxn & obstrxn of urinary system.

RENAL FAILURE

Fill in the symptoms of renal failure under the body systems on the figure below.

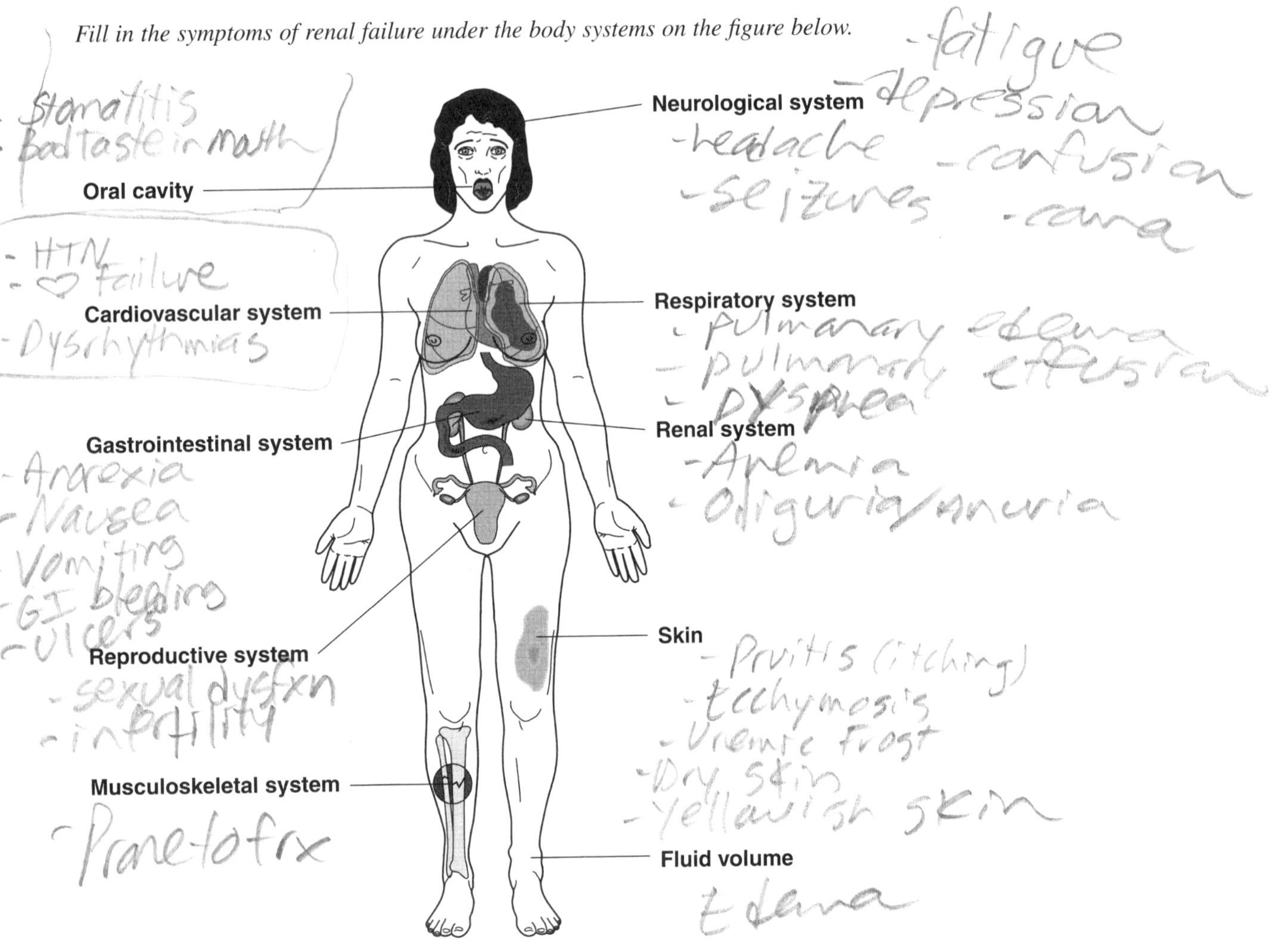

Choose the best answer unless directed otherwise.

1. A 72-year-old patient had a cystoscopy, which revealed bladder cancer. He is admitted to the hospital for a cystectomy and formation of an ileal conduit. The nurse should assess for the most common symptom of cancer of the bladder, which is which of the following?
   a. Nocturia
   b. Dysuria
   c. Urinary retention
   d. Hematuria

2. Postoperatively, the nurse notes the presence of mucus in the urinary drainage. Which of the following actions should the nurse take?
   a. Notify the physician.
   b. Collect a urine specimen for culture and sensitivity.
   c. Measure the specific gravity of the urine.
   d. Recognize that this is a normal occurrence.

3. A patient is admitted to intensive care in hypovolemic shock caused by gastrointestinal bleeding. It is determined that the patient is in acute renal failure. Which of the following is the most significant sign of acute renal failure that the nurse should observe for as part of the nursing assessment?
   a. A rise in blood pressure
   b. An elevation in body temperature
   c. A decrease in urine output
   d. An increase in urine specific gravity

4. When assessing the patient, the nurse notes the following diagnostic tests on the patient's chart. Which of the following diagnostic tests results is most indicative of acute renal failure?
   a. BUN 80 mg/100 mL (8 to 25 mg/100 L)
   b. 24-hour creatinine clearance of 5 mL/min (100 mL/min)
   c. Uric acid 8 ng/dL (2.5 to 5.5 ng/dL)
   d. Serum creatinine 1.7 mg/100 L (0.5 to 1.5 mg/100 L)

Multiple response item. Select all that apply.
5. Which of the following snacks is most appropriate for the nurse to serve a patient with acute renal failure to control potassium levels?
   a. Dried peanuts
   b. An orange
   c. Yogurt
   d. A gelatin dessert
   e. Cranberry juice

6. A patient with severe right flank pain, general weakness, and fever is hospitalized. He has a history of recurrent urinary tract infection, and renal calculi are suspected. On the second hospital day, the patient's urine output drops to 300 mL/24 hr, and he has distention and pain in the suprapubic area. The nurse would evaluate which of the following to be the most likely cause for this sudden change?
   a. Sudden decreased renal perfusion
   b. Inadequate fluid intake
   c. Interstitial fluid shift
   d. Urinary tract obstruction

7. Which of the following foods should the patient be taught to avoid for a kidney stone composed of calcium oxalate?
   a. Bread
   b. Beer
   c. Beef
   d. Beans

8. Which of the following is appropriate patient teaching to obtain a midstream urine specimen for culture and sensitivity?
   a. A second-voided specimen is preferred.
   b. The specimen should be collected early in the morning.
   c. The patient should begin voiding, collect the specimen, and then finish voiding in the toilet.
   d. A 24-hour urine specimen is needed; the first void should be discarded.

9. A patient is admitted in chronic renal failure. The patient has a potassium level of 6.4 mEq/L and is put on a cardiac monitor and given Kayexalate (sodium polystyrene sulfonate) by retention enema. Which of the following is the most significant symptom that the nurse should observe for?
   a. Diarrhea
   b. Irregular heart rhythm
   c. Increased blood pressure
   d. Increased respiratory rate

10. The patient in renal failure has the following symptoms: neck vein distention, periorbital edema, and crackles in the lungs. The nursing diagnosis of excess fluid volume is made. Which of the following nursing assessments is most important for this patient based on the symptoms?
    a. Intake and output
    b. Vital signs
    c. Daily weight
    d. Skin turgor

11. A patient with newly diagnosed chronic renal failure has elevated sodium, potassium, and serum creatinine levels. When the breakfast tray is served, there is a glass of orange juice on it. Which of the following actions should the nurse take first?
    a. Encourage the patient to drink the orange juice for vitamin C to help fight the infection.
    b. Take the orange juice off the tray because it is high in potassium.
    c. Give the patient a smaller glass of orange juice because the patient is on a fluid restriction.
    d. Check the kind of diet the patient is on to determine any restrictions.

12. A patient goes to surgery for a graft insertion for dialysis. The patient asks why it needs to be done. Which of the following is the best explanation by the nurse on the advantages of a graft over a two-tailed subclavian catheter?
    a. "There is a larger blood flow, and dialysis is more efficient."
    b. "There is less risk of clotting with the graft."
    c. "It is easier to access the graft than the two-tailed subclavian."
    d. "It is less likely to be damaged by trauma."

13. After hemodialysis, which of the following nursing interventions is imperative for the nurse to carry out?
    a. Measure stool output.
    b. Weigh the patient.
    c. Check for neck vein distention.
    d. Administer any insulin held previously.

14. The patient has a permanent peritoneal catheter inserted and is begun on continuous ambulatory peritoneal dialysis (CAPD). The patient asks how it works. Which of the following would be the best explanation of how this type of dialysis works?
    a. The peritoneum allows solutes in the dialysate to pass into the intravascular system.
    b. The peritoneum acts as a semipermeable membrane through which solutes move by diffusion and osmosis.
    c. The presence of excess metabolites causes increased permeability of the peritoneum and allows excess fluid to drain.
    d. The peritoneum permits diffusion of metabolites from the intravascular to the interstitial space.

15. A patient on dialysis has a severe cerebrovascular accident and is now semicomatose. His family decides that dialysis should be stopped. He is sent home with his daughter to die. As part of discharge planning, his daughter should be taught to expect which of the following symptoms of untreated end-stage renal failure?
    a. Polyuria, pruritus, and extreme irritability
    b. Dehydration with sunken eyeballs and oliguria
    c. Edema, possible convulsions, then coma
    d. Decreased respiratory rate and cyanosis

16. A patient is admitted who was involved in a motor vehicle accident resulting in trauma to the abdomen and back. He has a ruptured spleen and probable trauma to his kidneys. For which of the following changes in the patient's urine should the nurse observe?
    a. Dysuria
    b. Pyuria
    c. Polyuria
    d. Hematuria

17. A patient is admitted with symptoms of a recent weight gain, 3+ pitting edema of his feet, distended neck veins, and crackles in his lungs. Which of the following nursing diagnoses is most appropriate for this patient's plan of care?
    a. Deficient fluid volume
    b. Excess fluid volume
    c. Imbalanced nutrition, more than body requirements
    d. Noncompliance

UNDERSTANDING THE ENDOCRINE SYSTEM

CHECKLIST FOR LEARNING SUCCESS

Review of Anatomy and Physiology

- ❑ Antidiuretic hormone
- ❑ Growth hormone
- ❑ Thyroid-stimulating hormone
- ❑ Adrenocorticotropic hormone
- ❑ T_3 and T_4
- ❑ Calcitonin
- ❑ Parathyroid hormone
- ❑ Glucagon
- ❑ Insulin
- ❑ Norepinephrine
- ❑ Epinephrine
- ❑ Aldosterone
- ❑ Cortisol
- ❑ Aging changes

Major Disorders

- ❑ Diabetes insipidus
- ❑ Syndrome of inappropriate secretion of antidiuretic hormone
- ❑ Acromegaly
- ❑ Hypothyroidism
- ❑ Hyperthyroidism
- ❑ Goiter
- ❑ Thyroid cancer
- ❑ Hypoparathyroidism
- ❑ Hyperparathyroidism
- ❑ Pheochromocytoma
- ❑ Addison's disease
- ❑ Cushing's syndrome
- ❑ Diabetes mellitus
- ❑ Reactive hypoglycemia

Nursing Assessment

- ❑ Fluid balance
- ❑ Mood, affect
- ❑ Exophthalmos
- ❑ Tremor
- ❑ Polyuria, polydipsia, polyphagia
- ❑ Self-monitoring of blood glucose (SMBG)
- ❑ Knowledge of self-care

Diagnostic Tests

- ❑ 24-hour urine
- ❑ Hormone levels
- ❑ Stimulation tests
- ❑ Suppression tests
- ❑ Thyroid scan
- ❑ Blood glucose
- ❑ Glycohemoglobin
- ❑ Glucose tolerance test
- ❑ Ultrasound
- ❑ Biopsy

Interventions

- ❑ Monitoring of symptoms
- ❑ Pre- and postthyroidectomy care
- ❑ Teaching r/t self-care
- ❑ Diabetes education

Common Medications

- ❑ Hormone replacement
- ❑ Calcium
- ❑ Calcitonin
- ❑ Thyroid hormone
- ❑ Insulin
- ❑ Oral hypoglycemics

Endocrine System Function and Assessment

VOCABULARY

Complete the following sentences with the appropriate words.

1. Glucose is converted to _____________ for storage.
2. High blood glucose is called _____________.
3. Emotional tone is called _____________.
4. Bulging eyes, or _____________, is a symptom of hyperthyroidism.
5. Hormone secretion is regulated through a _____________ system.

glycogen
hyperglycemia
affect
exophthalmos
feedback

ENDOCRINE GLANDS AND HORMONES

Label the figure with the glands of the endocrine system. List the hormone(s) secreted by each gland.

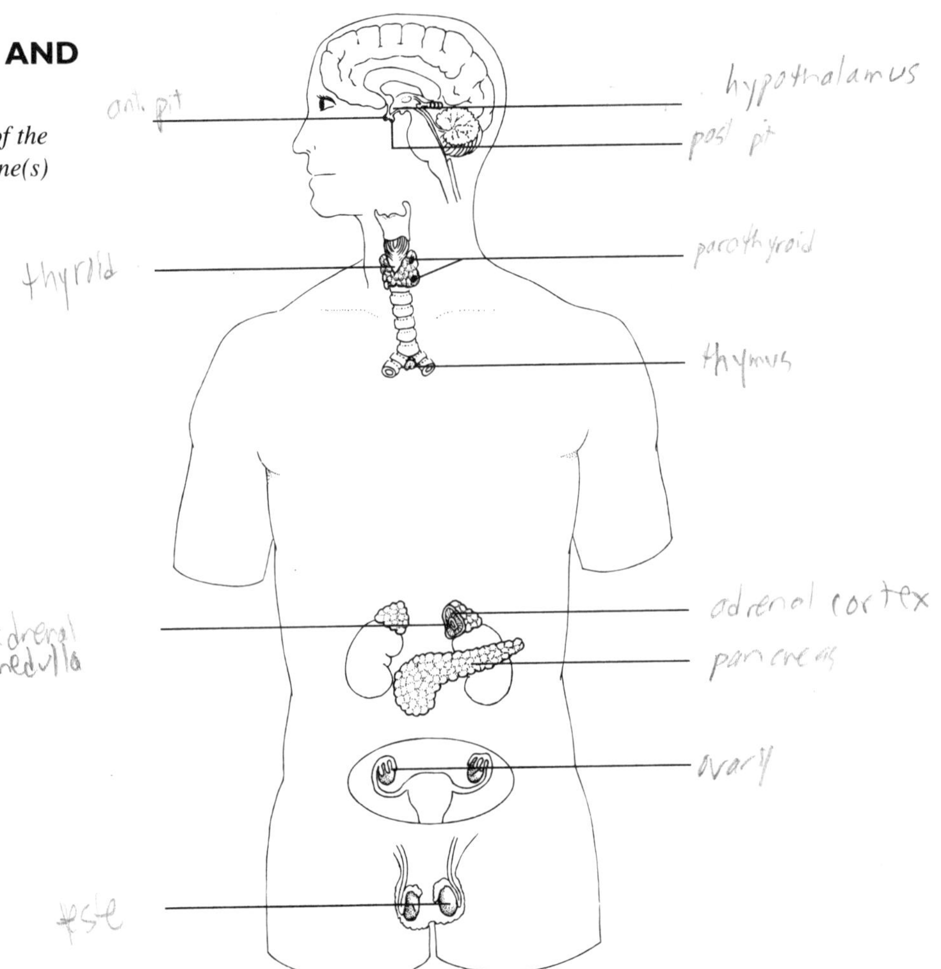

HORMONES

Match each hormone with its function. Use each letter only once.

1. _____ Antidiuretic hormone (ADH)
2. _____ Oxytocin
3. _____ Thyroid-stimulating hormone
4. _____ Adrenocorticotropic hormone
5. _____ Growth hormone (GH)
6. _____ Prolactin
7. _____ Follicle-stimulating hormone
8. _____ Luteinizing hormone
9. _____ Thyroxine
10. _____ Calcitonin
11. _____ Parathyroid hormone (PTH)
12. _____ Epinephrine
13. _____ Norepinephrine
14. _____ Cortisol
15. _____ Aldosterone
16. _____ Insulin
17. _____ Glucagon

A. Stimulates growth and secretions of the thyroid gland
B. Increases glucose intake by cells and glycogen storage in the liver
C. Decreases the resorption of calcium from bones; lowers blood calcium level
D. Increases the use of fats and amino acids for energy and has an anti-inflammatory effect
E. Stimulates mitosis and protein synthesis
F. Increases heart rate and force of contraction
G. Causes vasoconstriction throughout the body
H. Increases secretion of cortisol by the adrenal cortex
I. Increases energy production for a normal metabolic rate
J. Directly increases water resorption by the kidneys
K. In men, stimulates secretion of testosterone
L. Increases the conversion of glycogen to glucose in the liver between meals
M. Initiates milk production in the mammary glands
N. Increases the resorption of calcium from bones; raises blood calcium level
O. Increases the resorption of sodium by the kidneys
P. In women, initiates development of ova in ovaries
Q. Causes contraction of the myometrium during labor

REVIEW QUESTIONS

Choose the best answer.

1. Which two hormones help regulate the blood calcium level?
   a. Insulin and glucagon
   b. Calcitonin and PTH
   c. Thyroxine and epinephrine
   d. Cortisol and aldosterone

2. Which hormone is most important for day-to-day regulation of metabolic rate?
   a. Insulin
   b. Epinephrine
   c. GH
   d. Thyroxine

3. What happens when aldosterone increases the resorption of sodium ions by the kidneys?
   a. Water is also reabsorbed back to the blood.
   b. Bicarbonate ions are excreted in urine.
   c. More water is excreted in urine.
   d. Potassium ions are also reabsorbed back into the blood.

4. Which two hormones help maintain blood volume and blood pressure?
   a. Thyroxine and epinephrine
   b. Glucagon and insulin
   c. Aldosterone and ADH
   d. Cortisol and norepinephrine

5. Which of the following hormones has an anti-inflammatory effect?
   a. Epinephrine
   b. Cortisol
   c. Aldosterone
   d. Thyroxine

6. A patient is completing a 24-hour urine test. What should the nurse do to complete the test at the end of the 24 hours?
   a. Have the patient void exactly 24 hours after the test was begun and discard the specimen.
   b. Save the last specimen and send it in a separate container.
   c. Have the patient void exactly 24 hours after the test was begun, and add this urine to the remainder of the specimen.
   d. Send only the specimen voided at 24 hours.

7. A female patient is admitted to the hospital with hyperthyroidism. What related assessment should the nurse perform?
   a. Ask questions about symptoms of hyperthyroidism.
   b. Palpate thyroid gland for enlargement.
   c. Do a capillary blood glucose level.
   d. Observe for a "buffalo hump" on the patient's back.

8. A patient asks the nurse, "My doctor told me my thyroid scan showed a "cold spot." What does that mean?" Which of the following responses by the nurse is best?
   a. "That means you have cancer of the thyroid gland."
   b. "Cold spots are areas that have no living tissue."
   c. "A cold spot is an area that did not pick up the radioactive material they injected."
   d. "Nothing. A cold spot is just part of your thyroid gland."

Nursing Care of Patients with Endocrine Disorders

VOCABULARY

Use the following terms to fill in the blanks.

Polydipsia	Pheochromocytoma
Euthyroid	Amenorrhea
Polyuria	Goiter
Ectopic	Dysphagia
Nocturia	Myxedema

1. A normally functioning thyroid gland produces a ______________ state.

2. Enlargement of the thyroid gland is called a ______________.

3. Excessive thirst is called ______________.

4. Excessive urination is called ______________.

5. A ______________ is a tumor of the adrenal medulla.

6. Difficulty swallowing is called ______________.

7. Untreated hypothyroidism can lead to ______________ coma.

8. ______________ is the word for getting up to void during the night.

9. Absence of menses is called ______________.

10. Sometimes hormones are produced outside the endocrine gland in a/an ______________ site.

HORMONES

Match the disorder in column 1 to a hormone imbalance in column 2 and signs and symptoms in column 3.

Disorder	Hormone Problem	Major Signs and Symptoms
Diabetes insipidus	Antidiuretic hormone (ADH) deficiency	Polyuria
Syndrome of inappropriate ADH secretion (SIADH)	Growth hormone (GH) deficiency	Growing feet
Cushing's syndrome	High calcium	Moon face
Addison's disease	ADH excess	Labile hypertension
Graves' disease	Steroid excess	Tetany
Hypothyroidism	Deficient steroids	Muscle weakness, brittle bones
Pheochromocytoma	Epinephrine excess	Short stature
Hyperparathyroidism	GH excess	Water retention
Dwarfism	Low T_3 and T_4	Weight gain and fatigue
Acromegaly	Low calcium	Exophthalmos
Hypoparathyroidism	High T_3 and T_4	Hypotension

CRITICAL THINKING

Read the case studies and answer the following questions.

Sam is diagnosed with SIADH related to lung cancer. He enters the hospital for treatment of symptoms.

1. What (fluid-related) nursing diagnosis would be most appropriate for Sam? *Sam will be retaining H₂O; ∴ he'll be @ risk for fluid vol. EXCESS*

2. How will you monitor Sam's fluid balance? *Daily wts @ same time each day, on same scale, in & same amt (weight & clothing. Also, I&O, VS, urine spec. grav, lung sounds, skin turgor*

3. Why is Sam at risk for seizures? *Bec. of retaining H₂O, blood osmolality ↓'s. This can cause cerebral edema, intracranial pressure, & seizures.*

4. How will you reduce his risk for injury from seizures? *pad railings; ↓ stimulation; keep crash cart @ bedside *If seizure occurs, prevent Sam from hurting himself.*

5. What do you expect Sam's urine to look like? *cloudy, dark yellow/amber CONCENTRATED*

6. How will Sam's urine look after treatment is begun? *clear, more dilute, lighter yellow bec he'll be excreting ↑ H₂O.*

Judy is hospitalized following a motor vehicle accident in which she sustained a head injury. She develops diabetes insipidus (DI).

7. Why does head injury place Judy at risk for DI? *It can cause pituitary gland dysfnxn, leading to imbalance in ADH ie, a reduction of ADH production which causes DI.*

8. What symptoms do diabetes insipidus and diabetes mellitus have in common? *both have fluid excess/deficiency volume complications. polyuria & polydipsia*

9. Will Judy's urine specific gravity be high or low? *too low*

10. Will Judy's serum osmolality be high or low? *too high*

11. For which (fluid-related) nursing diagnosis is Judy at risk? *Fluid deficit*

12. Judy begins treatment with DDAVP. To what signs of overdose should she be alert? *S/S of fluid overload, such as ↑.ing weight & concentrated urine.*

THYROID DISORDERS

Label each symptom with an R if it suggests hyperthyroidism or an O if it suggests hypothyroidism.

1. _____ *O* Bradycardia
2. _____ *O* Lethargy
3. _____ *R* Restlessness
4. _____ *R* Frequent stools
5. _____ *O* Hypercholesterolemia
6. _____ *O* Dry hair
7. _____ *R* Tremor
8. _____ *R* Insomnia
9. _____ *O* Mental dullness, confusion
10. _____ *R* Warm, diaphoretic skin
11. _____ *R* Weight loss
12. _____ *O* Decreased appetite

REVIEW QUESTIONS

Choose the best answer.

1. A 42-year-old woman enters an outpatient clinic with symptoms of weight gain and fatigue. Laboratory studies are done, and she is diagnosed with primary hypothyroidism. She asks why her thyroid-stimulating hormone (TSH) level is elevated. Which of the following is the best response by the nurse?
   a. "The thyroid makes more TSH to take the place of the deficient T_3 and T_4."
   b. "The TSH tries to directly raise the metabolic rate when there is not enough T_3 and T_4."
   c. "The pituitary makes more TSH to try to stimulate the underactive thyroid."
   d. "The extra fat cells from your weight gain make excess TSH."

2. Which of the following nursing diagnoses would be most appropriate for a patient with weight gain and fatigue related to hypothyroidism?
   a. Imbalanced nutrition, more than body requirements, related to overeating
   b. Impaired gas exchange related to weight gain

c. Activity intolerance related to fatigue

d. Ineffective coping related to depression

3. A patient with hypothyroidism is started on levothyroxine (Synthroid), a synthetic thyroid hormone. You know that she understands the side effects of this medication when she makes the following statement:

a. "I know I should call my doctor if my heart races."

b. "I understand that I may develop a moon-shaped face."

c. "The sleepiness I experience when I start this medication will subside within 2 weeks."

d. "I'll have to watch my diet to avoid further weight gain while on this medication."

4. A 26-year-old female patient is hospitalized for radioactive iodine treatment for hyperthyroidism. Which of the following precautions by the nurse is appropriate?

a. Talk with the patient only over the intercom system.

b. Wear gloves when emptying her bedside commode.

c. Maintain reverse isolation for 3 months.

d. No precautions are necessary because the dose is so small.

5. Following surgery for thyroidectomy, the nurse watches carefully for which of the following signs and symptoms of tetany?

a. Numb fingers, muscle cramps

b. Weakness, muscle fatigue

c. Hallucinations, delusions

d. Dyspnea and tachycardia

6. What assessment findings should the nurse monitor to detect the onset of thyrotoxicosis?

a. Peripheral pulses

b. Serum sodium

c. Vital signs

d. Incision site

7. The nurse needs to accomplish all the following interventions for a patient who is 24 hours post-thyroidectomy. Place the interventions in the correct order in which they should be completed.

a. Check the surgical site dressing for signs of bleeding.

b. Verify that the airway is patent.

c. Assess vital signs.

d. Administer an analgesic for postoperative pain.

e. Teach the patient about Synthroid (levothyroxine) use after discharge.

f. Assist with range of motion exercises of the neck.

8. Which of the following dietary recommendations will reduce the risk of kidney stones in the patient with hyperparathyroidism?

a. Limit meat products

b. Limit bread products

c. Increase fluids

d. Increase citrus fruits

9. The nurse develops the nursing diagnosis of pain related to bone demineralization for a patient with hypoparathyroidism. Which of the following goals is most appropriate?

a. Serum calcium level will be <20 mg/dL

b. Patient will state correct dietary restrictions

c. Patient will perform activities of daily living (ADLs) without injury

d. Patient will verbalize acceptable pain level

10. An excess of which hormone is responsible for acromegaly?

a. TSH

b. Insulin

c. Growth hormone

d. Adrenocorticotropic hormone (ACTH)

11. A patient enters a clinic with possible Cushing's syndrome. Which of the following assessment findings support this diagnosis?

a. Weight loss, pale skin

b. Buffalo hump, easy bruising

c. Nausea, vomiting

d. Polyuria, polydipsia

12. Which assessment activity by the nurse is most important for the patient with a pheochromocytoma?

a. Vital signs

b. Daily weights

c. Peripheral pulses

d. Bowel sounds

13. Which of the following nursing diagnoses is most appropriate for the patient admitted in addisonian crisis?

a. Imbalanced nutrition: more than body requirements

b. Disturbed body image

c. Deficient fluid volume

d. Acute pain

VOCABULARY

Fill in the blanks.

1. Glucose in the urine is called ____________.
2. ____________ is too much sugar in the blood.
3. ____________ is too little sugar in the blood.
4. Deep, sighing respirations from diabetic acidosis are called ____________ respirations.
5. Excessive hunger is called ____________.
6. Excessive thirst is called ____________.
7. The patient who gets up to urinate at night has ____________.
8. The time when insulin is working its hardest after injection is called its ____________ action time.
9. The length of time insulin works is called its ____________.
10. The Diabetes Control and Complications Trial (DCCT) found that individuals who maintain ____________ control of their diabetes will have fewer long-term complications.

HYPOGLYCEMIA AND HYPERGLYCEMIA

Place an R in front of each symptom of hyperglycemia and an O in front of each symptom of hypo-glycemia.

1. ______ Tremor
2. ______ Polydipsia
3. ______ Polyuria
4. ______ Lethargy
5. ______ Irritability
6. ______ Fruity breath
7. ______ Sweating
8. ______ Abdominal pain

LONG-TERM COMPLICATIONS OF DIABETES

Match the complication with its signs and symptoms.

1. _______ Retinopathy   E
2. _______ Neuropathy   B
3. _______ Hyperosmolar, hyperglycemic, nonketotic syndrome   D
4. _______ Diabetic ketoacidosis (DKA)   A
5. _______ Nephropathy   G
6. _______ Gastroparesis   F
7. _______ Infection   C

A. Ketones in the blood and urine
B. Burning pain in legs and feet
C. Fever
D. Profound hyperglycemia without
   ketonemia
E. Impaired vision
F. Food intolerance
G. Microalbuminuria

CRITICAL THINKING

Read the case study and answer the following questions.

Jennie is a 56-year-old overweight woman admitted to your medical unit with cellulitis of the left leg. She has a history of diabetes mellitus; her blood sugar level is 436. She tells you that she takes insulin glargine *NPH* (Lantus) 18 units every bedtime and insulin lispro (Humalog) 10 units with each meal. *regular*

1. Chart the action of Jennie's insulins over the course of 24 hours.

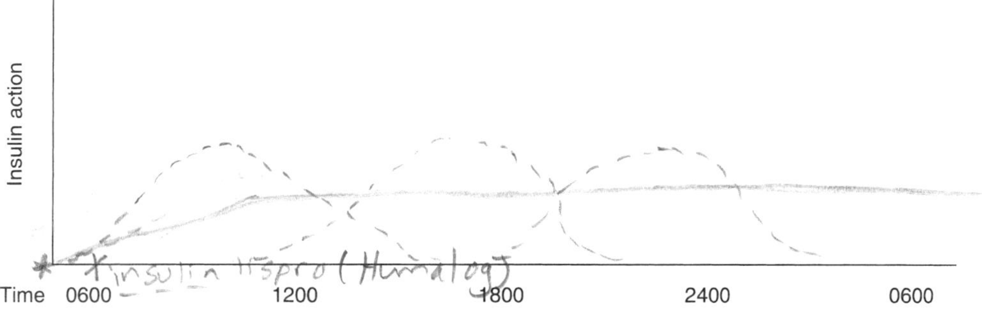

2. Jennie tells you that her physician wants her to keep her blood sugar level between 100 and 150 mg/dL. You know that a normal blood sugar level is 70 to 100. Why the discrepancy?

If her blood glucose gets too low, this puts her @ risk for hypoglycemia. If she has any autonomic neuropathy, s/s of hypogl may go unnoticed, making hypoglycemia even more risky. The physician should ALWAYS be consulted re: pt's desired bs range.

3. When you enter Jennie's room to check her 4 p.m. vital signs, she says she has a headache. By the time you finish taking her blood pressure, she has developed a cold sweat. What is happening? What should you do?

HYPOGLYCEMIC "attack" s/s. Follow facility policy re: protocol of care which usually directs a nurse to check blood sugar levels & provide quick source of glucose such as juice or glucose tablets. Notify charge RN per policy/procedure.

4. At 5 p.m., you check Jennie's blood sugar level and find that it is 80 mg/dL. What is your next step?

Evidently the tx was effective. 80mg/dL is probably OK, esp if a meal tray is to be served soon. CK to be sure meal is on its way, & WATCH for any further sx's. Consult c doc. before administering supper Humalog.

5. List three things that may have caused Jennie's blood sugar level to drop.

— eating less than rx'd @ a meal;
— skipping or delaying a meal;
— more exercise than usual

6. You explain to Jennie the importance of eating three meals a day on a regular schedule. She asks why. How do you explain this to her? _Bec she is receiving regularly sk'd insulin, it is important to eat regularly to prevent periods during which there is insulin but not enough glucose in her blood._

7. Jennie is discharged and follows her diet, exercise, and insulin regimen carefully. She even loses 50 lb. One year after her first admission, she is brought into the emergency department with a blood sugar level of 32. Why has her blood sugar level dropped? _Obesity ↑'s insulin resistance. ∴, losing wt can ↓ insulin resistance, making her insulin dose more effective._

8. Jennie's physician discontinues her insulin and starts her on glipizide (Glucotrol) 5 mg twice a day. What are two ways this oral hypoglycemic works? _Glucotrol stimulates insulin production AND ↑'s tissue sensitivity to insulin._

9. You teach Jennie to take her glipizide (Glucotrol) at what times each day? Why? _Sulfonyureas are administered 30 minutes before supper if BID dosing is ordered. This allows absorption of med before eating._

10. Does Jennie have type 1 or type 2 diabetes? How do you know? _Type 2. If she had type 1, she'd not be able to take oral hypoglycemics. Also, obesity is common in type2 DM._

REVIEW QUESTIONS

Choose the best answer.

1. A 56-year-old gentleman is admitted to the hospital with a blood glucose of 680 mg/dL, and ketones in his blood and urine. Which type of diabetes does he have?
   a. Type 1
   b. Type 2
   c. Prediabetes
   d. Gestational

2. In addition to stimulating insulin production, glyburide (Micronase) has which of the following effects?
   a. Stimulates gluconeogenesis
   b. Promotes fat breakdown
   c. Increases tissue sensitivity to insulin
   d. Enhances appetite

3. Which of the following symptoms do you expect if a patient with diabetes forgets to take a dose of glyburide (Micronase)?
   a. Cold, clammy sweat
   b. Tachycardia, nervousness, hunger
   c. Chest pain, shortness of breath
   d. Fatigue, thirst, blurred vision

4. Which of the following is an acceptable blood sugar range for a patient with diabetes?
   a. 46 to 98 mg/dL
   b. 90 to 130 mg/dL
   c. 180 to 250 mg/dL
   d. 350 to 600 mg/dL

5. By which routes can insulin be administered? Choose all correct answers.
   a. Oral
   b. Inhaled
   c. Intravenous
   d. Subcutaneous

6. Before giving insulin, the nurse always checks which test result?
   a. Recent potassium level
   b. Blood sugar level
   c. Urine ketones
   d. White blood cell count

7. A patient takes NPH insulin every morning. At which of the following times should the patient observe for signs and symptoms of low blood sugar level?
   a. 1 hour after administration of insulin
   b. 6 to 12 hours after administration of insulin
   c. 24 to 36 hours after administration of insulin
   d. NPH insulin does not cause low blood sugar level

8. At what point after injection does the peak action of regular insulin occur?
   a. 30 to 60 minutes
   b. 1 to 2 hours
   c. 2 to 5 hours
   d. 8 to 12 hours

9. Which of the following are symptoms of hypoglycemia?
   a. Nausea and vomiting
   b. Glycosuria
   c. Cold sweat and tremor
   d. Polyuria and polydipsia

10. Which of the following is an appropriate treatment for hypoglycemia?
    a. Raisins
    b. Cheese
    c. Tylenol
    d. Beef jerky

11. Some patients use subcutaneous glucagon for emergency episodes of which of the following conditions?
    a. Hyperglycemia
    b. Ketonuria
    c. Diabetic ketoacidosis
    d. Hypoglycemia

12. Which of the following is a major risk factor of type 2 diabetes?
    a. Obesity
    b. Viral infection
    c. Binge eating
    d. Hypertension

13. A patient on an American Diabetes Association diet receives a breakfast tray and does not care for the oatmeal. Which of the following foods can the nurse substitute for a half cup of oatmeal?
    a. 4 oz of orange juice
    b. Two strips of bacon
    c. 1 oz of cheese
    d. A slice of wheat toast

unit ELEVEN

UNDERSTANDING THE GENITOURINARY AND REPRODUCTIVE SYSTEM

CHECKLIST FOR LEARNING SUCCESS

Review of Anatomy and Physiology

- ❏ Female reproductive system
- ❏ Female hormones
- ❏ The menstrual cycle
- ❏ Male reproductive system
- ❏ Male hormones
- ❏ Aging changes

Major Disorders

- ❏ Breast cancer
- ❏ Menstrual disorders
- ❏ Infections
- ❏ Displacement disorders
- ❏ Fertility disorders
- ❏ Tumors of the cervix, uterus, and ovaries
- ❏ Prostatitis
- ❏ Benign prostatic hypertrophy (BPH)
- ❏ Prostate cancer
- ❏ Penile disorders
- ❏ Testicular disorders
- ❏ Erectile dysfunction
- ❏ Sexually transmitted diseases (STDs)

Nursing Assessment

- ❏ History
- ❏ Breast assessment
- ❏ Breast self-examination (BSE)
- ❏ Sexual function
- ❏ Testicular self-examination (TSE)

Diagnostic Tests

- ❏ Mammogram
- ❏ Biopsy
- ❏ Hormone tests
- ❏ Pelvic examination
- ❏ Papanicolaou (Pap) smear
- ❏ Swabs and smears
- ❏ Endoscopic examinations
- ❏ Cystourethroscopy
- ❏ Digital rectal examination (DRE)
- ❏ Prostate specific antigen (PSA)
- ❏ Fertility testing

Interventions

- ❏ Breast surgeries
- ❏ Hysterectomy
- ❏ Contraception
- ❏ Prostatectomy
- ❏ Transurethral resection of the prostate (TURP)
- ❏ Teaching

Common Medications

- ❏ Antibiotics
- ❏ Hormone replacement therapy
- ❏ Oral contraceptives

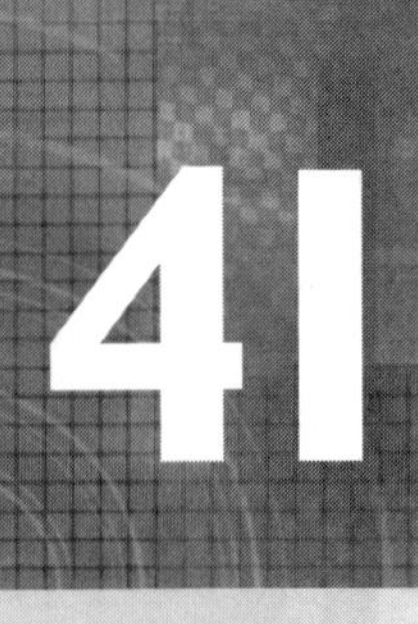

Genitourinary and Reproductive System Function and Assessment

VOCABULARY

Complete the following sentences with the correct term from the chapter.

1. A _hysteroscopy_ may be done to view the inside of the uterus with an endoscope.
2. During some diagnostic procedures, a body cavity is filled with carbon dioxide to make it easier for the physician to view structures. This is called _insufflation_.
3. A male patient should have a yearly _digital_ _rectal_ _exam_ to detect prostate cancer.
4. Some men have excessive breast tissue, or _gynecomastia_.
5. If the urethral opening is on the underside of the penis, it is called _hypospadias_.
6. Fluid in the scrotum is called a _hydrocele_.
7. If the scrotum feels like a bag of worms when palpated, it is called a _varicocele_.
8. Another word for sexual desire is _libido_.
9. The beginning of menstruation in the female is called _menarche_.
10. X-ray examination of the breasts is called _mammography_.

ANATOMY AND PHYSIOLOGY

Label the structures of the male and female reproductive systems.

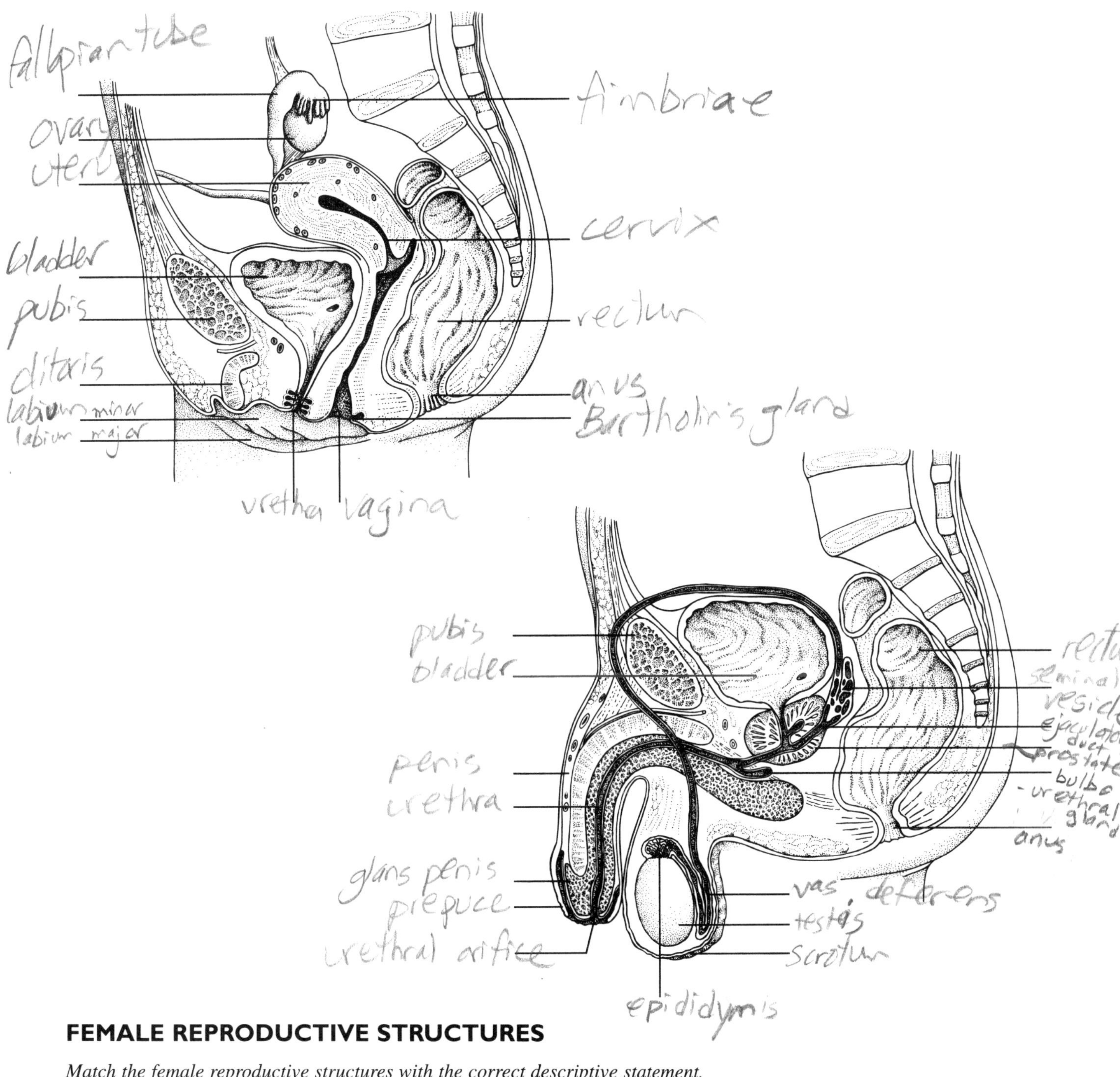

FEMALE REPRODUCTIVE STRUCTURES

Match the female reproductive structures with the correct descriptive statement.

1. _____ E _____ Fallopian tube
2. _____ G _____ Myometrium
3. _____ F _____ Bartholin's glands
4. _____ C _____ Vestibule
5. _____ B _____ Endometrium
6. _____ A _____ Ovarian follicle
7. _____ D _____ Corpus luteum

A. Site of development of an ovum
B. Becomes the maternal side of the placenta
C. Contains the urethral and vaginal openings
D. Secretes progesterone and estrogen after ovulation
E. The usual site of fertilization
F. Secrete mucus at the vaginal orifice
G. Contracts for labor and delivery

MALE REPRODUCTIVE SYSTEM

Number the following in proper sequence with respect to the pathway sperm travel from the testes.

____4____ Ejaculatory duct

____2____ Epididymis

____5____ Urethra

____1____ Seminiferous tubules

____3____ Ductus deferens

DIAGNOSTIC TESTS

Match the following tests with their descriptions.

1. ___B___ Cytology
2. ___A___ Colposcopy
3. ___C___ Sonography
4. ___F___ Computed tomographic (CT) scan
5. ___D___ Magnetic resonance imaging
6. ___E___ Testicular self-examination (TSE)

A. Scope examination of the vagina

B. Examination of cells using a microscope

C. Mapping of tissues according to their densities using sound waves

D. Mapping of tissue by using radiofrequency radiation and magnetic fields

E. Self-examination of the male testicles

F. Computer-assisted recording of very precise x-ray pictures of layers of tissue

CRITICAL THINKING

Read the case studies and answer the following questions.

1. Mr. White comes to see his physician for a yearly checkup. As you are taking his blood pressure, he says, "I don't need that rectal examination, do I? I had prostate surgery last year." How do you respond?

____

____

____

2. Mrs. Bitner has just returned from having an endoscopic examination. She says, "Something went wrong, I just know it. Look at my belly. I look like I'm 9 months pregnant." How do you respond?

____

____

____

3. Ms. Wilson comes to the clinic with complaints of excessive vaginal discharge. While asking her some initial questions, you learn that she has multiple sex partners. How do you set up for the examination? What teaching is important? _____________________

____

____

4. Mr. Brown is being admitted to the hospital for complications of diabetes. While collecting initial data, you learn that although he is married, he is no longer sexually active. How do you respond? _____________________

____

____

Choose the best answer.

1. Which of the following male reproductive structures carries semen through the penis to the exterior?
   a. Urethra
   b. Epididymis
   c. Ductus deferens
   d. Ejaculatory duct

2. Which layer of the uterus will become the maternal portion of the placenta?
   a. Myometrium
   b. Endometrium
   c. Epimetrium
   d. Serosa

3. Which of the following descriptions best describes the position of the uterus?
   a. Superior to the bladder with the fundus most anterior
   b. Anterior to the bladder with the cervix most inferior
   c. Inferior to the bladder with the cervix most superior
   d. Posterior to the bladder with the fundus most inferior

4. Which of the following hormones stimulates the mammary glands to produce milk after pregnancy?
   a. Progesterone
   b. Estrogen
   c. Oxytocin
   d. Prolactin

5. Strong contractions of the smooth muscle of the uterus for labor and delivery are brought about by which of the following hormones?
   a. Progesterone
   b. Follicle-stimulating hormone (FSH)
   c. Oxytocin
   d. Luteinizing hormone (LH)

6. According to the American Cancer Society, how often should breast self-examination be done?
   a. Weekly
   b. Monthly
   c. Yearly
   d. Semiannually

7. When should men over age 40 have digital rectal examinations?
   a. Weekly
   b. Monthly
   c. Every other month
   d. During yearly physician visit

8. A patient being prepared for cystourethrography asks what is going to be done to him. Which is the best explanation by the nurse?
   a. "The doctor will put an endoscope into your bladder."
   b. "You will have a catheter put in, then a dye will be injected and x-rays will be taken."
   c. "You will have a small needle inserted through your lower abdomen and into your bladder."
   d. "You will have an intravenous injection of dye, then x-rays will be taken as it travels through your kidneys."

9. How should the nurse prepare a patient for a routine Pap smear?
   a. Give her an enema.
   b. Ask her to empty her bladder.
   c. Ask her to take a deep breath and hold it.
   d. Set out a suture tray and local anesthetic.

10. Which of the following positions is advised for doing a portion of the breast self-examination?
    a. Supine
    b. Simm's
    c. Kneeling
    d. Fowler's

11. Which supplies should the nurse set out when assisting with collecting gonorrhea bacteria for culture?
    a. Clear swab
    b. *Chlamydia* kit
    c. Charcoal swab
    d. Viral collection kit

12. Why are additional tests used to verify mammography findings?
    a. The mammogram needs no other verification.
    b. Mammograms are unable to show lesions in breast tissue.
    c. The mammogram can show only breast cysts, not cancers.
    d. Many things can cause shadows on a mammogram besides cancer.

13. What danger does magnetic resonance imaging pose?
    a. It can cause radiation poisoning.
    b. High frequency sound waves can damage hearing.
    c. Metal objects in the body can become heated or dislodged.
    d. The contrast that is used to outline body cavities can be toxic.

14. A nurse practitioner completes a wet mount specimen on a patient with a suspected STD, then leaves the room. As the assisting LPN prepares to take the slide to the lab, the patient says, "I'm really scared that I have something serious. What do you think I should do?" Which response by the LPN is best?
    a. Sit next to the patient and say, "What frightens you the most?"
    b. Stand at the foot of the examination table and say, "There is nothing to be worried about until we get the test results."
    c. Give the patient time to verbalize concerns, then advise that she have her partner tested.
    d. Touch her lightly on the arm and say, "Let me get this slide to the lab, then I'll come back and we'll talk."

Nursing Care of Women with Reproductive System Disorders

VOCABULARY

Match the term with its definition.

1. __C__ Imperforate
2. __D__ Colporrhaphy
3. __B__ Dysmenorrhea
4. __J__ Cryotherapy
5. __E__ Agenesis
6. __G__ Dyspareunia
7. __A__ Cystocele
8. __F__ Rectocele
9. __H__ Anteversion
10. __I__ Salpingo-oophorectomy

A. Bladder sags into vaginal space
B. Painful menstruation
C. Not having expected opening
D. Surgical repair of a part of the vagina
E. Undeveloped
F. Rectum sags into the vagina
G. Painful intercourse
H. Forward turning
I. Removal of fallopian tubes and ovaries
J. Freezing of tissue

BREAST SURGERIES

Match the following breast surgery terms with their descriptions.

1. __E__ Mastopexy
2. __A__ Mastectomy
3. __C__ Reduction mammoplasty
4. __B__ Augmentation mammoplasty
5. __D__ Reconstructive mammoplasty

A. Surgery to remove a breast
B. Surgery to increase the size of the breasts
C. Surgery to decrease the size of the breasts
D. Surgery to rebuild a breast after mastectomy
E. Surgery to change the position of the breasts

MENSTRUAL DISORDERS

Match the following menstrual disorders with their description.

1. __E__ Amenorrhea
2. __C__ Menorrhagia
3. __A__ Dysmenorrhea
4. __B__ Polymenorrhea
5. __D__ Hypomenorrhea

A. Difficult or painful menstruation
B. Menses more often than every 21 days
C. Passing more than 80 mL of blood per menses
D. Less than expected amount of menstrual bleeding
E. Absence of menstrual periods for 6 months or three previous cycle lengths once cycles have been established

MASTECTOMY CARE

Circle the errors in the following scenario and write the correct information in the space provided.

You are assigned to care for Mrs. Joseph, who is 1 day postoperative following a right radical mastectomy. You know that she is not anxious, because she had a left mastectomy a year ago and knows everything to expect. You listen to her breath sounds and find them clear, so it is not necessary to have her cough and deep breathe. You encourage her to lie on her right side to prevent bleeding. You use her right arm for blood pressures, because both arms are affected and the right one is more convenient. You also encourage her to avoid use of her right arm to prevent injury to the surgical site. You provide a balanced diet and plenty of fluids to aid in her recovery.

____

____

____

____

____

CRITICAL THINKING

Read the case study and answer the following questions.

A 21-year-old female college student comes in to the physician's office where you work and comments with evident frustration that she has a yeast infection again. She has type 1 diabetes mellitus and takes her insulin routinely. However, she seldom tests her blood glucose level, because, she says, "I don't have time to mess with that stuff as often as I should." She comments that every time she goes home on weekends to visit her parents (a 3-hour bus trip), she develops a very uncomfortable vaginal yeast infection.

1. What factors may be contributing to her frequent yeast overgrowths? _________________________

____

2. What suggestions can you give her to help prevent this problem? _________________________

____

Choose the best answer.

1. A nurse is teaching a patient about use of a condom with spermicide for contraception. Which statement by the patient indicates the need for further teaching?
   a. "This method will be affordable."
   b. "I am glad that barrier methods are 100% effective."
   c. "I'm glad there are fewer side effects than there are with the pill."
   d. "I know that both I and my husband will need to be diligent to use the method all the time."

2. Place the following nursing diagnoses for the woman who has just had a mastectomy for breast cancer in correct priority order.
   a. Ineffective tissue perfusion
   b. Risk for ineffective coping
   c. Ineffective breathing pattern
   d. Anxiety

3. How will a douche affect a vaginal examination to determine the type of pathogen present?
   a. Helps clear the area for better visualization
   b. Does not affect the outcome negatively or positively
   c. May wash away evidence of the pathogen, making diagnosis difficult
   d. Baking soda douche must be done before the examination to neutralize the pH

4. In which patient is it most important to teach about risks of receiving estrogen without progestins?
   a. The patient with a family history of cancer
   b. The patient whose grandmother died of heart disease
   c. The patient who has been diagnosed with osteoporosis
   d. The patient who is exhibiting signs of atrophic vaginitis

5. Which of the following nursing interventions will help prevent swelling after a radical mastectomy with lymph node removal?
   a. Restricting all movement of the affected arm
   b. Raising the affected arm above the heart on pillows
   c. Applying warm moist heat to the arm
   d. Holding the arm close to the body with a sling

6. Which of the following is a known risk factor for cervical cancer?
   a. Tight clothing
   b. A high-sodium diet
   c. Multiple sexual partners
   d. Beginning sexual activity late in life

7. A patient who had a panhysterectomy 4 days ago for endometrial cancer learns that she has metastases to her lungs. When asked about her plans after discharge, she answered sharply that she "cannot plan for any future, because there isn't going to be any!" She then started to cry. Which of the following nursing diagnoses best fits this situation?
   a. Anticipatory grieving
   b. Body image disturbance
   c. Sleep pattern disturbance
   d. Noncompliance

8. Which of the following is a risk factor for development of breast cancer?
   a. Late menarche
   b. No pregnancies
   c. Early menopause
   d. Early first pregnancy

9. A patient with breast cancer is being treated with tamoxifen citrate, which deprives cancer cells of the estrogen that makes them grow. This is an example of which mode of therapy?
   a. Hormonal therapy
   b. Radiation therapy
   c. Cytotoxic chemotherapy
   d. Biological response modifier therapy

10. If a patient is taking cytotoxic chemotherapy drugs to fight cervical cancer, maintaining adequate nutrition is often a problem because of nausea and mouth sores. Which of the following nursing actions will best help increase the patient's food intake?
    a. Provide very hot or cold foods.
    b. Provide a bland diet.
    c. Avoid fresh fruits and vegetables.
    d. Administer antiemetic medications before meals.

11. A 38-year-old patient had a reduction mammoplasty 4 days ago. When changing her dressing the home care nurse notes redness, swelling, and some thick yellow drainage escaping from areas of the incision line around her left nipple. Which of the following nursing interventions is appropriate?
    a. Monitor it for 24 hours, and if there is no improvement, notify the registered nurse or physician.
    b. Inform the patient that the incision is not healing properly, and that she should see her physician as soon as possible.
    c. Clean the incision with normal saline and redress it, and recheck it the following day.
    d. Promptly report the situation to the registered nurse or physician and document it in the patient's chart.

12. Which of the following lifestyle habits is most likely to increase premenstrual syndrome symptoms?
    a. Restricting alcohol intake
    b. Avoiding smoking
    c. Drinking coffee
    d. Eating a low-salt diet

Nursing Care of Male Patients with Genitourinary Disorders

43

VOCABULARY

Fill in the blanks in the following sentences with words from the chapter.

1. When semen goes into the bladder during intercourse, it is called _retrograde ejaculation_.
2. An erection that lasts too long is called _priapism_.
3. _Phimosis_ is the term used to describe uncircumcised foreskin that cannot be extended over the head of the penis.
4. _Smegma_ is a cottage cheese–like secretion made by the gland of the foreskin.
5. Surgical removal of the foreskin is called _circumcision_.
6. _Cryptorchidism_ is a birth condition in which one or both of the testicles have not descended into the scrotum.
7. Inflammation or infection of a testicle is called _orchitis_.
8. The correct term for male impotence is _ED_.
9. A _varicocele_ is varicose veins of the scrotum.
10. Surgical cutting of the vas deferens as a method of birth control is called a _vasectomy_.

DISORDERS OF THE MALE REPRODUCTIVE SYSTEM

Match the disorder with its definition.

1. __C__ Benign prostatic hypertrophy (BPH)
2. __E__ Hydronephrosis
3. __A__ Hematuria
4. __B__ Peyronie's disease
5. __J__ Priapism
6. __G__ Epididymitis
7. __D__ Infertility
8. __F__ Orchitis
9. __H__ Dysuria
10. __I__ Reflux

A. Blood in the urine
B. Curved penis
C. Noncancerous overgrowth of prostate tissue
D. Inability to reproduce
E. Distention of kidney with retained urine
F. Inflammation of the testicles
G. Inflammation or infection of the tube where sperm matures
H. Painful or difficult urination
I. Backward flow of urine
J. Prolonged erection

ERECTILE DYSFUNCTION

Unscramble the causes of erectile dysfunction.

aeiioctdmn _medication_
sssrte _stress_
eeiophysnntr _hypertension_
PRUT _TURP_
threa flraeiu _heart failure_
tiellpum lersssoic _multiple sclerosis_

CRITICAL THINKING

Read the case study and answer the following questions.

Mr. Washington is a 62-year-old retired teacher who comes to the urgent care center complaining that he "can't pass water."

1. What initial questions do you ask to further assess Mr. Washington's problem? ______________________
____
____

2. What do you think is happening? ______________
____
____

3. What care do you anticipate as the physician examines him? ______________________
____
____

4. What can result if the problem continues untreated?
____
____

Mr. Washington is transferred to the local hospital where BPH is confirmed. He is scheduled for a transurethral resection of the prostate (TURP). He asks the nurse, "What's a TURP?"

5. How would the nurse explain a TURP to Mr. Washington? ______________________
____

6. Following surgery, Mr. Washington has a three-way Foley catheter. What is the purpose of this type of catheter? How does the nurse total intake and output (I&O) at the end of the shift? ______________________
____
____

7. Bladder spasms are common after TURP. How will the nurse know if this is happening? What interventions will help? ______________________
____
____

8. Mr. Washington is discharged. The next day he calls the nursing unit and says in a panicky voice, "I just wet my pants! I can't hold my urine! This is worse than not being able to go at all!" How should the nurse respond? What can he do? ______________________
____
____

REVIEW QUESTIONS

Choose the best answer.

1. The nurse completes a nursing history on a patient admitted for a TURP. What symptoms are typically seen with BPH? Choose all answers that are correct.
   - a. A feeling of incomplete bladder emptying after voiding
   - b. Difficulty maintaining an erection
   - c. Difficulty urinating
   - d. Grossly bloody urine
   - e. Pain in the lower back that radiates to the hips during urination
   - f. Nocturia

2. A patient tells his nurse that he has delayed having a TURP because he is afraid it will affect his sexual function. Which response by the nurse is most appropriate?
   - a. "Don't worry about sterility; sperm production is not affected by this surgery."
   - b. "Would you like some information about implants used for impotence?"
   - c. "This type of surgery rarely affects the ability to have an erection or ejaculation."
   - d. "There are many methods of sexual expression that are alternatives to sexual intercourse."

3. A patient returns from surgery following a TURP with a three-way Foley catheter and continuous bladder irrigation. Postoperative orders include meperidine (Demerol) 75 mg IM q3h as needed for pain, belladonna and opium (B&O) suppository q4h as needed, and strict I&O. The patient complains of painful bladder spasms, and the nurse observes blood-tinged urine on the sheets. Which action should the nurse take?
   a. Give the Demerol.
   b. Give the B&O suppository.
   c. Warm the irrigation solution to body temperature.
   d. Notify the physician stat.

4. A patient who has just had a TURP asks his nurse to explain why he has to have the bladder irrigation because it seems to increase his pain. Which of the following explanations by the nurse is best?
   a. "The bladder irrigation is needed to stop the bleeding in the bladder."
   b. "Antibiotics are being administered into the bladder to prevent infection."
   c. "The irrigation is needed to keep the catheter from becoming occluded by blood clots."
   d. "Normal production of urine is maintained with the irrigations until healing can occur."

5. A post-TURP patient experiences dribbling following removal of his catheter. Which action should the nurse take?
   a. Have him restrict fluid intake to 1000 mL/day.
   b. Teach him to perform Kegel's exercises 10 to 20 times per hour.
   c. Reinsert the Foley catheter until he regains urinary control.
   d. Reassure him that incontinence never lasts more than a few days.

6. A 36-year-old man is scheduled for a unilateral orchiectomy for treatment of testicular cancer. He is withdrawn and does not interact with the nurse. Which action is most appropriate?
   a. Identify the problem with a nursing diagnosis of impaired communication related to the diagnosis of cancer.
   b. Set a patient outcome that the patient will verbalize his concerns about his diagnosis.
   c. Ask the patient whether he is worried about future sexual functioning.
   d. Say, "You seem quiet. Are you feeling concerned about your diagnosis or treatment?"

7. A 28-year-old man is diagnosed with acute epididymitis. Which of the following symptoms supports this diagnosis?
   a. Burning and pain on urination
   b. Severe tenderness and swelling in the scrotum
   c. Foul-smelling ejaculate and severe scrotal swelling
   d. Foul-smelling urine and pain on urination

8. A man with a history of diabetes and chronic lung disease is admitted to the hospital with prostate cancer. He has all the following symptoms. Which should the nurse address first?
   a. Fever of 101°F (38.3°C)
   b. Respiratory rate 36 per minute
   c. Difficulty urinating
   d. Painful legs and feet

9. Which of the following nursing actions is most appropriate when doing perineal care on an uncircumcised male patient?
   a. Leave the foreskin retracted so air can keep the area dry.
   b. Do not retract the foreskin during washing.
   c. Replace the foreskin over the head of the penis after washing.
   d. Use alcohol and a cotton swab to clean under the foreskin.

10. What is the best way to detect testicular cancer early?
    a. Monthly testicular self-examination (TSE)
    b. Yearly digital rectal examination (DRE)
    c. Annual physician examination
    d. Annual ultrasonography

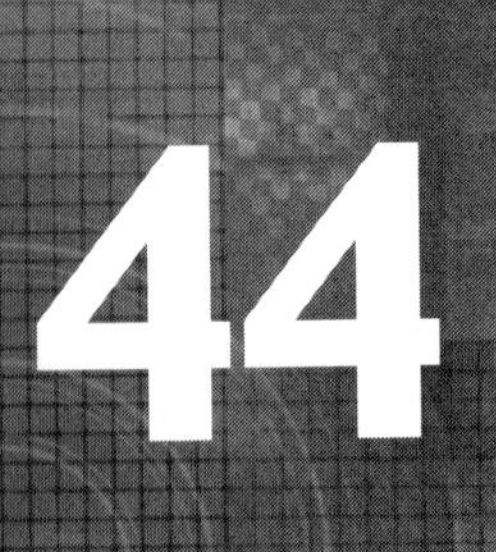

Nursing Care of Patients with Sexually Transmitted Diseases

VOCABULARY

Match the term with its definition.

1. _D_ Condylomatous
2. _B_ Gumma
3. _C_ Chancre
4. _E_ Cytotoxic
5. _A_ Herpetic
6. _F_ Puerperal

A. Relating to herpes
B. Rubbery tumor
C. Red ulcer from syphilis
D. Wartlike
E. Poison to cells
F. Time following childbirth

INFLAMMATORY DISORDERS

Match the following inflammation words with their definitions.

1. _A_ Proctitis
2. _C_ Urethritis
3. _B_ Cervicitis
4. _E_ Endometritis
5. _D_ Conjunctivitis

A. Inflammation of the rectum and anus
B. Inflammation of the cervix
C. Inflammation of the urethra
D. Inflammation of parts of the eye
E. Inflammation of the lining of the uterus

BARRIER METHODS FOR SAFER SEX

List the teaching that should accompany each of the following barriers against STDs.

1. Male condoms

2. Female condoms

3. Diaphragms

4. Rubber gloves ____

5. Double condoms ____

CRITICAL THINKING

Read the case study and answer the following questions.

James, 32 years old, arrives at an outpatient clinic requesting STD testing for him and his fiancée. You learn that he met his fiancée through an international dating agency and that she has come here to marry him. She does not speak English. He asks you to give him the paperwork for both of them to get the blood test for STDs—just to make sure they don't have anything contagious. He seems in a hurry and asks if they can have their blood drawn first and then he could come back in an hour or two and see the doctor for the results for both of them.

1. What misunderstandings does James have about STD diagnosis? _____________________________________
____

2. Legally and ethically, does James have a right to be told his fiancée's test results? ___________________
____
____

3. What procedures should occur before any testing is done? ____
____
____

4. Is James likely to get his answer about whether either he or his fiancée has a contagious STD today?
____
____
____

REVIEW QUESTIONS

Choose the best answer.

1. A 36-year-old woman who has had no prenatal care comes into the hospital in active labor for her fourth child. She has vesicles evident on her perineum. Which of the following nursing actions are appropriate to protect the unborn baby and the staff? Choose all answers that are correct.
   a. Maintain standard precautions.
   b. Reprimand the mother for putting her baby at risk for herpes.
   c. Prepare for the possibility that the baby may be delivered by cesarean section.
   d. Notify the obstetrician or nurse midwife about the vesicles as soon as possible.
   e. Apply antibiotic ointment to the vesicles.
   f. Place the mother in reverse isolation.

2. A 23-year-old woman is seen at an outpatient clinic for a routine Papanicoloau (Pap) smear. When questioned, she states she is deciding whether to engage in sexual activity with a man she is just getting to know. She asks how she can tell if he has an STD. Which response by the nurse is best?
   a. "If the man appears clean and has been conscientious about using condoms, he is likely infection free."
   b. "Look carefully for signs of lesions before engaging in sexual activity."
   c. "Be sure to use either a male or female condom to protect against possible transmission of infection."
   d. "An examination by a physician with diagnostic testing is the only way to know if he is infection free."

3. A college student goes to the college clinic and asks the best way to avoid contracting an STD. The nurse provides the clinic's standard STD teaching. Which statement by the student indicates the need for additional instruction?
    a. "There is no guarantee that I won't contract an STD if I choose to be sexually active."
    b. "Abstinence is the only sure way to avoid an STD."
    c. "If I use a condom with spermicide, I will be safer than if I don't use one."
    d. "If I question my partner about past sexual encounters, I can avoid STDs."

4. What equipment should the nurse prepare for the primary care provider when a woman says she is concerned about possible *Chlamydia* infection?
    a. *Chlamydia* slide
    b. *Chlamydia* swab
    c. *Chlamydia* collection kit
    d. *Chlamydia* wet mount

5. While bathing an 82-year-old man hospitalized with pneumonia, a nurse notes an ulcerated area on his penis. What action should the nurse take first?
    a. Report the ulcer to the admitting care provider.
    b. Teach the man about STD prevention.
    c. Ask the man if he has a history of syphilis.
    d. Clean the ulcer; reporting is not necessary because an STD is unlikely in a man this age.

6. A 16-year-old girl is diagnosed with genital herpes. She has vesicles on her genitals and urethritis. She is tearful as she asks what she can do to prevent complications of the disease. Based on the data provided, which nursing diagnosis is appropriate for her plan of care?
    a. Risk for transmission of infection
    b. Health-seeking behaviors
    c. Pain
    d. Ineffective sexuality pattern

7. Which virus causes genital warts?
    a. Cytomegalovirus
    b. Herpes simplex virus type II
    c. Human papillomavirus
    d. Human immunodeficiency virus

8. A patient has cloudy penile discharge. For which additional symptoms of urethritis should the nurse assess?
    a. Throat or rectal infection
    b. Chancres or vesicles on the genitals
    c. Painful and frequent urination
    d. Oliguria and flank pain

9. A woman with pelvic inflammatory disease complains of lower abdominal pain. Which action should the nurse take first?
    a. Have her rate her pain on a 0 to 10 scale.
    b. Administer antibiotics as ordered.
    c. Administer an analgesic as ordered.
    d. Teach the patient about causes and prevention of STDs.

10. The nurse needs to administer an intramuscular injection of 2.4 million units of penicillin G. It is supplied in a vial of 5,000,000 units of powder for injection. Instructions state to dilute with 8 mL of sterile water. How many mL should the nurse draw up? _______

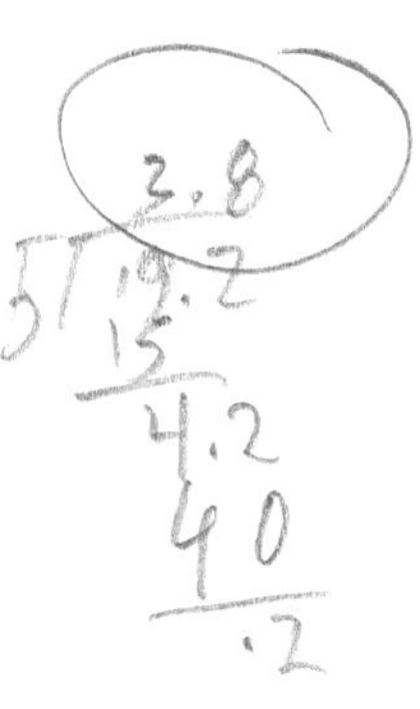

UNDERSTANDING THE MUSCULOSKELETAL SYSTEM

CHECKLIST FOR LEARNING SUCCESS

Review of Anatomy and Physiology

- ❑ Skeletal system
- ❑ Muscular system
- ❑ Aging effects

Major Musculoskeletal Disorders

- ❑ Osteoarthritis
- ❑ Rheumatoid arthritis
- ❑ Gout
- ❑ Systemic lupus erythematosus
- ❑ Muscular dystrophy
- ❑ Carpal tunnel syndrome
- ❑ Fractures
- ❑ Complications of fractures
- ❑ Rhabdomyolysis
- ❑ Osteomyelitis
- ❑ Osteoporosis
- ❑ Paget's disease
- ❑ Bone cancer

Nursing Assessment

- ❑ Medical history
- ❑ Medications
- ❑ Vital signs
- ❑ Physical assessment
- ❑ Deformities/limb length
- ❑ Crepitation
- ❑ Swelling
- ❑ Range of motion
- ❑ Muscle strength
- ❑ Pain
- ❑ Neurovascular checks

Diagnostic Tests

- ❑ Alkaline phosphatase
- ❑ Erythrocyte sedimentation rate
- ❑ Serum calcium/phosphorus/uric acid
- ❑ Creatinine kinase
- ❑ Myoglobin
- ❑ Rheumatoid factor
- ❑ Arthrocentesis
- ❑ Arthrography
- ❑ Arthroscopy
- ❑ Bone scan
- ❑ Electromyography (EMG)
- ❑ Magnetic resonance imaging (MRI)
- ❑ Myelogram
- ❑ X-rays

Interventions

- ❑ Amputation
- ❑ Prosthesis
- ❑ Casts
- ❑ Closed reduction
- ❑ Continuous passive motion machine
- ❑ Diet therapy
- ❑ External fixation
- ❑ Heat and cold
- ❑ Hip protectors
- ❑ Open reduction/internal fixation
- ❑ Rest, ice, compression, elevation
- ❑ Total joint replacement
- ❑ Traction

Common Medications

- ❑ Allopurinol (Zyloprim)
- ❑ Analgesics
- ❑ Anticoagulants
- ❑ Antirheumatic drugs
- ❑ Biophosphonates
- ❑ Calcitonin (Calcimar)
- ❑ Corticosteroid
- ❑ Cox-2 selective inhibitors
- ❑ Muscle relaxants
- ❑ Nonsteroidal anti-inflammatory drugs (NSAIDs)
- ❑ Raloxifene (Evista)

Musculoskeletal Function and Assessment

STRUCTURE OF NEUROMUSCULAR JUNCTION AND SARCOMERES

Label the structures from the following word list.

Acetylcholine
Acetylcholine receptors
Actin filament
Axon terminal
Myosin filament
Sarcolemma
Sarcomere
Synaptic cleft
Vesicle of acetylcholine

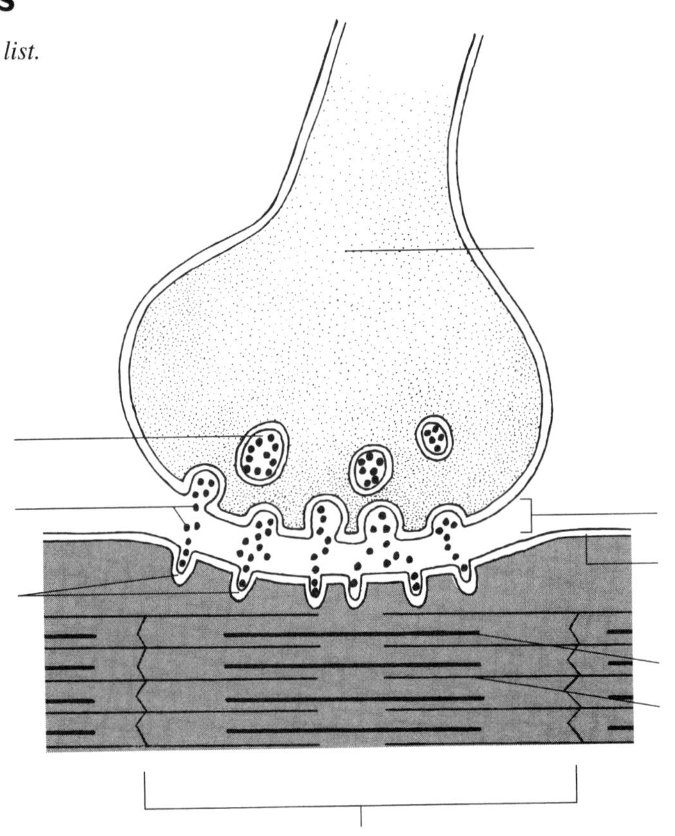

NEUROMUSCULAR JUNCTION

Match each part of the neuromuscular junction with the proper descriptions. Each part will have two correct answers.

1. _______ Synapse
2. _______ Axon terminal
3. _______ Sarcolemma

A. Contains the transmitter acetylcholine
B. The cell membrane of the muscle fiber
C. The space between the muscle fiber and the motor neuron
D. Has receptors for acetylcholine
E. An impulse is transmitted by the diffusion of acetylcholine
F. The end of the motor neuron

SYNOVIAL JOINTS

Match each part of a synovial joint with the correct description.

1. _______ Articular cartilage
2. _______ Joint capsule
3. _______ Synovial membrane
4. _______ Synovial fluid
5. _______ Bursae

A. Lines the joint capsule and secretes synovial fluid
B. Prevents friction within the joint cavity
C. Encloses the joint similar to a sleeve
D. Permit tendons to slide easily across a joint
E. Provides a smooth surface on the joint surfaces of bones

VOCABULARY

Match the word with its definition.

1. _______ Symphysis
2. _______ Ball and socket
3. _______ Hinge
4. _______ Condyloid
5. _______ Pivot
6. _______ Gliding
7. _______ Saddle
8. _______ Bursa
9. _______ Crepitation
10. _______ Synovitis

A. Movement in all planes
B. Rotation
C. Disk of fibrous cartilage between bones
D. Movement in one plane
E. Hinge with some lateral movement
F. Side-to-side movement
G. Small sacs of synovial fluid between joints and tendons
H. Movement in several planes
I. Swollen synovial tissue within the joint
J. Grating sound as joint or bone moves

DIAGNOSTIC TESTS

Match the diagnostic tests to the appropriate description.

1. _______ X-ray
2. _______ Arthrogram
3. _______ MRI
4. _______ Arthroscopy
5. _______ Arthrocentesis
6. _______ Bone scan
7. _______ Alkaline phosphatase
8. _______ Calcium
9. _______ Phosphorus
10. _______ Erythrocyte sedimentation rate
11. _______ Uric acid

A. Dye required to view joint structures: tendons, ligaments, cartilage
B. Radio waves and magnetic field view of soft tissue
C. Bones show up as white areas
D. Insertion of a needle into a joint space to remove fluid, obtain a specimen, or instill medication
E. An endoscopy of joints with local or general anesthesia
F. Serum level of enzyme that is made by osteoblasts to mineralize bone
G. After being injected, the radioisotope Napertechnate is taken up by bone and 2 hours later a camera scans the body front and back
H. Serum level of substance stored in bone that makes bone rigid
I. Serum test for inflammation
J. Serum level of substance that mineralizes bones and teeth
K. Serum level for end product of purine metabolism

CRITICAL THINKING

Read the case study and answer the questions.

Mr. John Allen, age 45, was in an automobile accident and comes to the emergency department with a fractured femur.

1. What information should the nurse include in Mr. Allen's history? _______________________________
____

2. What areas should Mr. Allen's physical assessment focus on first? _______________________________
____

3. What tests can the nurse anticipate will be done on Mr. Allen? _______________________________
____

4. What types of teaching should the nurse do? _______
____

REVIEW QUESTIONS

Choose the best answer unless directed otherwise.

1. Absorbing shock between adjacent vertebrae is the function of disks made of which of the following?
   a. Smooth muscle
   b. Synovial fluid
   c. Fibrous cartilage
   d. Adipose tissue

2. Which of the following is the transmitter at neuromuscular junctions?
   a. Sodium ions
   b. Acetylcholine
   c. A nerve impulse
   d. Cholinesterase

3. Muscles are attached to bones by which of the following?
   a. Tendons
   b. Ligaments
   c. Fascia
   d. Other muscles

4. Which of the following is the part of the brain that initiates muscle contraction?
   a. Parietal lobe
   b. Cerebellum
   c. Frontal lobe
   d. Temporal lobe

5. Which of the following organ systems is not considered directly necessary for muscle contraction?
   a. Circulatory system
   b. Digestive system
   c. Respiratory system
   d. Nervous system

6. The nurse is inspecting the knee of a patient who reports pain and stiffness in it. As the patient moves the knee the nurse hears a grating sound. The nurse documents the grating sound as which of the following?
   a. Friction rub
   b. Crepitation
   c. Effusion
   d. Subcutaneous emphysema

7. When the nurse observes a joint that has a grating sound with movement, which of the following actions should the nurse take next?
   a. Adduct the extremity.
   b. Flex the joint.
   c. Avoid joint movement.
   d. Abduct the extremity.

8. The nurse is gathering functional data on a patient with rheumatoid arthritis. Which of the following areas would the nurse include in the assessment?
   a. Response to treatment
   b. Ability to prepare food
   c. Appearance of joints
   d. Lung sounds

9. Following a patient's bone biopsy, the nurse inspects the biopsy site. The nurse is assessing for which of the following complications that may occur immediately following a biopsy?
   a. Joint dislocation
   b. Crackles
   c. Infection
   d. Hematoma formation

10. The nurse understands that increased pain that is unresponsive to analgesic medication in a patient who has had a biopsy may indicate which of the following biopsy complications?
    a. Bleeding in soft tissue
    b. A low pain tolerance
    c. An allergic reaction
    d. Inadequate analgesic dose

11. A patient, age 66, has rheumatoid arthritis. Which of the following symptoms would the nurse most likely be told was the first symptom that caused the patient to seek health care?
    a. Cold intolerance
    b. Stiff, sore joints
    c. Shortness of breath
    d. Crepitation

Multiple response item. Select all that apply.

12. The nurse is seeing a patient in preadmission testing who will have an arthroscopy of the knee. Which of the following would be included in nursing preoperative care for this patient?
    a. A soft breakfast
    b. No food after midnight
    c. Explaining the surgical procedure
    d. Explaining the anesthetic agents
    e. Explaining coughing and deep breathing exercises

Nursing Care of Patients with Musculoskeletal and Connective Tissue Disorders

46

VOCABULARY

Fill in the blank with the word that is formed by the word building.

1. _____________ arthro—joint + itis—inflammation
2. _____________ arthro—joint + plasty—creation of
3. _____________ synovia—synovial fluid or tissue + itis—inflammation
4. _____________ arthro—joint + centesis—puncture of a cavity
5. _____________ hyper—excessive + uric—uric acid + emia—in blood
6. _____________ sclero—hardening + derma—skin
7. _____________ vascul—blood vessel + itis—inflammation
8. _____________ poly—many + myo—muscle + itis—inflammation
9. _____________ a—without + vascular—blood + necrosis—death
10. _____________ re—again + plant—to plant + tion—process
11. _____________ hemi—half + pelv—pelvis + ectomy—removal of
12. _____________ fascia—fibrous tissue + otomy—opening into
13. _____________ osteo—bone + myel—bone marrow + itis—inflammation
14. _____________ osteo—bone + sarco—flesh + oma—tumor

FRACTURES

Match the type of fracture with its definition.

1. _______ More than two fragments that appear to float
2. _______ Fragment overrides the other fragment
3. _______ Splintered and bent, occurring mainly in children
4. _______ More than two fragments driven into each other
5. _______ Extends into articular surface
6. _______ Runs along axis of bone
7. _______ Oblique fracture line
8. _______ Spontaneous fracture from bone disease
9. _______ Fracture spirals around shaft of bone
10. _______ From repeated stress (jogging)
11. _______ At right angle to bone

A. Transverse
B. Stress
C. Spiral
D. Pathological
E. Oblique
F. Longitudinal
G. Interarticular
H. Impacted
I. Greenstick
J. Displaced
K. Comminuted

PROSTHESIS CARE EDUCATION

Indicate whether the statement is true or false, and correct false statements.

1. _______ Replace shoes when they wear out with new ones of a different height and type.

2. _______ Clean the prosthesis socket with alcohol and water, and dry it completely.

3. _______ Replace worn inserts and liners when they become too soiled to clean adequately.

4. _______ Use garters to keep socks or stockings in place.

5. _______ Oil the mechanical parts as instructed by the physician.

HEALTH PROMOTION FOR PATIENTS WITH GOUT

Fill in the blanks.

1. Avoid high _____________ foods, such as organ meats, shellfish, and oily fish such as _____________.

2. _____________ alcohol.

3. Drink plenty of _____________, especially water.

4. Avoid all forms of _____________ and drugs containing _____________.

5. _____________ diuretics.

6. Avoid excessive physical or emotional _____________.

CRITICAL THINKING

Complete the nursing diagnosis of impaired physical mobility for a patient with a hip replacement.

NURSING DIAGNOSIS
Impaired Physical Mobility Related to Hip Precautions and Surgical Pain

Interventions	Rationale	Evaluation
_____________ _____________ _____________	Activity is restricted due to hip precautions and weight-bearing limitations.	_____________ _____________ _____________
Place overhead frame and trapeze on bed; teach patient how to use it.	_____________ _____________	Does patient use overbed frame and trapeze for movement?
Assess the patient for and take measures to prevent complications of immobility: _____________ _____________ _____________ _____________ _____________	_____________ _____________	Does patient experience complications of immobility?

REVIEW QUESTIONS

Choose the best answer unless directed otherwise.

1. A patient is in skin traction using a foam boot with Velcro fasteners for a fractured hip. The nurse would document this type of skin traction as which of the following?
   a. Gardner's tongs
   b. Buck's traction
   c. Crutchfield's tongs
   d. Steinmann's pin

2. A patient sustains a closed fracture of the right tibia and is placed in a long-leg plaster cast, which is still damp. Which of the following methods should the nurse use to move the cast without causing complications?
   a. Have the patient move own leg.
   b. Palm the cast to move it.
   c. Use fingertips to grasp cast.
   d. Avoid moving the cast until it is dry.

Multiple response item. Select all that apply.

3. A patient is being treated with gold therapy for rheumatoid arthritis. Which of the following interventions is essential when gold therapy is started?
   a. Removing all metal objects patient is wearing
   b. Assessing allergies to iodine
   c. Giving a test dose of gold
   d. Planning a biweekly dosing schedule
   e. Monitoring the patient after the injection

4. Which of the following is the recommended protocol for caring for a severed body part that may be replanted?
   a. Cover it with a warm dry towel.
   b. Wrap it in a cool moist cloth.
   c. Place it on dry ice.
   d. Wrap it in a dry sterile dressing.

5. The nurse is caring for a patient who has a fractured ankle that is in a cast. The patient has morphine 10 to 15 mg intramuscularly ordered every 3 to 4 hours. The patient received morphine 10 mg 2 hours and 45 minutes ago and is rating the pain at 10+ and moans that leg hurts. The patient has good capillary refill. Which of the following actions is most appropriate for the nurse to take next?
   a. Apply ice to the cast.
   b. Notify the physician immediately.
   c. Remove the pillow under the cast.
   d. Prepare morphine 15 mg for administration.

6. The nurse turns a 2-day postoperative patient with a right total hip replacement using three pillows between the legs. The nurse later returns and finds the patient lying supine with legs crossed. Which of the following should the nurse assess to determine whether a complication has developed?
   a. The right knee for crepitation
   b. The left leg for internal rotation
   c. The left leg for loss of function
   d. The right leg for shortening

7. Discharge teaching for patients who have gout includes diet teaching. The patients will require additional teaching if they say they will be eating which one of the following?
   a. Cod
   b. Chicken
   c. Eggs
   d. Liver

8. Which of the following medications should a patient with gout be encouraged to avoid to prevent a gout attack?
   a. Aspirin
   b. Tylenol
   c. Nonsteroidal anti-inflammatory drugs
   d. Narcotics

9. The nurse is reviewing an erythrocyte sedimentation rate (ESR) for a patient. Which of the following does the nurse understand is the purpose of an ESR test?
   a. To identify the number of red blood cells the patient has
   b. To determine sedimentation found in red blood cells
   c. To identify the presence of systemic inflammation
   d. To diagnose various types of arthritis

10. Which of the following is a common nursing diagnosis that the nurse will include in the plan of care for a patient with lupus?
    a. Fatigue
    b. Impaired mobility
    c. Impaired swallowing
    d. Impaired tissue perfusion

11. A patient asks why he must receive a test dose of gold therapy. Which of the following is the most appropriate response by the nurse?
    a. To avoid waste of expensive gold
    b. To determine the necessary dose
    c. To determine the therapeutic response
    d. To assess for an allergic reaction

UNDERSTANDING THE NEUROLOGICAL SYSTEM

CHECKLIST FOR LEARNING SUCCESS

Review of Anatomy and Physiology

- ❏ Central nervous system (CNS)
  - ❏ Brain
  - ❏ Spinal cord
- ❏ Peripheral nervous system (PNS)
  - ❏ Cranial nerves
  - ❏ Spinal nerves
  - ❏ Sympathetic
  - ❏ Parasympathetic
- ❏ Aging changes

Major Disorders

- ❏ CNS infections
- ❏ Headaches
- ❏ Transient ischemic attack (TIA)
- ❏ Stroke
- ❏ Aneuryms
- ❏ Seizures
- ❏ Traumatic brain injury (TBI)
- ❏ Hematomas
- ❏ Brain tumors
- ❏ Herniated disk
- ❏ Spinal cord injury
- ❏ Parkinson's disease
- ❏ Alzheimer's disease
- ❏ Multiple sclerosis
- ❏ Myasthenia gravis
- ❏ Amyotrophic lateral sclerosis (ALS)
- ❏ Guillain-Barré
- ❏ Postpolio syndrome
- ❏ Cranial nerve disorders

Nursing Assessment

- ❏ Level of consciousness (LOC) (Glasgow coma scale)
- ❏ Pupils
- ❏ Muscle function
- ❏ Cranial nerves
- ❏ Intracranial pressure (ICP)

Diagnostic Tests

- ❏ Lumbar puncture
- ❏ Computed tomographic (CT) scan
- ❏ Magnetic resonance imaging (MRI)
- ❏ Angiogram
- ❏ Myelogram
- ❏ Electroencephalogram (EEG)

Interventions

- ❏ Positioning
- ❏ Nutrition
- ❏ Interventions for swallowing
- ❏ Activities of daily living (ADLs)
- ❏ Communication
- ❏ Rehabilitation
- ❏ Intacranial pressure (ICP) monitoring
- ❏ Intracranial surgery

Common Medications

- ❏ Anticoagulants
- ❏ Thrombolytics
- ❏ Corticosteroids
- ❏ Platelet aggregation inhibitors
- ❏ Diuretics
- ❏ Anticonvulsants

Neurological Function, Assessment, and Therapeutic Measures

VOCABULARY

Fill in the blank with the correct term.

1. Difficulty swallowing is called ____________.
2. An ____________ is a test that uses scalp electrodes to evaluate brain activity.
3. A patient might say his leg feels like it is asleep to describe a ____________.
4. Abnormal flexion posturing when eliciting best motor response is called ____________ posturing.
5. Abnormal extension posturing when eliciting best motor response is called ____________ posturing.
6. ____________ is the term that describes unequal pupils.
7. Involuntary eye movement is called ____________.
8. Permanent muscle contractions are called ____________.
9. Difficulty speaking because of muscle dysfunction is called ____________.
10. Patients who have difficulty speaking after a stroke are experiencing ____________.

DIAGNOSTIC TESTS

Describe the procedure and preprocedure and postprocedure care for each of the following diagnostic tests.

1. Myelogram ____

____

2. EEG ____

____

3. Lumbar puncture ____

____

4. MRI ____

____

5. CT scan ____

____

ANATOMY

Label the parts of the sensory and motor measures.

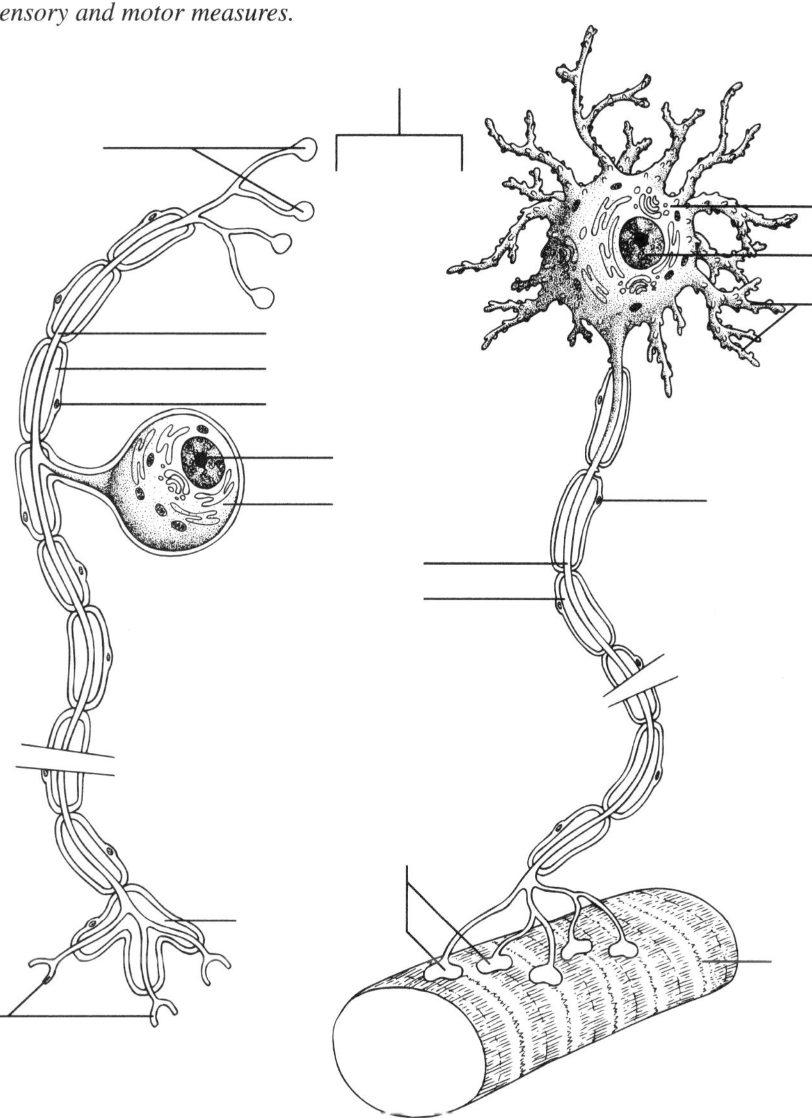

Label the parts of the brain.

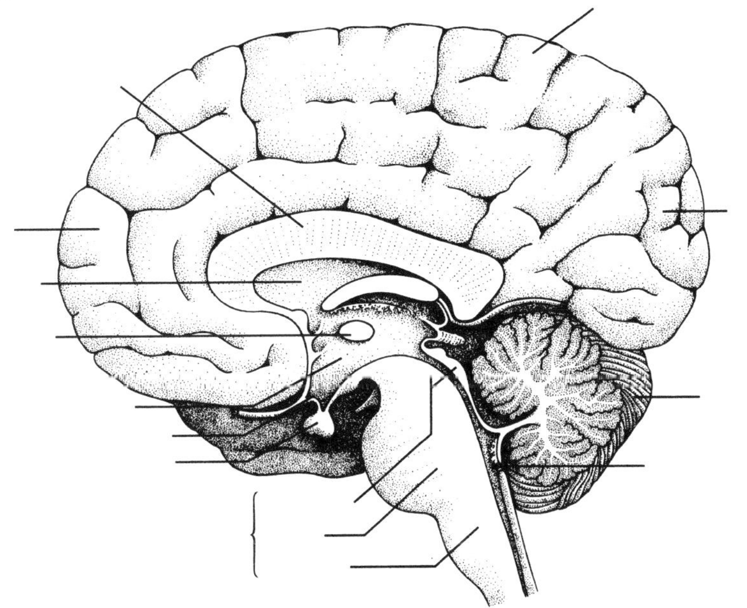

ANATOMY REVIEW

Match the part of the brain with the function it controls.

1. _______ Cerebrum
2. _______ Medulla oblongata
3. _______ Occipital lobe
4. _______ Cerebellum
5. _______ Temporal lobe

A. Vision center
B. Speech
C. Equilibrium and coordination
D. Respiratory center
E. Information storage

ASSESSMENT OF CRANIAL NERVES

Match the following assessment tools with the nerve to be tested.

1. _______ Cotton ball
2. _______ Snellen chart
3. _______ Use of hands to check neck/shoulder strength
4. _______ Tuning fork or whisper
5. _______ Tongue blade and cotton swab

A. Acoustic (VIII)
B. Spinal accessory (XI)
C. Trigeminal (V)
D. Optic (II)
E. Vagus (X)

CRITICAL THINKING

Read the case study and answer the following questions.

Mrs. Pickett is admitted to the nursing home where you work as a nurse. She had a stroke 2 weeks ago and is not strong enough to go to a rehabilitation facility. She has left-sided weakness. You collect admitting data to help determine her plan of care.

1. Mrs. Pickett tells you she needs to get up to go to the bathroom. What are some things you can do to determine if she is able to do this? ____
   ____
   ____

2. Mrs. Pickett's first meal is served. What do you do to assess her ability to eat safely? ____________
   ____
   ____

3. Mrs. Pickett says, "Will you go to the kitchen and get me one of those cookies I like?" How do you assess whether she is confused? ____
   ____
   ____

4. Mrs. Pickett is weak on her left side. Why do you think her blood pressure will be more accurate in her right arm? ____
   ____
   ____

REVIEW QUESTIONS

Choose the best answer.

1. Which of the following parts of a neuron transmits impulses away from the cell body?
   a. Dendrite
   b. Axon
   c. Neurolemma
   d. Synapse

2. Which type of neuron transmits impulses from the central nervous system to the muscles and glands?
   a. Afferent
   b. Efferent

3. Which part of the body is supplied by nerves from the thoracic cord?
   a. Head
   b. Trunk
   c. Pelvis
   d. Coccyx

4. Which part of the brain controls breathing?
   a. Medulla
   b. Cerebellum
   c. Cerebrum
   d. Thalamus

5. When a neurologist asks a patient to smile, which cranial nerve is being tested?
   a. II optic
   b. VII facial
   c. X vagus
   d. XI accessory

6. The neurologist tests the fourth (trochlear) and sixth (abducens) cranial nerves together by having a patient do which of the following?
   a. Turn his head to the right and left.
   b. Identify whispering in his ears.
   c. Say "ahhh."
   d. Follow his finger with his eyes.

7. Which of the following responses indicates sympathetic nervous system function?
   a. Tachycardia, dilated pupils
   b. Increased peristalsis, abdominal cramping
   c. Hypoglycemia, headache
   d. Pupil constriction, bronchoconstriction

8. Which neurotransmitter mediates the sympathetic response?
   a. Norepinephrine
   b. Acetylcholine
   c. Prostaglandin
   d. Serotonin

9. Which of the following nursing actions prepares a patient for a lumbar puncture?
   a. Administering enemas until clear
   b. Removing all metal jewelry
   c. Positioning the patient on his or her side
   d. Removing the patient's dentures

10. Which of the following nursing interventions is appropriate after a lumbar puncture?
    a. Have the patient lie flat for 6 to 8 hours.
    b. Keep the patient from eating or drinking for 4 hours.
    c. Monitor the patient's pedal pulses q4h.
    d. Keep the head of the bed elevated 30 degrees for 24 hours.

11. A patient is scheduled for an MRI and asks what to expect. Which of the following responses by the nurse is best?
    a. "It is the measurement of muscle contraction after stimulation by tiny needle electrodes."
    b. "Electrodes will be placed on your scalp to measure activity of the brain."
    c. "A scan of the brain will be done after injection of a radioisotope."
    d. "It is a noninvasive test that uses magnetic energy to visualize internal parts."

Nursing Care of Patients with Central Nervous System Disorders

VOCABULARY

Match the term with the correct definition.

1. _______ Contralateral hemiparesis
2. _______ Ipsilateral hemiplegia
3. _______ Quadriplegia
4. _______ Paraplegia
5. _______ Photophobia
6. _______ Bradykinesia
7. _______ Craniotomy
8. _______ Encephalitis
9. _______ Nuchal rigidity
10. _______ Prodromal

A. All four extremities paralyzed
B. Sensitive to light
C. Inflammation of the brain
D. Slow movement
E. Surgical opening in the skull
F. Paralyzed on same side
G. Paralyzed lower extremities
H. Neck pain and stiffness
I. Weak on opposite side
J. Warning sign

DRUGS USED FOR CENTRAL NERVOUS SYSTEM DISORDERS

Match the drug with its action.

1. _______ Mannitol
2. _______ Tacrine (Cognex)
3. _______ Carbamazepine (Tegretol)
4. _______ Dexamethasone (Decadron)
5. _______ Levodopa/carbidopa (Sinemet)

A. Anticonvulsant
B. Osmotic diuretic
C. Cholinesterase inhibitor
D. Converts to dopamine in the brain
E. Corticosteroid

ALZHEIMER'S DISEASE

Match the stage of disease with its primary symptom.

1. _______ Stage 1
2. _______ Stage 2
3. _______ Stage 3
4. _______ Stage 4

A. Terminal
B. Confused
C. Forgetful
D. Ambulatory dementia

CENTRAL NERVOUS SYSTEM DISORDERS

Match the signs and symptoms with the correct disorders.

1. _________ Unconscious at accident scene
2. _________ Polyuria and polydipsia following head injury
3. _________ Hypotension, loss of sympathetic function
4. _________ Nuchal rigidity
5. _________ High blood pressure, bradycardia, diaphoresis
6. _________ Brief period of staring
7. _________ Automatic repetitive movement such as picking or lip smacking
8. _________ Status epilepticus
9. _________ Rising weakness
10. _________ Numbness, weakness, spasticity

A. Spinal shock
B. Absence seizure
C. Multiple sclerosis
D. Guillain-Barré syndrome
E. Meningitis
F. Diabetes insipidus
G. Autonomic dysreflexia
H. Complex partial seizure
I. Epidural bleed
J. Continuous seizure

SPINAL DISORDERS

Determine whether each of the following symptoms is associated with lumbar spine or cervical spine dysfunction.

_________ Radiating pain to the ankle
_________ Deltoid weakness
_________ Diminished triceps reflex
_________ Footdrop
_________ Inability to walk on the toes

CRITICAL THINKING: SPINAL CORD INJURY

Mr. Granger is a 23-year-old admitted to your unit with a C5–C6 spinal cord injury following an auto accident. You collect the following data:

Subjective Data
Pain in cervical spine

Objective Data
No sensation or movement below the level of the injury
Blood pressure 80/60
Pulse 45
Respirations shallow
Temperature 97°F (36.1°C)

1. Explain Mr. Granger's hypotension, hypothermia, and bradycardia. ____

2. Why are Mr. Granger's respirations shallow? ____

3. Explain the purpose of each of the following therapies. How will they benefit Mr. Granger? _________

   Cervical traction: _________________________

   Vasopressor administration: _________________

   Insertion of a urinary catheter: _____________

4. Mr. Granger suddenly becomes anxious and dyspneic. He is using his accessory muscles with each breath. Explain what might be happening. _____________

5. What treatment would you expect for the dyspnea, and why will it be beneficial to Mr. Granger? _________

6. List two priority nursing diagnoses and goals for the acute stage of Mr. Granger's injury. _________

7. What are two health learning needs Mr. Granger faces in his acute stage? _________

REVIEW QUESTIONS

Choose the best answer.

1. A 90-year-old nursing home resident with stage 2 Alzheimer's disease is found alone and crying in the dining room. She says she lost her mother and doesn't know what to do. Which response by the nurse will help calm the resident?
   a. "Remember your mother has been dead for 30 years. You forgot again, didn't you?"
   b. "I'm sorry you lost your mother; let's go and try to find her."
   c. "Are you feeling frightened? I'm here and I will help you."
   d. "You are 90 years old. It is impossible for your mother to still be living. I know if you try, you can figure out what to do."

2. A patient asks the nurse what side effects to expect from a muscle relaxant medication that has been prescribed. Which of the following side effects should the nurse relate?
   a. Hypoglycemia
   b. Hypotension
   c. Drowsiness
   d. Dyspnea

3. A nurse caring for a patient with a herniated lumbar disk develops a plan of care for impaired mobility related to nerve compression. Which patient outcome indicates that the plan has been successful?
   a. The patient rates the pain at 3 to 4 on a 0 to 10 scale.
   b. The patient has full range of motion of the upper extremities.
   c. The patient demonstrates correct self-administration of analgesics.
   d. The patient is able to ambulate 25 feet without pain.

4. Which of the following problems during the immediate postoperative course following lumbar microdiskectomy should be reported to the physician immediately?
   a. Incisional pain
   b. Two-inch area of bleeding on dressing
   c. Inability to move affected leg
   d. Muscle spasm of affected leg

5. A patient with a brain tumor is admitted to the medical unit to begin radiation treatments. Which nursing action should take priority?
   a. Pad the patient's side rails.
   b. Assess the patient's pain level.
   c. Teach the patient what to expect during radiation treatments.
   d. Place the patient in isolation.

6. Which of the following settings is most therapeutic for an agitated head-injured patient?
   a. A day room with family visitors and a variety of caregivers
   b. A semiprivate room with one or two consistent caregivers
   c. A ward with other head-injured patients and volunteers to assist with needs
   d. A hallway near the nurse's station with adequate sensory stimulation

7. Decreasing level of consciousness is a symptom of which of the following physiological phenomena?
   a. Increased intracranial pressure (ICP)
   b. Sympathetic response
   c. Parasympathetic response
   d. Increased cerebral blood flow

8. Which of the following blood pressure changes alerts the nurse to increasing ICP, and should be reported immediately?
   a. Gradual increase
   b. Rapid drop followed by gradual increase
   c. Widening pulse pressure
   d. Rapid fluctuations

9. Which of the following nursing interventions will help prevent a further increase in ICP?
   a. Encourage fluids.
   b. Elevate the head of the bed.
   c. Provide physical therapy.
   d. Reposition the patient frequently.

10. Which nursing interventions can help prevent falls in a patient with Parkinson's disease? Choose all answers that are correct.
    a. Keep the patient's call light within reach.
    b. Apply a soft vest restraint when the patient is in bed.
    c. Avoid use of throw rugs.
    d. Maintain the patient's bed in a low position.
    e. Encourage the patient to be independent for as long as possible.
    f. Provide a cane or walker for ambulation.

Nursing Care of Patients with Cerebrovascular Disorders

VOCABULARY

Match the term with the correct definition.

1. _________ Thrombotic
2. _________ Aphasia
3. _________ Dysphagia
4. _________ Hemianopsia
5. _________ Flaccid

A. Difficulty swallowing
B. Caused by a clot
C. Inability to speak or understand language
D. Vision lost in half of visual field
E. Without muscle tone

DRUGS USED FOR CEREBROVASCULAR DISORDERS

Match the drug with its action.

1. _________ Heparin
2. _________ Clopidogrel (Plavix)
3. _________ Tissue plasminogen activator (tPA)
4. _________ Cyclandelate (Cyclospasmol)
5. _________ Simvastatin (Zocor)

A. Anticoagulant
B. Peripheral vasodilator
C. Antiplatelet
D. Thrombolytic
E. Cholesterol-lowering agent

CRITICAL THINKING: STROKE

Read the case study and answer the questions.

Mrs. Saunders is a 70-year-old retired secretary admitted to your unit from the emergency department with a diagnosis of stroke (cerebrovascular accident). She has a history of hypertension and atherosclerosis, and she had a carotid endarterectomy 6 years ago. She is 40% over her ideal body weight and has a 20-pack-year smoking history. Her daughter says her mother has been having short episodes of confusion and memory loss for the past few weeks. This morning she found her mother slumped to the right in her recliner, unable to speak.

1. Explain the pathophysiology of a cerebrovascular accident. Which type of stroke is most likely the cause of Mrs. Saunders' symptoms? _________________________ _________________________ _________________________

2. Mrs. Saunders is flaccid on her right side. What is the term used to describe this? _________________________ _________________________

3. Which hemisphere of Mrs. Saunders' brain is damaged? _________________________

4. List four risk factors for stroke evident in Mrs. Saunders' history. _________________________ _________________________ _________________________

5. Mrs. Saunders appears to understand when you speak to her but is only able to speak in garbled words. What is the term for this? ___________________

6. Neurological checks are ordered every 2 hours for 24 hours, then every 4 hours. When you enter her room and call her name, she opens her eyes. She is able to squeeze your hand with her left hand when you ask her to but is only able to make incomprehensible sounds. What is her score on the Glasgow Coma Scale? ___________ List seven symptoms of rising intracranial pressure (ICP) that you will watch for.

____

____

____

7. List two medications that the physician may order. Why might they be used? ___________________

____

____

8. Identify a nursing diagnosis related to Mrs. Saunders' right-sided paralysis. List three interventions to prevent complications. ___________________

____

____

9. How will you protect Mrs. Saunders' skin? List at least three interventions. ___________________

____

____

10. As you enter Mrs. Saunders' room on her third day on your unit, you find her agitated, trying to speak, and trying to get out of bed. List at least three ways to try to find out what she wants. ___________________

____

____

11. Before feeding Mrs. Saunders for the first time, what reflex do you check? How do you do this? ___________

____

____

12. Mrs. Saunders has some difficulty swallowing and pockets her food in her right cheek. List three interventions you can try. ___________________

____

____

13. Mrs. Saunders begins to move her right hand slightly and is able to say her daughter's name when she enters the room. She is prepared for discharge to a rehabilitation facility. List three ways you can prepare her family for her move and her eventual discharge home.

____

____

____

14. What class of drugs might be ordered for Mrs. Saunders to prevent another stroke? ___________________

____

____

REVIEW QUESTIONS

Choose the best answer.

1. A 46-year-old woman is admitted to the rehabilitation unit with left-sided hemiparesis resulting from a subarachnoid hemorrhage. She is not oriented to her surroundings or situation, but she does recognize her family. On admission, she tells her nurse that she can walk to the bathroom without assistance. Which of the following responses by the nurse is best?
   a. Allow her to ambulate unassisted, to encourage positive self-esteem.
   b. Ask her to demonstrate her ability to ambulate.
   c. Explain that someone will assist her as long as she is in the rehabilitation facility.
   d. Ask another staff member to help ambulate the patient the first time.

2. A patient who is recovering from a stroke becomes easily frustrated when unable to complete a task. Which of the following responses by the nurse will best help the patient get the task done?
   a. Perform the task for the patient.
   b. Tell the patient not to worry about it.
   c. Break the task down into simple steps.
   d. Have another patient demonstrate how to perform the task.

3. A nurse approaches a hospitalized poststroke patient from the patient's left side to do an assessment. The patient is staring straight ahead, and does not respond to the nurse's presence or voice. Which action should the nurse take first?
   a. Walk to the other side of the bed and try again.
   b. Speak more loudly and clearly.
   c. Wave his or her fingers in front of the patient's face.
   d. Use a picture board to explain to the patient what the nurse is going to do.

4. A 72-year-old man is admitted to a skilled care facility following a stroke. When the nursing assistant is bathing him, he makes a sexual remark and tries to touch her inappropriately. The assistant finishes the bath, then tells the LPN in charge, "I refuse to take care of that dirty old man!" Which response by the nurse is best?
   a. "The next time he tries to touch you inappropriately, lightly smack his hand and tell him no!"
   b. "His stroke has made him less inhibited. We'll see if we can find a male assistant to help him."
   c. "We have to take care of all patients equally, even the dirty old men."
   d. "He didn't mean anything by it; just ignore it."

5. A patient is having difficulty swallowing following a stroke, and a swallowing evaluation is ordered. Which nursing interventions might be recommended to help prevent aspiration during eating? Choose all answers that are correct.
   a. Place the patient in a semi-Fowler's position.
   b. Encourage the use of a straw for liquids.
   c. Provide clear liquids only until the patient can swallow solid foods.
   d. Have the patient swallow twice after each bite.
   e. Place food on the unaffected side of the patient's mouth.
   f. Check the patient's mouth for pocketing of food.

6. A patient is unable to control his bowels following a subarachnoid hemorrhage. Which intervention by the nurse can help reduce episodes of bowel incontinence?
   a. Ask the patient frequently if he has to have a bowel movement.
   b. Place incontinence pads on the patient's bed and chair.
   c. Toilet the patient according to his pre-illness schedule, whether or not he feels the urge.
   d. Take care not to embarrass the patient when incontinent episodes occur.

7. The nurse needs to administer aspirin 62 mg to a poststroke patient. It is supplied in 1-g tablets. How many tablets should the nurse prepare? ___________

8. A patient is hospitalized following a stroke. Three days after admission, the patient is able to converse clearly with the nurse during the morning assessment. Early in the afternoon, the patient's daughter runs out of the room and says, "My mother can't talk. Somebody help!" Which response by the nurse is best?
   a. Explain to the daughter that this is not uncommon, especially in the afternoon when the patient is tired from morning care activities.
   b. Do a quick assessment to confirm the change in the patient's status, then notify the RN or physician.
   c. Call the speech therapist to come and do a comprehensive speech assessment.
   d. Show the daughter how to do the speech exercises with her mother that were provided by the therapist.

50 Nursing Care of Patients with Peripheral Nervous System Disorders

VOCABULARY

Fill in the blanks with the correct terms.

1. Muscles that are not used become wasted, or ____________.
2. Some diseases are characterized by remissions and ____________.
3. Tic douloureux causes nerve pain, or ____________.
4. An early symptom of myasthenia gravis is drooping eyelids, also called ____________.
5. Symptoms of Guillain-Barré syndrome are caused by ____________ of axons.
6. Myasthenia gravis is sometimes treated with ____________, which separates blood cells from plasma to remove antibodies.
7. Muscle twitching, or ____________, occur in amyotrophic lateral sclerosis.
8. Medications for myasthenia gravis that can increase acetylcholine at the neuromuscular junction are called ____________ agents.

PERIPHERAL DISORDERS

Underline incorrect information in the following case studies. Write the correct information in the space provided.

1. Miss Mary Garvey sees her physician because she has been seeing double off and on for several weeks and has been fatigued. Her physician suspects myasthenia gravis and schedules her for a carotid ultrasound. He confirms his suspicions with a Tensilon test. He explains to Miss Garvey that she has a disease that is characterized by a decrease in the neurotransmitter norepinephrine. He begins her on Mastadon and prednisone. Her nurse teaches her the importance of getting regular exercise and recommends joining a local health and exercise club. ____

____

2. Mr. Tom Newby has a history of trigeminal neuralgia. He enters the emergency department with severe pain in his left wrist. The physician orders a narcotic analgesic because Mr. Newby's third cranial nerve is inflamed. Once the acute pain has subsided, Mr. Newby is discharged with instructions to get plenty of fresh air and to take his phenytoin (Dilantin) as ordered.

____

3. Mrs. Mattie Schultz is admitted with exacerbated multiple sclerosis. Her legs are becoming weaker, causing difficult walking, and she has been having difficulty swallowing. You know that build-up of myelin on her neurons is responsible for her weakness. You assess her for stressors that might have caused her exacerbation, such as a urinary tract infection (UTI) or upper respiratory tract infection (URI). Mrs. Schultz is started on thyroid-stimulating hormone (TSH) to stimulate her thyroid, which will help reduce her symptoms. She is also placed on trimethoprim/sulfamethoxazole (Bactrim) for the UTI you identified through your excellent assessment and on diazepam (Valium) for urinary retention.

____

CRITICAL THINKING

Read the case study and answer the following questions.

Reverend Wilson is a 50-year-old minister who sees his physician when he develops weakness in his arms and legs and has difficulty carrying out his job duties. He is diagnosed with amyotrophic lateral sclerosis (ALS).

1. Mrs. Wilson asks what ALS is. How do you describe it for her? ___________________________

2. Reverend Wilson returns to the physician's office several months after his initial diagnosis because he fell walking to the podium to preach. What is happening? What can he do about it? ___________________________

3. Reverend Wilson is concerned about continuing in his job and asks if his mind is going to be affected. How do you respond? ___________________________

4. He develops painful muscle spasms. What medications might be ordered to help relieve them? ___________

5. Reverend Wilson stabilizes for a while. A year later he is admitted to the hospital with aspiration pneumonia. What probably happened? What nursing diagnosis is appropriate in this situation? List an appropriate goal and two or three interventions. ___________

6. Reverend Wilson's condition deteriorates, and he has to retire. He becomes confined to a wheelchair. He has a gastrostomy tube inserted because he is no longer able to swallow. What additional nursing diagnoses are now appropriate? ___________________________
____

Choose the best answer.

1. A 32-year-old male patient is admitted to a medical unit with a diagnosis of Guillain-Barré syndrome. His legs are weak, and he is unable to walk without assistance. Which of the following is most likely responsible for this syndrome?
   a. Bacterial infection
   b. Heredity
   c. High-fat diet
   d. Autoimmune reaction

2. Patients with Guillain-Barré syndrome should be closely monitored. Which of the following parameters is most important to be checked regularly for acute complications?
   a. Blood urea nitrogen (BUN) and creatinine
   b. Arterial blood gases (ABG)
   c. Hemoglobin (Hgb) and hematocrit (Hct)
   d. Serum potassium

3. A woman sees her primary care provider because of extreme fatigue for the past 2 months; she has difficulty lifting even light objects. Her physician suspects myasthenia gravis. Which of the following tests should the nurse anticipate assisting with to confirm this diagnosis?
   a. Mestinon test
   b. Quinine tolerance test
   c. Pulmonary function studies
   d. Tensilon test

4. Which drug class is used to reduce symptoms of muscle weakness from myasthenia gravis?
   a. Anticholinesterase drugs
   b. Anticholinergic drugs
   c. Adrenergic drugs
   d. Beta-blocker drugs

5. A 39-year-old homemaker sees her physician after she falls twice for seemingly no reason. Diagnostic tests are done, and she is diagnosed with multiple sclerosis. Which of the following explanations will help her understand her disease?
   a. "You have a build-up of myelin in your nervous system, causing congestion and muscle weakness."
   b. "You are missing a neurotransmitter that is important to muscle contraction."
   c. "The receptor sites on your muscles are damaged, so they can't contract correctly."
   d. "The insulation on your nerve cells is damaged, which slows the impulses to the muscles."

6. Which of the following medications might be ordered to help control symptoms of multiple sclerosis, and possibly induce a remission?
   a. Acyclovir (Zovirax)
   b. Adrenocorticotropic hormone (ACTH)
   c. Thyrotropin
   d. Diphenhydramine (Benadryl)

7. Many neuromuscular disorders can impair respiratory function. What intervention can a home care nurse recommend to help prevent complications in patients with impaired respiratory function?
   a. Antibiotics as needed
   b. Elevate the head of the bed
   c. Bedrest
   d. Suction q4hr

8. Which of the following nursing interventions will help prevent complications in the patient with Bell's palsy?
   a. Megavitamin therapy
   b. Elastic bandages
   c. Application of ice to the affected area
   d. Lubricating eye drops

9. Which assessment action will help the nurse determine if the patient with Bell's palsy is receiving adequate nutrition?
   a. Monitor meal trays.
   b. Measure intake and output.
   c. Check twice-weekly weights.
   d. Assess swallowing reflex.

10. A nurse is preparing an intramuscular injection of prednisolone acetate, 30 mg. It is supplied as 50 mg/mL. How many milliliters should the nurse prepare? ________

11. The nurse notes frequent muscle twitching when collecting admission data on a patient admitted for increasing muscle weakness. Which of the following terms should the nurse use to document this?
    a. Fasciculations
    b. Atrophy
    c. Chorea
    d. Neuropathy

12. A 19-year-old student develops trigeminal neuralgia. Which of the following actions will most likely aggravate her pain?
    a. Sleeping
    b. Eating
    c. Reading
    d. Cooking

UNDERSTANDING THE SENSORY SYSTEM

CHECKLIST FOR LEARNING SUCCESS

Review of Sensory Anatomy and Physiology
- ❑ Eye structures
- ❑ Eye function
- ❑ Ear structures
- ❑ Ear function
- ❑ Aging effects

Major Sensory Disorders
- ❑ Vision
  - ❑ Eye infections/inflammation
  - ❑ Refractive errors
  - ❑ Blindness
  - ❑ Diabetic retinopathy
  - ❑ Retinal detachment
  - ❑ Glaucoma
  - ❑ Cataracts
  - ❑ Macular degeneration
- ❑ Hearing
  - ❑ Hearing loss
  - ❑ Infection
  - ❑ Otosclerosis
  - ❑ Ménière's disease

Nursing Assessment
- ❑ Medical history
- ❑ Psychosocial history
- ❑ Medications
- ❑ Physical assessment
- ❑ Vision:
  - ❑ Pupillary reflexes
  - ❑ Accommodation
  - ❑ Romberg's test
- ❑ Hearing:
  - ❑ Rinne test
  - ❑ Weber test

Diagnostic Tests
- ❑ Vision
  - ❑ Amsler grid
  - ❑ Angiography
  - ❑ GDx access
  - ❑ Intraocular pressure
  - ❑ Ophthalmoscopy
  - ❑ Slit lamp
  - ❑ Visual acuity
- ❑ Hearing
  - ❑ Audiometric
  - ❑ Caloric test
  - ❑ Otoscopic
  - ❑ Tympanometry

Interventions
- ❑ Corrective eyewear
- ❑ Trabeculoplasty
- ❑ Trabeculectomy
- ❑ Cyclocryotherapy
- ❑ Iridotomy/iridectomy
- ❑ Scleral buckling
- ❑ Supportive services
- ❑ Postoperative eye care
- ❑ Irrigation
- ❑ Hearing aids
- ❑ Myringotomy
- ❑ Stapedectomy
- ❑ Postoperative ear care

Common Medications
- ❑ Cycloplegics
- ❑ Cholinergics (miotics)
- ❑ Acetazolamide (Diamox)
- ❑ Timolol (Timoptic)
- ❑ Ceruminolytics

51 Sensory System Function, Assessment, and Therapeutic Measures: Vision and Hearing

STRUCTURES OF THE EYE

Label the following structures.

Anterior chamber
Aqueous humor
Canal of Schlemm
Choroid layer
Ciliary body
Conjunctiva
Cornea

Fovea
Inferior rectus muscle
Iris
Lens
Optic disc
Optic nerve
Posterior chamber

Pupil
Retina
Retinal artery and vein
Sclera
Superior rectus muscle
Suspensory ligaments
Vitreous humor

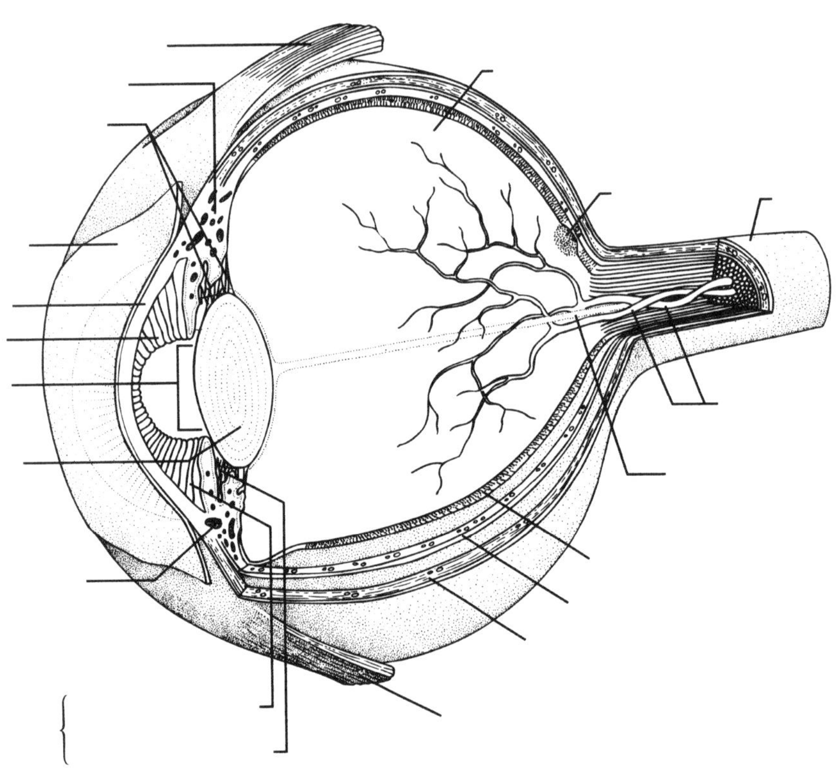

STRUCTURES OF THE EAR

Label the following structures.

Auricle
Cochlea
Ear canal
Eighth cranial nerve
Eustachian tube

Incus
Malleus
Semicircular canals
Stapes
Tympanic membrane (eardrum)

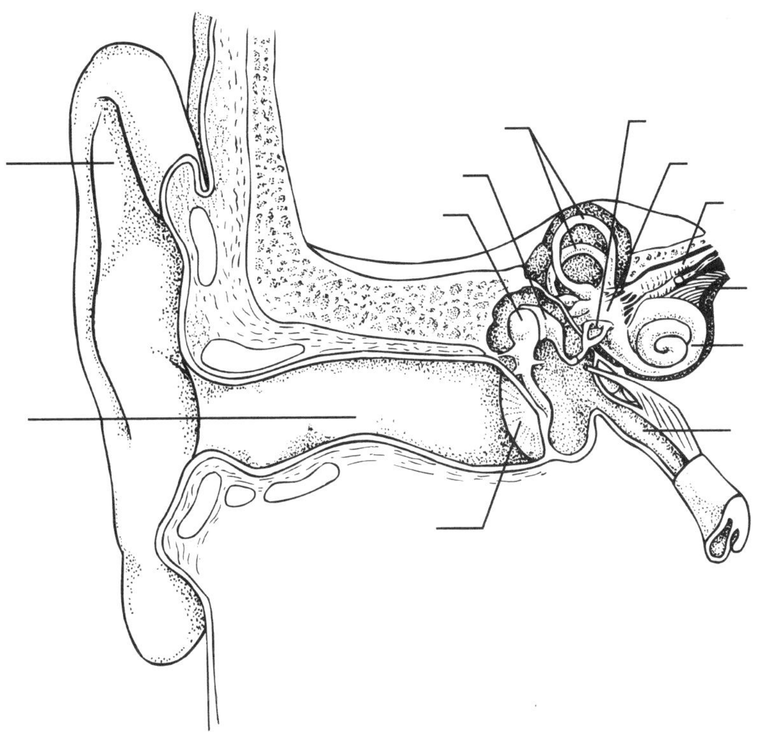

VISION

Number the following in the proper sequence as they are involved in the process of vision.

________ A. Cornea

________ B. Vitreous humor

________ C. Optic nerve

________ D. Aqueous humor

________ E. Occipital lobe

________ F. Lens

________ G. Retina

HEARING

Number the following in the order they function in the process of hearing when sound waves enter the ear canal.

________ A. Eardrum

________ B. Oval window

________ C. Incus

________ D. Eighth cranial nerve

________ E. Malleus

________ F. Stapes

________ G. Fluid in the cochlea

________ H. Hair cells in the organ of Corti

________ I. Temporal lobes

VOCABULARY

Define the following terms and use them in a sentence.

Nystagmus

Definition: ____

Sentence: ____

Tropia

Definition: ____

Sentence: ____

Accommodation

Definition: ____

Sentence: ____

Ptosis

Definition: ____

Sentence: ____

Arcus senilis

Definition: ____

Sentence: ____

Ophthalmologist

Definition: ____

Sentence: ____

Optometrist

Definition: ____

Sentence: ____

Optician

Definition: ____

Sentence: ____

DIAGNOSTIC TESTS

Fill in the table.

Assessment Test	Purpose of Test	Normal Test Results
___________	___________	OD 20/20, OS 20/20, OU 20/20
Visual fields	___________	___________
___________	Extraocular movement	___________
Accommodation	___________	Eyes turn inward and pupils constrict when focusing on a near object
___________	___________	Air conduction more than bone conduction
Weber	___________	___________
___________	Balance/vestibular function	___________
___________		___________

CRITICAL THINKING

Read the case study and answer the following questions.

Ms. Sally Little Thunder works on a computer as a data processor. She is complaining of recurring eye discomfort about 2 hours after she begins work each day.

1. What do you suspect is occurring with Ms. Little Thunder? ___________________________
   ____

2. For what environmental factors should the nurse assess? ______________________________
   ____

3. To protect Ms. Little Thunder from eyestrain, what safety measures should be implemented in her office? ____
   ____

REVIEW QUESTIONS

Choose the best answer unless directed otherwise.

1. Which of the following would the nurse explain to the patient is indicated by a Snellen chart finding of 20/80?
   a. The eye can see at 80 feet what the normal eye can see at 20 feet.
   b. The eye can see at 20 feet what the normal eye can see at 80 feet.
   c. The eye can see four times what the normal eye can see.
   d. The eye sees normally.

2. Which of the following would indicate that the patient has a normal corneal light reflex?
   a. The eye focuses the image in the center of the pupil.
   b. The eyes converge to focus on the light.
   c. Constriction of both pupils occurs in response to bright light.
   d. Light is reflected at the same spot in both eyes.

3. The examiner shines a light in the patient's eyes and notes that the pupils are round and constrict from 4 to 2 mm bilaterally. Next, the examiner asks the patient to focus on a far object, then on the examiner's finger as it is brought from 3 feet distance to 5 inches distance. The pupils constrict bilaterally and the eyes turn inward. Which of the following would be the correct documentation of these findings?
   a. Pupils 2 mm
   b. Pupils constricted
   c. Pupils equal, round, and reactive to light and accommodation (PERRLA)
   d. Pupils normal

4. When testing visual fields, the nurse is assessing which of the following parts of vision?
   a. Peripheral vision
   b. Near vision
   c. Distance vision
   d. Central vision

5. In planning safe care for the older adult, which of the following conditions does the nurse recognize would not cause visual problems?
   a. Glaucoma
   b. Cataracts
   c. Macular degeneration
   d. Arcus senilis

6. Which of the following statements does the nurse understand is true concerning air conduction of sound in the ear?
   a. It is caused by the vibration of bones in the skull.
   b. It is less efficient than bone conduction.
   c. It is heard longer than bone conduction.
   d. It is caused by transmission of heat through the air.

Multiple response item. Select all that apply.

7. Which of the following data collection findings could indicate to the nurse that the patient has a hearing loss?
   a. Patient converses easily with nurse.
   b. Patient answers questions appropriately.
   c. Patient's face is relaxed during conversation.
   d. Patient speaks in a very loud voice.
   e. Patient turns toward person speaking.
   f. Patient is withdrawn.

8. Which of the following statements would the nurse understand is true when assessing normal auditory acuity using the Rinne test?
   a. The patient perceives sound equally in both ears.
   b. Air conduction is heard longer than bone conduction in both ears.
   c. Bone conduction is heard longer than air conduction in both ears.
   d. The patient's left ear will perceive the sound better than the right ear.

9. Which of the following terms would indicate to the nurse that a substance is toxic to the ear?
   a. Otoplasty
   b. Otalgia
   c. Ototoxic
   d. Tinnitus

10. Which of the following subjective data questions would assist the nurse in assessing the patient's eye health?
    a. "Have you had any recent upper respiratory infections?"
    b. "Have you ridden in a car recently?"
    c. "Have you been scuba diving lately?"
    d. "Have you seen halos around lights?"

11. When assessing the external ear, the nurse palpates a small protrusion of the helix called a Darwin tubercle. The nurse would document this finding as which of the following?
    a. A normal finding
    b. An abnormal finding
    c. A normal finding only in the older adult
    d. An abnormal finding only in the older adult

12. Which of the following tests would the nurse use as an initial screening test to determine hearing loss?
    a. Romberg test
    b. Otoscopic examination
    c. Caloric test
    d. Whisper voice test

13. Which of the following would the nurse use to document a finding that the patient's ear is draining?
    a. Otorrhea
    b. Otalgia
    c. Ototoxic
    d. Tinnitus

14. Which of the following terms indicates that the patient has a hearing loss caused by aging?
    a. Otoplasty
    b. Otalgia
    c. Presbycusis
    d. Tinnitus

Nursing Care of Patients with Sensory Disorders: Vision and Hearing

VOCABULARY

Match the following terms with the appropriate definition.

1. _______ Carbuncle
2. _______ Cholesteatoma
3. _______ Mastoiditis
4. _______ Barotrauma
5. _______ Labyrinthitis
6. _______ Presbycusis

A. Hearing loss caused by aging
B. Inflammation or infection of the inner ear
C. Complication of otitis media
D. Epithelial cystlike sac filled with skin and sebaceous material
E. Several hair follicles forming an abscess
F. Pressure in the middle ear caused by atmospheric changes

ERRORS OF REFRACTION

Draw a picture showing the eye size and focal point differences in (a) hyperopia and (b) myopia.

PRESBYOPIA

Circle the seven errors in the following paragraph, and insert the correct information.

Presbyopia is a condition in which the lenses increase their elasticity resulting in a decrease in ability to focus on far objects. The loss of elasticity causes light rays to focus in front of the retina, resulting in hyperopia. This condition usually is associated with aging and generally occurs before age 40. Because accommodation for close vision is accomplished by lens contraction, people with presbyopia exhibit the ability to see objects at close range. They often compensate for blurred close vision by holding objects to be viewed closer. Complaints of eye strain and mild occipital headache are common.

VISUAL AND HEARING DATA COLLECTION

Describe how you would know that a patient has the following condition based on data collection (include diagnostic tests and examinations).

Macular degeneration (dry type) ___________________________

____

Cataract ____

____

Hordeolum ____

____

Acute angle-closure glaucoma ____________________________

____

External otitis _______________________________________

____

Impacted cerumen ____________________________________

____

Otitis media ____

____

Otosclerosis ____

____

GLAUCOMA

Circle the seven errors in the following paragraph, and insert the correct information.

Glaucoma is characterized by abnormal pressure outside the eyeball. This pressure causes damage to the cells of the acoustic nerve, the structure responsible for transmitting visual information from the ear to the brain. The damage is evident, progressive, and reversible until the end stages when initially loss of central vision occurs, and then eventually blindness. Once glaucoma occurs, the patient can be cured.

CONDUCTIVE HEARING LOSS

Circle the six errors in the following paragraph, and insert the correct information.

Conductive hearing loss is interference with conduction of light waves through the external auditory canal, the eardrum, or the middle ear. The inner ear is involved in a pure conductive hearing loss. Conductive hearing loss is a neural problem. Causes of conductive hearing loss include cerumen, foreign bodies, infection, perforation of the tympanic membrane, trauma, fluid in the middle ear, cysts, tumor, and otosclerosis. Many causes of conductive hearing loss, such as infection, foreign bodies, or impacted cerumen, cannot be corrected. Hearing devices may not improve hearing for conditions that cannot be corrected. Hearing devices are most effective with conductive hearing loss when inner ear and nerve damage are present.

OTOSCLEROSIS

Circle the nine errors in the following paragraph, and insert the correct information.

Otosclerosis results from the formation of new bone along the incus. With new bone growth, the incus becomes mobile and causes conductive hearing loss. Hearing loss is most apparent after the sixth decade. Otosclerosis usually occurs less often in women than in men. The disease usually affects one ear. It is thought to be a hereditary disease. The primary symptom of otosclerosis is rapid hearing loss. The patient usually experiences bilateral conductive hearing loss, particularly with soft, high tones. Otoectomy is the treatment of choice.

CRITICAL THINKING

Read the case study and answer the following questions.

Mr. Nyugen, age 70, reports that he has difficulty seeing at night, so much so that he has given up driving. When questioned further, he also states, "I used to be an avid reader, but I guess I'm getting too old to read, the words aren't very clear." The nurse examines his eye and finds that he is sensitive to light, has opacity of both lenses, and denies any pain.

1. What do you suspect is occurring with Mr. Nyugen?

____

____

2. For which diagnostic tests should you prepare Mr. Nyugen? _______________________________________

____

3. After the physician has made a definitive diagnosis, Mr. Nyugen asks you to explain the surgical procedure and recovery regimen to him. Outline your teaching plan.

____

____

____

REVIEW QUESTIONS

Choose the best answer unless directed otherwise.

Multiple response item. Select all that apply.

1. Which of the following would be a symptom the nurse would expect to find during assessment of a patient with macular degeneration?
   a. Decreased ability to distinguish colors
   b. Sudden loss of vision
   c. Loss of near vision
   d. Loss of central vision
   e. Loss of peripheral vision

2. Which of the following type of eyedrops does the nurse understand is given to constrict the pupil, permitting aqueous humor to flow around the lens?
   a. Osmotic
   b. Myotic
   c. Mydriatic
   d. Cycloplegic

3. Which of the following safety instructions should the nurse give a patient who has temporarily dilated pupils?
   a. Keep eyes closed.
   b. Do not drive for 8 hours.
   c. Wear sunglasses.
   d. Avoid caffeinated beverages.

4. Which of the following procedures does the nurse understand is used to correct otosclerosis?
   a. Myringotomy
   b. Myringoplasty
   c. Mastoidectomy
   d. Stapedectomy

5. The nurse understands that labyrinthitis is treated primarily with which of the following drug categories?
   a. Antihistamines
   b. Antispasmotics
   c. Anti-inflammatories
   d. Antiemetics

6. Which of the following types of hearing loss does the nurse understand is most improved with the use of a hearing aid?
   a. Conductive
   b. Sensorineural
   c. Mixed
   d. Central

7. Which of the following would the nurse explain to a patient is the main purpose of a hearing aid?
   a. Amplify background noise
   b. Occlude the ear
   c. Amplify musical sounds
   d. Improve ability to hear

8. Which of the following would the nurse explain to the patient is the triad of symptoms associated with Ménière's disease?
   a. Hearing loss, vertigo, and tinnitis
   b. Nystagmus, headache, and vomiting
   c. Nausea, vomiting, and pain
   d. Nystagmus, vomiting, and pain

9. Which of the following actions would the nurse include in the plan of care to reduce the symptoms of the patient who has vertigo?
   a. Avoid noises.
   b. Avoid sudden movements.
   c. Encourage fluid intake.
   d. Administer analgesics.

10. A patient is diagnosed with acute bacterial conjunctivitis. In providing patient teaching the nurse would tell the patient that this condition is more commonly known as which of the following?
    a. Glaucoma
    b. Astigmatism
    c. Color blindness
    d. Pinkeye

11. Which of the following is usually the first symptom of a cataract that the nurse would expect a patient to report during assessment?
    a. Dry eyes
    b. Eye pain
    c. Blurring of vision
    d. Loss of peripheral vision

12. Which of the following would the nurse teach the patient is the most common site for ear infections?
    a. Outer ear
    b. Inner ear
    c. Middle ear
    d. Semicircular canal

13. Which of the following nursing interventions would have the highest priority in the plan of care for the postoperative eye patient?
    a. Do not leave the patient unattended at any time.
    b. Teach the patient not to bend over.
    c. Report sudden onset of acute pain.
    d. Apply sandbags to either side of the head.

14. Which of the following descriptions by the nurse would best explain glaucoma to a patient?
    a. "There is an increase in the amount of vitreous humor."
    b. "There is an increase in the intraocular pressure."
    c. "There is a decrease in the amount of aqueous humor."
    d. "There is a decrease in the intraocular pressure."

15. Which of the following is a symptom that the nurse would expect to find during assessment of a patient experiencing acute angle-closure glaucoma?
    a. Flashing lights
    b. Lens opacity
    c. Halos around lights
    d. Vertigo

16. Which of the following activities would the nurse teach a patient to avoid so that intraocular pressure is not increased after eye surgery?
    a. Sitting upright in bed
    b. Coughing
    c. Chewing food vigorously
    d. Reading a book

UNDERSTANDING THE INTEGUMENTARY SYSTEM

CHECKLIST FOR LEARNING SUCCESS

Review of Anatomy and Physiology	Major Disorders	Nursing Assessment	Diagnostic Tests	Interventions	Common Medications
❑ Epidermis	❑ Pressure ulcers	❑ History	❑ Cultures	❑ Dressings	❑ Antibiotics
❑ Dermis	❑ Dermatitis	❑ Color	❑ Biopsy	❑ Balneotherapy	❑ Antivirals
❑ Appendages	❑ Herpes simplex	❑ Lesions	❑ Wood's light	❑ Topical medications	❑ Corticosteroids
❑ Subcutaneous tissue	❑ Herpes zoster	❑ Moisture	❑ Skin tests	❑ Plastic surgery	❑ Analgesics
❑ Aging changes	❑ Fungal infections	❑ Edema			❑ Chemotherapy
	❑ Cellulitis	❑ Vascular markings			
	❑ Acne	❑ Integrity			
	❑ Parasites	❑ Cleanliness			
	❑ Pemphigus				
	❑ Malignant lesions				
	❑ Burns				

53 Integumentary Function, Assessment, and Therapeutic Measures

INTEGUMENTARY STRUCTURES

Match each integumentary structure with its proper description.

1. _______ Epidermis
2. _______ Dermis
3. _______ Subcutaneous tissue
4. _______ Collagen fibers
5. _______ Eccrine glands
6. _______ Receptors
7. _______ Melanin
8. _______ Stratum corneum
9. _______ Stratum germinativum

A. If unbroken, prevents entry of pathogens
B. Give strength to the dermis
C. Detect changes in the external environment
D. Contains the accessory structures of the skin, such as glands
E. Made of both living and nonliving cells
F. Mitosis takes place to produce new epidermis
G. Stores fat
H. Acts as a barrier to ultraviolet light
I. Stimulated by exercise or heat

VOCABULARY

Match the word with its definition.

1. _______ Absence or loss of hair
2. _______ Blue-black bruise, changing to greenish-brown or yellow with time
3. _______ Diffuse redness over the skin
4. _______ Small, purplish, hemorrhagic spots on the skin
5. _______ Measure of skin elasticity

A. Ecchymosis
B. Erythema
C. Petechiae
D. Turgor
E. Alopecia

PRIMARY SKIN LESIONS

Match the lesion with its description.

1. _______ Macule
2. _______ Papule
3. _______ Vesicle
4. _______ Bulla
5. _______ Pustule
6. _______ Wheal
7. _______ Plaque
8. _______ Cyst

A. Vesicle or blister larger than 1 cm
B. Flat, nonpalpable change in skin color
C. Round, transient elevation of the skin caused by dermal edema and surrounding capillary dilation
D. Patch or solid, raised lesion on the skin or mucous membrane that is greater than 1 cm
E. Palpable solid raised lesion
F. Small elevation of skin or vesicle or bulla that contains pus
G. Closed sac or pouch tumor that consists of semisolid, solid, or liquid material
H. Small raised area that contains serous fluid, less than 0.5 cm

DIAGNOSTIC SKIN TESTS

Match the test with its definition.

1. _________ Skin biopsy
2. _________ Wood's light examination
3. _________ Scratch test
4. _________ Patch test

A. Superficial testing with allergen for immediate reaction
B. Excision of small piece of tissue for microscopic assessment
C. Superficial testing with allergen for delayed hypersensitivity reaction
D. Use of ultraviolet rays to detect fluorescent materials in skin and hair

CRITICAL THINKING

Read the case study and answer the questions.

Mr. Carr is admitted to a medical unit after having a hemorrhagic stroke. His vital signs are stable, but he is disoriented except to person. He is on bedrest and is often restless. He responds appropriately to questions intermittently. His left side is flaccid, but he can move his right side. The nurse notes that Mr. Carr rarely moves himself into a different position. He is of thin build. He is receiving 5% dextrose/0.9% normal saline intravenously. He has difficulty swallowing and has not eaten. Mr. Carr is diaphoretic and his gown is damp.

1. Why is Mr. Carr at high risk for developing pressure ulcers? _________________________________
____
____

2. How many calories is Mr. Carr receiving? ____
____
____

3. What are priority nursing diagnoses and nursing interventions for Mr. Carr related to his skin needs?
____
____
____

REVIEW QUESTIONS

Choose the best answer.

1. How do arterioles in the dermis respond to a cold environment?
   a. Dilate to release heat
   b. Constrict to release heat
   c. Dilate to conserve heat
   d. Constrict to conserve heat

2. Which of the following tissues stores fat in subcutaneous tissue?
   a. Fibrous connective tissue
   b. Stratified squamous epithelium
   c. Adipose tissue
   d. Areolar connective tissue

3. Which substances are formed when the ultraviolet rays of the sun strike the skin?
   a. Vitamin A and keratin
   b. Melanin and vitamin D
   c. Sebum and vitamin A
   d. Keratin and melanin

4. Which layer of skin, if unbroken, prevents the entry of most pathogens?
   a. Stratum corneum
   b. Papillary layer
   c. Stratum germinativum
   d. Dermis

5. White blood cells, which destroy pathogens that enter breaks in the skin, are found in which of the following structures?
   a. Stratum corneum
   b. Keratinized layer
   c. Subcutaneous tissue
   d. Adipose cells

6. In which of the following developmental age-groups would less elasticity and moisture of the skin be a normal finding?
   a. Adolescent
   b. Young adult
   c. Middle-aged adult
   d. Elderly adult

7. Which of the following terms is used to document a bluish discoloration of the skin?
   a. Cyanosis
   b. Erythema
   c. Jaundice
   d. Pallor

8. The nurse understands that an elderly person may be more sensitive to cold temperatures due to which of the following changes?
   a. Slower cell division in the epidermis
   b. Deterioration of collagen and elastin fibers
   c. Less fat in the subcutaneous layer
   d. Death of melanocytes in the skin

9. The nurse is caring for a patient with a skin tear. Which of the following dressing types is most appropriate for the nurse to apply to a skin tear?
   a. Moist sterile gauze
   b. Hydrocolloid
   c. Paste
   d. Transparent dressing

10. Which of the following actions should the nurse take when new petechiae are observed on the patient's skin?
    a. Cleanse the skin.
    b. Apply cool compresses.
    c. Inform the registered nurse or physician.
    d. Apply heat to the area.

Nursing Care of Patients with Skin Disorders

VOCABULARY

Match the word with its definition.

1. ________ To lose color		A. Seborrhea
2. ________ Inflammation of cellular or connective tissue		B. Pyoderma
3. ________ Skin lesion that occurs in acne vulgaris		C. Purulent
4. ________ Inflammation of the skin		D. Psoriasis
5. ________ A fungal infection of the skin		E. Pruritus
6. ________ The growth of skin over a wound		F. Pemphigus
7. ________ Thickened or hardened from continued irritation		G. Pediculosis
8. ________ Disease of the nails due to fungus		H. Onychomycosis
9. ________ Infestation with lice		I. Lichenified
10. ________ Acute or chronic serious skin disease characterized by bullae on skin and mucous membranes		J. Epithelialization
11. ________ Severe itching		K. Dermatophytosis
12. ________ Chronic inflammatory skin disorder in which epidermal cells proliferate abnormally quickly		L. Dermatitis
13. ________ Describes fluid that contains pus		M. Comedo
14. ________ Any acute, inflammatory, purulent bacterial dermatitis		N. Cellulitis
15. ________ Disease of the sebaceous glands marked by increase in the amount, and often alteration of the quality, of sebaceous secretion		O. Blanch

BENIGN SKIN LESIONS

Match the lesion with its definition.

1. ________ Cyst		A. Small, common growths caused by a virus
2. ________ Seborrheic keratosis		B. Vascular tumors of dilated blood vessels
3. ________ Keloid		C. Saclike growth with a definite wall
4. ________ Pigmented nevi		D. Scar formation at site of trauma or surgical incision
5. ________ Warts		E. Light brown to dark brown patches, plaques, or papules that occur mainly in older patients
6. ________ Hemangiomas		F. Flesh colored to dark brown macule or papule

PLASTIC SURGERY PROCEDURES

Fill in the blanks.

1. A ______________ is done to correct nasal septal defects.

2. A ______ ______ is referred to as a rhytidoplasty.

3. Removal of bags under the eyes is known as ______________ .

CRITICAL THINKING

Read the case study and answer the questions.

Mrs. Miller, age 59, is admitted for a femoral-popliteal bypass graft. She has type 2 diabetes mellitus. After surgery, she is in the intensive care unit (ICU) and is hypotensive for 24 hours. Her operative leg is painful and she barely moves. During her bath, the nurse notes a dark red-black area 4 inches in diameter and 2 inches deep on her sacral area and a reddened oozing area on the heel of her right foot.

1. Why did these dark red-black and red areas develop?

   ____

   ____

2. To plan Mrs. Miller's care, what stage are these discolored areas? ______________________

   The surgeon is notified of these areas and orders turning every 2 hours, elevation of the right foot, and a sheepskin pad.

3. What is the benefit and effectiveness of each of these ordered interventions? ______________

   ____

4. Why should the nurse discuss the use of the sheepskin with the surgeon? ______________

   ____

Choose the best answer.

1. Which of the following activities creates a mechanical force that can lead to the formation of a pressure ulcer?
   a. Massaging nonreddened areas
   b. Whirlpool baths
   c. Pulling a patient up in bed
   d. Range-of-motion exercises

2. A nurse is caring for a nursing home resident with a red, pruritic skin rash. The patient is confused and scratches the rash, which results in broken skin. Which interventions will help the rash heal? Select all answers that apply.
   a. Pat the skin dry after bathing.
   b. Leave topical agent as ordered at the bedside so the patient can apply when itching is severe.
   c. Place a transparent dressing on the rash to prevent scratching.
   d. Place gloves or mits on the patient.
   e. Keep the patient's fingernails short.

3. Which of the following dressings should a nurse choose for a deep pressure ulcer that has purulent drainage?
   a. Sterile gauze
   b. Transparent film (Opsite)
   c. Hydrocolloid (DuoDERM)
   d. Occlusive

4. A patient has a wound with moderate blood-tinged fluid draining from it. Which of the following would be an appropriate description of this drainage for the nurse to document?
   a. Purulent drainage
   b. Serosanguineous drainage
   c. Copious drainage
   d. Serous drainage

5. Which of the following cleansing methods is most appropriate for the nurse to use on a noninfected pressure ulcer?
   a. 45 psi pressure flushing
   b. Gentle flushing with a needleless 30-mL syringe.
   c. Gentle scrubbing with gauze and normal saline
   d. Flushing with a 30-mL syringe with an 18-gauge needle

6. A 62-year-old woman is admitted to the hospital with a lesion on her face that is a small, pearly papule. It has a rolled, waxy edge with crusting and ulceration. Which action by the nurse is best?
   a. Notify the physician.
   b. Clean the lesion.
   c. Place a gauze dressing on the lesion.
   d. Place an occlusive dressing on the lesion.

7. Place the wounds in correct order from stage I to stage IV.
   a. Skin appears abraded
   b. Skin red, intact
   c. Full-thickiness skin loss, muscle and bone showing
   d. Full-thickness skin loss, no muscle or bone involvement

8. A 92-year-old woman is admitted from a nursing home to the hospital for a colon resection. Four days postoperatively she reports that her perineum is sore. It is reddened and has whitish discharge. She has been on three intravenous antibiotics. Which of the following problems does the nurse suspect?
   a. Monilial intertrigo
   b. Psoriasis
   c. Herpes zoster
   d. Contact dermatitis

55 Nursing Care of Patients with Burns

VOCABULARY

Match the word with its definition.

1. _________ Leathery skin, usually painless
2. _________ Pink to red moist skin, blisters may be present
3. _________ The growth of skin over a wound
4. _________ Removal of a slough or scab formed on skin and underlying tissue of severely burned skin
5. _________ Epidermis and dermis involved, pain from exposed nerve endings
6. _________ Hard scab or dry crust from necrotic tissue

A. Escharotomy
B. Eschar
C. Epithelialization
D. Superficial burn
E. Partial-thickness deep burn
F. Full-thickness burn

CRITICAL THINKING

Read the case study and answer the questions.

Mr. Patel is a 45-year-old patient in County General Hospital's Burn Unit. He was admitted with a 20% electrical burn over his right arm, right shoulder, right leg, and right foot. The entry wound is on his right shoulder and the exit wound is on his right foot. When you check on him at the beginning of your shift, you find his right radial pulse is diminished and his right forearm has a small spot that is beginning to change color to a whitish gray.

1. What might be causing his change in circulation? ____

2. What additional data should you collect? ____

3. What interventions are important right away? ____

Choose the best answer.

1. The nurse finds the skin on the arms of a burn patient to be white and hard. It is inelastic and insensitive to pressure. Which of the following does the nurse understand this burn would be classified as?
   a. Superficial
   b. Superficial partial thickness
   c. Deep partial thickness
   d. Full thickness

2. A patient with full-thickness burns has surgery for skin grafting. One day postoperatively, the area around the graft is red and warm, and there is a foul smell under the dressing. Which of the following actions would be most appropriate by the nurse?
   a. Remove the dressing.
   b. Apply an occlusive dressing.
   c. Apply an antibiotic ointment dressing.
   d. Notify the registered nurse and physician.

3. During morning report, a nurse learns she will be caring for a patient who is in stage III burn care. What care can the nurse anticipate providing during the shift?
   a. Dressing changes
   b. Debridement
   c. Pain management
   d. Exercises

4. A patient is brought to the emergency department with burns over 40% of his body from a fire in his apartment. Which assessment should take priority?
   a. Burn depth
   b. Percent of body surface burned
   c. Respiratory status
   d. Circulatory status

5. A home care nurse visits an 82-year-old man. On entering his home, the nurse finds that he has just dropped a pot of boiling water on his legs. What action should the nurse take first?
   a. Call 911.
   b. Remove the man's trousers.
   c. Pour cold water over the affected area.
   d. Assess the extent of the burn.

6. A patient has a burn encircling her left thigh from a motorcycle accident. When the nurse enters her room during rounds, the patient appears very anxious and says her left foot feels funny. What should the nurse do first?
   a. Check circulatory status in her foot and report changes.
   b. Explain that some numbness and tingling in the affected extremity is normal following a burn.
   c. Check the burn dressing for an increase in drainage.
   d. Assess for the cause of the patient's anxiety.

7. A homebound patient is receiving IV antibiotics for an infected burn site. Instructions are to use gravity to infuse 100 mL over 1 hour. How many drops per minute should the nurse administer if the tubing has a drip factor of 15? _________

unit SIXTEEN

UNDERSTANDING MENTAL HEALTH CARE

CHECKLIST FOR LEARNING SUCCESS

Review of Basic Concepts
- ❑ Mental health
- ❑ Mental illness
- ❑ Nature vs nurture
- ❑ Psychoanalytic theory
- ❑ Psychobiological theory
- ❑ Coping

Major Disorders
- ❑ Anxiety disorders
- ❑ Mood disorders
- ❑ Somatoform disorders
- ❑ Schizophrenia
- ❑ Substance abuse disorders

Nursing Assessment
- ❑ Appearance and behavior
- ❑ Awareness and orientation
- ❑ Thinking
- ❑ Memory
- ❑ Speech
- ❑ Mood and affect
- ❑ Judgment
- ❑ Perception

Diagnostic Tests
- ❑ DSM-IV
- ❑ Blood tests
- ❑ Computed tomographic (CT) scan
- ❑ Positron emission therapy (PET) scan

Interventions
- ❑ Therapeutic communication
- ❑ Milieu therapy
- ❑ Psychoanalysis
- ❑ Behavior management
- ❑ Cognitive therapies
- ❑ Person-centered therapy
- ❑ Counseling
- ❑ Group therapy
- ❑ Electroconvulsive therapy (ECT)
- ❑ Relaxation therapy

Common Medications
- ❑ Antipsychotics
- ❑ Antianxiety agents
- ❑ Antidepressants
- ❑ Stimulants
- ❑ Antiparkinsonism agents

56 Mental Health Function, Assessment, and Therapeutic Measures

VOCABULARY

Fill in the blanks with the correct terms.

1. _____________ is the way one adapts to a stressor.
2. The ability to think rationally and process thoughts is referred to as _____________ ability.
3. _____________ is the use of medication to treat psychological disorders.
4. _____________ _____________ uses electric shocks to stimulate neurotransmitters in severely depressed patients.
5. A therapeutic _____________ is a structured environment that aids in treatment of mental health disorders.
6. Psychoanalytic therapy can help clarify the meaning, and therefore help the patient gain _____________ into an event or feeling.
7. _____________ is assessed by asking a patient questions such as, "Where are you now?" and "What year is it?"
8. The outward expression of feelings is called _____________.

DEFENSE MECHANISMS

Name the defense mechanism being used in each of the following statements.

1. A patient with cancer says, "I know if I take my vitamins I'll be fine." _____________

2. A student comes unprepared to class and says, "I woke up late because my instructor gave us too much work to do and I had to stay up all night, and my kids are sick and the car isn't working." _____________

3. A man who always wanted to be a lawyer but was not accepted into law school says, "Lawyers are all crooked. I would never trust one." _____________

4. A teen who didn't make the football team says, "I've decided to give up trying to play in sports. I'm much better at piano." _____________

5. A woman who was raped says, "Why are you calling me to set up rape counseling? I was not raped and I do not need counseling." _____________

6. A man who is passed over for a promotion yells at his son for a minor mistake, "You messed up again. You never do anything right." _____________

7. An adolescent says to his mother, "I got a B on my project because you told me to do it all wrong." _____________

8. The woman who cheated on an examination turns in extra work and states, "Here is some extra work I did. I really want to learn this material." _______________

9. A teen tells her date, "I'm sorry I can't go out tonight; I have to wash my hair." _______________

10. The student nurse tells the instructor, "I don't think I can do that catheter. I am feeling sick to my stomach. I think I ate some bad food in the cafeteria." _______________

CRITICAL THINKING

Read the case study and answer the following questions.

Mrs. Jewel is a 48-year-old woman admitted to your unit with cellulitis of her lower legs and diabetes mellitus. She is disabled because of arthritis and morbid obesity. As you collect some initial data, you notice that her hair is dirty and unkempt, her clothes are dirty, and she has an unpleasant body odor. You also find that she does not appear to have a good understanding of her health or self-care needs. You decide to assess her mental status.

1. What factors related to Mrs. Jewel's appearance provide information about her mental status? How can you find out if this is unusual behavior for her? _______________

2. Mrs. Jewel is alert. What questions can you ask to assess orientation? _______________

3. How might you determine whether Mrs. Jewel's thought processes are intact? _______________

4. What questions can you ask to assess Mrs. Jewel's recent and remote memory? _______________

5. How do you assess speech and ability to communicate? _______________

6. You determine that Mrs. Jewel's affect is inappropriate. What does this mean? _______________

7. How can you assess Mrs. Jewel's judgment? _______________

8. How can perception be assessed? _______________

REVIEW QUESTIONS

REVIEW QUESTIONS

Choose the best answer.

1. Which behavior in a patient with a chronic physical illness alerts the nurse to possible mental health concerns?
   a. He prays for healing from his illness.
   b. He reads self-help books to gain insight into his problems.
   c. He has developed ways to cope with his chronic illness.
   d. He does not have any close friends.

2. Which defense mechanism is being used by the person who always seems to blame others for his problems?
   a. Denial
   b. Projection
   c. Rationalization
   d. Transference

3. Which of the following nursing actions is necessary for therapeutic interventions to be effective?
   a. Encourage the patient to repress negative feelings.
   b. Punish inappropriate behavior.
   c. Establish a therapeutic nurse-patient relationship.
   d. Give the patient ideas for to how to solve a problem.

4. Which of the following nursing actions is appropriate immediately following electroconvulsive therapy?
   a. Restrain the patient's extremities.
   b. Monitor the patient closely until he or she is oriented.
   c. Discharge the patient to home with instructions to rest.
   d. Administer oxygen at 4 L per minute.

5. The nurse is collecting admission data on a new patient with a long health history. Which of the following life events is considered a stressor?
   a. Gallbladder surgery at age 46
   b. Divorce at age 50
   c. Loss of job at age 55
   d. Whatever the patient says is stressful

6. A patient is admitted to the hospital mental health unit for behavior changes. The patient asks why an MRI has been ordered. Which response by the nurse is best?
   a. "MRI can determine levels of important neurotransmitters, so the doctor will know how to treat your problem."
   b. "MRI is used to rule out physical problems that could be causing your symptoms."
   c. "MRI uses magnetic energy to treat certain psychiatric disorders."
   d. "MRI can monitor electrical activity in the brain, which helps diagnose mental health problems."

7. A patient with panic disorder tells the nurse that she has a lot of job-related stress. Which response by the nurse is most therapeutic for this patient?
   a. "I'm really sorry you have so much job stress."
   b. "Can you identify some of the things in your job that are causing you to feel stressed?"
   c. "It is important to eliminate stressful situations so you can reduce your panic attacks."
   d. "You need to avoid stressful situations—it would be wise to start looking for another job."

8. A patient who quit drinking four months earlier tells the nurse that he is thinking about entering an inpatient alcohol rehabilitation program, and asks for the nurse's opinion. Which response by the nurse is best?
   a. "That is an excellent idea. I will help you start the paperwork."
   b. "Why do you think you need a rehabilitation program?"
   c. "What do you think you should do?"
   d. "You have done so well to be alcohol-free for four months."

Nursing Care of Patients with Mental Health Disorders

57

VOCABULARY

Fill in the blanks with the correct terms.

1. A patient with schizophrenia who is unable to speak is experiencing _____________.
2. A situation in which family members exist in order to enable a substance abuser is called

    _____________.

3. An irrational fear is called a/an _____________.
4. A repetitive thought or urge is called a/an _____________.
5. Manic-depressive illness is more appropriately called _____________ depression.
6. Physical symptoms that have no known organic cause may indicate the presence of a/an

    _____________ disorder.

7. People with _____________ cannot distinguish between their reality and society's reality.
8. Abrupt withdrawal from alcohol may cause a disorder called _____________ _____________.
9. _____________ is the repeated compulsive use of a substance in spite of negative consequences.
10. _____________ refers to the loss of ability to enjoy things that are usually pleasurable.

CRITICAL THINKING

Read the case study and answer the following questions.

You are caring for Mr. Joers, a 72-year-old man admitted to your surgical unit from a nursing home after he fell and broke his hip. He is scheduled for surgery this morning at 8 a.m. During morning report, you learn that he has a history of Parkinson's disease, schizophrenia, and anxiety, but that he was oriented and appropriate during admission and throughout the night. When you enter his room to check his vital signs and complete his preoperative checklist, he has a wild look in his eyes, and says, "Don't come near me! They told me what you're up to!"

1. What is your initial response to Mr. Joers? _____________
____
____

2. What implications does his behavior have for surgery this morning? _____________________________
____
____

3. What may have precipitated his worsening symptoms?
____
____

4. What actions do you need to take after your initial response to Mr. Joers? _____________________
____
____

5. What safety concerns do you have? _____________

REVIEW QUESTIONS

Choose the best answer.

1. A patient being treated with lorazepam (Ativan) during alcohol withdrawal becomes sleepy after the first two doses, then becomes difficult to arouse when the nurse attempts to give the third dose. Which of the following actions should the nurse take first?
   a. Hold the dose and notify the RN or physician.
   b. Understand that tolerance will occur with benzodiazepines and give the drug.
   c. Get the patient up and have him walk with assistance until he is more alert.
   d. Administer an antidote.

2. Which of the following responses to anxiety is a cause for concern?
   a. A student studies late into the night to prepare for a difficult examination.
   b. A woman takes deep breaths before going into the grocery store because shopping makes her nervous.
   c. A nurse has a glass of wine before a stressful night shift.
   d. A young man gets the opinions of several of his friends before asking a woman out.

3. A patient calls a nurse into her room and says, "Quick, nurse, there is a dog in the corner. Please get him out. I am terrified of dogs." The nurse sees no dog in the corner. Which of the following responses is best?
   a. "You know we don't allow dogs in the hospital."
   b. "We have been through this before. You know full well that there is no dog in the corner."
   c. "I do not see a dog. Let's take a walk down to the snack room."
   d. "What kind of a dog is it? What makes you so scared of dogs?"

4. A patient is starting on lithium for bipolar disorder. Which of the following nutrients should the nurse teach about maintaining in his diet?
   a. Potassium
   b. Sodium
   c. Selenium
   d. Tyramine

5. A nurse is making a home visit to a patient with schizophrenia who has been noncompliant with taking medications. Which of the following sources of data is most reliable when determining if the patient has been taking medications as prescribed?
   a. Ask the patient.
   b. Ask the significant other.
   c. Count pills in the bottles.
   d. Check with the pharmacy to see if refills have been picked up.

6. Which of the following is the most effective treatment for alcoholism?
   a. Group support, such as Alcoholics Anonymous
   b. Drug therapy
   c. Electroconvulsive therapy
   d. Slowly reducing amount of alcohol consumption

7. Which of the following behaviors by a nurse may aggravate the behavior of a patient with schizophrenia?
   a. Providing written instructions on when to take medications
   b. Speaking in short, simple sentences
   c. Maintaining a structured environment
   d. Speaking quietly to other staff members when the patient is present

8. A patient has an order for carbamazepine (Tegretol) 150 mg bid for bipolar disorder. It is supplied as a suspension, 100 mg in 5 mL. How many milliliters should the nurse prepare? _____________ mL

9. Which statement by a patient with depression indicates that nursing interventions have been helpful?
   a. "His comment upset me, but I took a deep breath and reminded myself that it really isn't true."
   b. "I feel so hopeless about everything, but I am glad you are a good listener."
   c. "I feel so much better now that I know how to control my husband's behavior."
   d. "I am really trying to understand why everyone is against me."

10. A patient is beginning treatment with paroxetine (Paxil) for unipolar depression, but after 10 days is still withdrawn and unable to participate in therapy. Which action by the nurse is best?
    a. Contact the ordering physician for an increase in the dose.
    b. Contact the ordering physician for an alternative antidepressant.
    c. Continue to support the patient while waiting for symptoms to subside.
    d. Encourage the patient to include St. John's wort, an herbal supplement, in the treatment regimen.

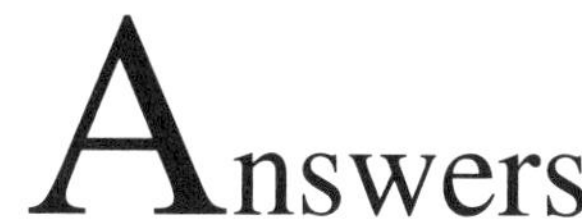

Answers

CHAPTER 1

VOCABULARY

Nursing Process
Definition: An organizing framework that links thinking with nursing actions. Steps include assessment/data collection, nursing diagnosis, planning, implementation, and evaluation.

Critical thinking
Definition: Use of knowledge and skills to make the best decisions possible that increase the probability of a desirable outcome.

Assessment
Definition: Exploring a situation to gather information and data.

Objective data
Definition: Factual information obtained through physical assessment and diagnostic tests. Objective data are observable or knowable through the health-care worker's five senses. Referred to as *signs*.

Subjective data
Definition: Information that is provided verbally by the patient and referred to as *symptoms*.

Evaluation
Definition: Examination of outcomes and interventions to determine progress toward desired outcomes and effectiveness of interventions.

SUBJECTIVE AND OBJECTIVE DATA

1. Subjective (symptom)
2. Subjective (symptom)
3. Objective (sign)
4. Objective (sign)
5. Subjective (symptom)
6. Objective (sign)
7. Subjective (symptom)
8. Objective (sign)
9. Subjective (symptom)
10. Subjective (symptom)
11. Objective (sign)
12. Objective (sign)
13. Subjective (symptom)
14. Objective (sign)
15. Objective (sign)

CRITICAL THINKING

This is just one possible way to complete a cognitive map.

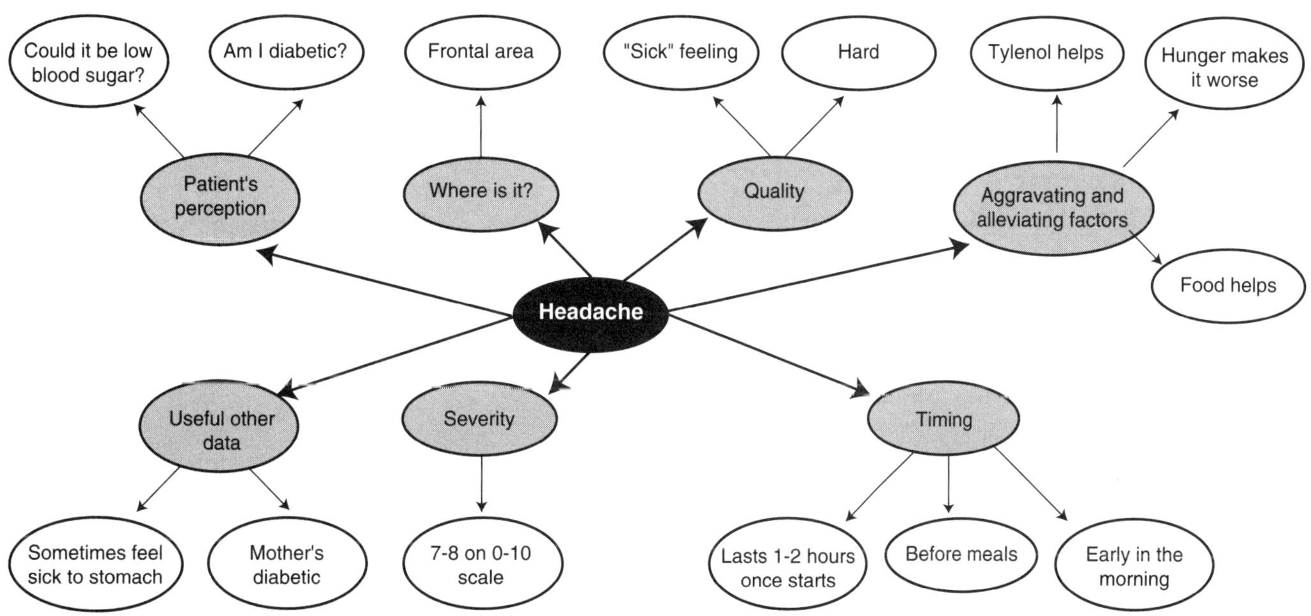

REVIEW QUESTIONS

*The correct answers are in **boldface.***

1. (**c**) is a nursing diagnosis. (a, b, d) are medical diagnoses.
2. (**a**) is a medical diagnosis. (b, c, d) are nursing diagnoses.
3. (**a**) the nurse who is not afraid to ask questions is demonstrating intellectual humility. (b, c, d) are incorrect.
4. (**c, d, e, a, b**)
5. (**a**) is the best definition. (b, c, d) do not define critical thinking, but are examples of good thinking.
6. (**d**) Evaluation determines whether goals are achieved and interventions effective. (a, b, c) are initial steps in developing the nursing care plan.
7. (**a**) The licensed practical nurse/licensed vocational nurse (LPN/LVN) can collect data. (b, c, d) are all steps in the nursing process for which the registered nurse (RN) is responsible; the LPN/LVN may assist the RN with these.
8. (**c**) is data the nurse can collect through use of the five senses. (a, b, d) are subjective data that the patient must report.
9. (**b**) indicates that the patient is concerned about freedom from injury and harm. (a) relates to basic needs such as air, oxygen, and water. (c) relates to feeling loved. (d) is related to having a positive self-esteem.
10. (**d**) is objective, realistic, and measurable with a time frame. (a, b, and c) are all good outcomes, but they relate to airway clearance, nutrition, and strength, not directly to swallowing.

CHAPTER 2

VOCABULARY

1. (**B**)
2. (**A**)
3. (**E**)
4. (**C**)
5. (**D**)
6. (**F**)

NURSING PRACTICE, ETHICAL AND LEGAL PRINCIPLES

1. high-level, life
2. state, protect, quality
3. Caring
4. dignity, maintaining
5. knowledgeable, role models, humor, respect

REVIEW QUESTIONS

*The correct answers are in **boldface.***

1. (**d**) the client is chronically ill but able to meet most goals so has moderate wellness. (a) the client is not near death, (b) since the client can not meet all goals high-level wellness is not achieved, (c) the client is not in poor health since most goals are met through adaptation.
2. (**b**) The nurse-patient relationship is based on trust that the nurse will maintain all patient's rights. (a) is a constitutional right, not an ethical issue. (c) is a legal issue. (d) is not an ethical principle.
3. (**c**) is correct. (a, b, d) are incorrect.
4. (**a**) is correct. (b, c, d) are incorrect.
5. (**d**) is correct. (a, b, c) are incorrect.
6. (**b**) is the first step. (a, c, d) are incorrect.
7. (**a**) is correct. (b, c, d) are incorrect.
8. (**c**) is correct. (a, b, d) are incorrect.
9. (**b**) is correct. (a, c, d) are incorrect.
10. (**a**) is correct. (b, c, d) are incorrect.
11. (**d**) Criminal punishment can result in loss of freedom; (a, b, c) are related to civil liability.
12. (**a**) is correct. (b, c, d) are intentional torts.
13. (**c**) is correct; health care and legal systems can enforce treatment for contagious disease. (a) Generally patients can refuse any or all treatments, except in cases such as contagious disease. (b) The Patient's Self-Determination Act generally guarantees the right to refuse all treatments, except in certain cases. (d) Health care systems along with legal systems can force patients to take medications for contagious diseases.
14. (**a, b, d, e**) These are all part of the 5 steps of delegation. (c) In delegation it is the right person not right patient that is considered. (f) The right route relates to medication administration.

CHAPTER 3

VOCABULARY

1. (**B**)
2. (**C**)
3. (**K**)
4. (**H**)
5. (**E**)
6. (**F**)
7. (**G**)
8. (**L**)
9. (**I**)
10. (**A**)
11. (**D**)
12. (**J**)

CULTURAL CHARACTERISTICS

1. Primary characteristics of culture include nationality, race, skin color, gender, age, and religious affiliation.
2. Secondary characteristics of culture include socioeconomic status, education, occupation, military status, political beliefs, length of time away from the country of origin, urban versus rural residence, marital status, parental status, physical attributes, sexual orientation, and gender issues.
3. Traditional practitioners are health-care practitioners who are not native to the United States. They are native to some other country, although they may practice in the

United States. Examples include curanderos, espirituistas, sobadors, acupuncturists, and crystal gazers.

4. Present-oriented people accept the day as it comes with little regard for the past—the future is unpredictable. Past-oriented people may worship ancestors. Future-oriented people anticipate a bigger and better future and place a high value on change. Some individuals balance all three views; they respect the past, enjoy living in the present, and plan for the future.

CRITICAL THINKING: IMMIGRANTS AND PERSONAL INSIGHTS

There are no right or wrong answers to these two exercises.

CRITICAL THINKING: BATHING

1. In this patient's culture, it is improper for someone of the opposite sex to help with bathing. It is important to assess whether this is the case with this gentleman.
2. Find a male nurse's aide, ask a family member to help, or skip the bath again.
3. Having a male aide do the bath is the best solution. If no male aide is available, the family may be approached for help, although this is not the best solution. Because this is the fourth day without a bath, skipping the bath is not a good option.

REVIEW QUESTIONS

*The correct answers are in **boldface**.*

1. (**a**) is correct. Many Native Americans are not time conscious. She may not keep her appointment if you reschedule, so give the immunizations now. (b) is incorrect; she may not keep her appointment. (c) is incorrect; she may not return to have her stitches removed. (d) is incorrect; to ensure that the children get the immunizations, give them now.
2. (**c**) is correct. Many Hispanics are openly expressive of their grief. Her bereavement behaviors are culturally congruent. Remaining with her is supportive. (a) is incorrect; there is no need to call the cardiac arrest team. (b) is incorrect; lying on the floor is more disconcerting to the nurse than it is to the bereaved woman. (d) is incorrect. This is not the best intervention. Expressive bereavement is normal. However, a later strategy may include a sedative.
3. (**b**) is correct. Cupping is a traditional Chinese practice that is harmless in most cases. (a) is incorrect. Cupping is not considered child abuse. (c) is incorrect. The situation should be reported to the mother by the school nurse. (d) is incorrect. The nurse has acted in good faith and has done nothing wrong.
4. (**a**) is correct. In certain Arabic countries, organs can be purchased for transplantation. This is currently illegal in the United States. (b) is incorrect. The patient does not have an ethical dilemma; however, the nurse may have one. (c) is incorrect. There is no need to call the supervisor. (d) is incorrect. Although there is no harm in giving him the telephone number, this does not take care of the immediate response. The organ center will tell him the same thing.

5. (**c**) is correct. Initially you must assess how traditional the family's food practices are before a dietary regimen can be set up. (a) is incorrect. Giving a traditional ethnic individual an exchange list of foods does not ensure that he or she will change dietary practices to an American food-exchange list. (b) is incorrect. Being able to calculate calories does not ensure that the family knows how to balance a diabetic diet. (d) is incorrect. Although this is certainly an option for the future, the initial step is to obtain a dietary assessment.

6. (**d**) is correct. Patients are allowed to have a Santero visit as long as he or she does not do anything to interfere with treatment or cause a safety problem. (a) is incorrect. It is not necessary to get the supervisor's permission. However, it is a good idea to let the supervisor know that a Santero is going to visit. (b) is incorrect. All religious counselors are allowed to visit. (c) is incorrect. The patient has the right to see her own religious counselor.

7. (**d**) is correct because family is usually very important to Hispanic patients' spirituality. (a) is incorrect. Large numbers of family members in the cafeteria may cause further disruption in the cafeteria. (b) is incorrect. Large groups in the lobby may cause overcrowding for other families. (c) is incorrect. All family members should be allowed to visit. It may help to have them choose a spokesperson to control visiting for this patient.

8. (**b**) is correct. Reducing portion size decreases the overall calorie and fat consumption. (a) is incorrect; telling a patient to not purchase lard does not mean she will comply. (c) is incorrect; rarely does a person bake two separate pies. The goal is to reduce overall fat and calorie consumption. (d) is incorrect; it is inconsistent with the goal of reducing fat and calories.

9. (**b**) is correct. She has to make her own decision, but she should be fully aware of the consequences. (a) is incorrect. Scare tactics are not appropriate; she may live whether or not she receives radiation therapy. (c) is incorrect; it borders on harassment by the staff. (d) is incorrect; radiation therapy may be the best choice for this type of cancer.

10. (**b**) is correct. Changing the schedule slightly is preferable to omitting the medication. (a) is incorrect. Blood levels can be maintained on a different schedule, as long as the doses are reasonably spread out. (c) is incorrect. Omitting the medication will alter blood levels. (d) is incorrect. It does not respect the patient's religious beliefs.

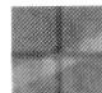

CHAPTER 4

VOCABULARY

1. (E)
2. (D)
3. (F)
4. (B)
5. (A)
6. (C)

COMPLEMENTARY THERAPY: PROGRESSIVE MUSCLE RELAXATION

Purpose: To help the patient use mental images to reduce stress and promote changes in attitude or behavior. May be useful in treating stress-related conditions such as high blood pressure or insomnia, and may even boost the immune system.

Teaching Plan: See Box 4.1 in your textbook.

CRITICAL THINKING

1. Feverfew is used for migraine headaches, inflammation, and menstrual problems, among other things.
2. Capsaicin is used for pain associated with a variety of disorders.
3. Several sources should be consulted before taking herbs. The Internet has a lot of good information, but the source should be carefully evaluated. A pharmacist knowledgeable in herbs and herb-drug interactions, as well as the primary physician or care provider, should be consulted.
4. "Mrs. Lawless, I am concerned that your herbs could interact with your heart failure medications. I will check with your doctor and the hospital pharmacist to be sure they are safe before you take them."

REVIEW QUESTIONS

*The correct answers are in **boldface**.*

1. (**d**) is correct. Progressive muscle relaxation is being added to a traditional therapy, making it complementary. (a) is incorrect. Inhalers and oral medications are both traditional therapies for asthma. (b) is incorrect. Cardiac rehabilitation is a traditional therapy. (c) would be considered an alternative therapy because the echinacea is being used in place of a traditional therapy.
2. (**a**) is correct. Hydrotherapy would be considered alternative because it is being used in place of nonsteroidal anti-inflammatory drugs. (b) is incorrect. Because chemotherapy is still being used, the addition of the spiritual healer would be considered complementary.

(c) is incorrect. Antibiotics and bronchodilators are both traditional medical therapy. (d) is incorrect. Aspirin is traditional therapy for a headache.
3. (**d**) is correct. The patient should keep his or her eyes closed during imagery, so this statement indicates more teaching is needed. (a, b, c) are all parts of guided imagery.
4. (**c**) is correct. Allopathy is the proper term for traditional Western medicine. (a, b, d) are all nontraditional medical practices.
5. (**b**) is correct. Chiropractors do not perform surgery. (a, c, d) are potentially true, but the nurse needs to safeguard the patient by informing her that a chiropractor is not trained or qualified to do surgery.
6. (**a**) is correct; echinacea has been shown in some studies to be potentially effective against colds and viruses. (b) is incorrect. Feverfew is used for headaches and inflammation, among other things. (c) is incorrect. Chamomile is used for anxiety. (d) is incorrect. Ginger is used for nausea.
7. (**b**) is correct. The primary care practitioner can help determine which alternative therapies are safe. (a) is incorrect. Any therapy can be potentially unsafe. (c) is incorrect. Many alternative therapies are safe when used correctly. (d) is incorrect. Alternative and complementary therapies can be effective for chronic pain.
8. (**c**) is correct. It is least appropriate to tell the patient he will be able to reduce his pain medications; this is a possibility, but not a guarantee. (a, b, d) are all appropriate measures to take before beginning to practice any new alternative therapy.

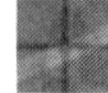

CHAPTER 5

VOCABULARY

1. diffusion
2. isotonic
3. hypertonic
4. hypovolemia
5. cations
6. hypernatremia
7. hypokalemia
8. hypocalcemia
9. acidosis
10. alkalosis

DEHYDRATION

*Corrections are in **boldface**.*

Mrs. White is a 78-year-old woman admitted to the hospital with a diagnosis of severe dehydration. The licensed practical nurse/licensed vocational nurse (LPN/LVN) assigned to

Mrs. White is asked to collect data related to fluid status. The LPN expects Mrs. White's blood pressure to be **elevated because of the shift of fluid from tissues to her bloodstream.** The nurse also finds Mrs. White's skin to be **taut and firm,** and she notes that the **urine is copious** and dark amber. The nurse asks Mrs. White if she knows where she is and what day it is because severe dehydration may cause confusion. In addition, the nurse initiates **intake and output measurements** because this is the most accurate way to monitor fluid balance.

- Blood pressure will be low, not elevated, due to loss of intravascular volume.
- The skin will have poor turgor and will tent when pinched. Remember, the best place to check for tenting in the elderly patient is over the sternum or forehead.
- Urine volume will be diminished as the body attempts to conserve fluid.
- Daily weights are the most reliable indicator of fluid loss or gain.

ELECTROLYTE IMBALANCES

1. (**D**)   4. (**C**)
2. (**E**)   5. (**A**)
3. (**B**)

CRITICAL THINKING

1. Check Mr. James' vital signs. Elevated blood pressure, bounding pulse, and shallow, rapid respirations are common signs of fluid overload. If he is able to stand, weigh him to see if his weight has increased since yesterday. Auscultation of his lungs may reveal new-onset or worsening crackles (he may have had crackles on admission related to his bronchitis).
2. Kidney function declines in the elderly, and the intravenous (IV) fluids may have been too much for him. Regular assessment and caution with IV therapy can prevent overload from occurring.
3. The registered nurse (RN) may decide to reduce the IV infusion rate until orders are obtained. The LPN can elevate the patient's head to ease breathing. Make sure oxygen therapy is being administered as ordered. Stay with him to help him feel less anxious. Anticipate a possible diuretic order. Continue to monitor fluid balance.
4. If a diuretic is administered, urine output should increase, but this does not signal resolution of the problem. It is probably unrealistic to expect Mr. James' lungs to clear because he was admitted with bronchitis. However, return of lung sounds to admission baseline would signal resolution of the acute overload. Other signs would include return to admission vital signs and weight and ability to walk to the bathroom again without excessive shortness of breath.

REVIEW QUESTIONS

*The correct answers are in **boldface**.*

1. (**b**) is the correct answer; 0.9% is isotonic, making 0.45% hypotonic. (a) is isotonic; (c, d) are hypertonic.
2. (**c**) is the correct answer. Aldosterone retains sodium and therefore water in the body. (b) Thyroid hormone and (d) insulin do not affect sodium; (a) antidiuretic hormone (ADH) retains water.
3. (**b**) is the correct answer. Failing kidneys cannot effectively excrete water, making the patient at risk for overload. (a) Meningitis, (c) psoriasis, and (d) influenza do not cause fluid retention. Influenza can cause fluid loss if vomiting or diarrhea is present.
4. (**a**) is the correct answer. The patient with an ileostomy loses large amounts of water with continuous liquid stools. (b) Asthma, (c) diabetes (as long as it is stable), and (d) fractures do not cause fluid loss.
5. (**b**) is the correct answer. Cheeses are high in sodium. (a) Apples, (c) chicken, and (d) broccoli are not high in sodium.
6. (**c**) is the correct answer. Potatoes are high in potassium. (a) Bread, (b) eggs, and (d) cereal are not high in potassium.
7. (**b**) is the correct answer. Fluid gains and losses are evidenced in weight gains and losses. (a) Intake and output (I&O), (c) vital signs, and (d) skin turgor are all ways to monitor fluid balance, but they are not as reliable. I&O may be inaccurate, vital signs may be affected by other factors, and measurement of skin turgor is subjective.
8. (**a**) is the correct answer. Hyponatremia accompanied by fluid loss results in dehydration and mental status changes. (b) Hyperkalemia, (c) hypercalcemia, and (d) hypomagnesemia are not as likely to affect fluid balance and mental status.
9. (**c**) is the correct answer. Ambulation can help prevent bone loss. Because the patient is weak and is at risk for falls and fractures, assistance should be provided. (a) Bedrest promotes bone loss, (b) fluids will not help bone or calcium levels, and (d) the patient needs calcium, not protein.
10. (**d**) is the correct answer. The heart is most at risk for dysrhythmias. (a) Lungs, (b) kidneys, and (c) liver are not as affected.
11. (**b**) is the correct answer. He is probably hyperventilating because of the anxiety. Rebreathing carbon dioxide exhaled into a paper bag can temporarily relieve symptoms of alkalosis until the underlying cause is corrected. (a) Oxygen, (c) positioning, and (d) coughing and deep breathing all help increase oxygenation, which is not needed at this time.
12. (**b**) is the correct answer. Hypoventilation related to lung disease causes retention of carbon dioxide, which causes acidosis. (a) Hyperventilation causes alkalosis, (c) loss of acid causes alkalosis, and (d) loss of base causes acidosis, but it is not the cause in this case.

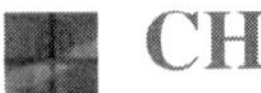# CHAPTER 6

VOCABULARY

1. **(H)**   5. **(E)**
2. **(F)**   6. **(C)**
3. **(A)**   7. **(D)**
4. **(G)**   8. **(B)**

PERIPHERAL VEINS

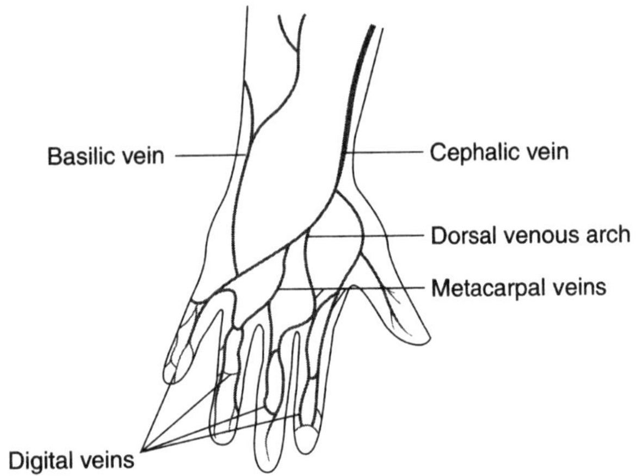

COMPLICATIONS OF IV THERAPY

1. Phlebitis
2. Infection
3. Extravasation
4. Circulatory overload
5. Infiltration
6. Septicemia
7. Catheter embolism
8. Air embolism

CRITICAL THINKING

Begin with mechanical problems such as positioning of catheter by moving the extremity around to see if the intravenous (IV) is simply "positional." Check the tubing for kinks, and the clamp to be sure it is open. Next, assess the infusion site: Look for redness and signs of infiltration (such as coolness and swelling), compare extremities, and check catheter/administration hub connection to make sure it is secure. If the infusion is still not running, the catheter may be occluded with a fibrin or blood clot. The catheter may need to be discontinued. Attempts should not be made to flush the catheter because this could dislodge a clot into the circulation. The role of the LPN varies by state. In many states, the RN would need to be consulted before discontinuing and restarting a new IV site. The RN may attempt to withdraw a clot by aspiration.

CALCULATION PRACTICE

1.

83 mL	1 hour	15 gtt	=	21 gtt
1 hour	60 minutes	mL		minute

2.

50 mL	10 gtt	=	25 gtt
20 minutes	mL		minute

3.

1 L	1000 mL	=	83 mL
12 hours	1 L		hour

4.

800 units	500 mL	=	8 mL
1 hour	50,000 units		hour

5.

1000 mL	1 hour	60 gtt	=	42 gtt
24 hours	60 minutes	1 mL		minute

REVIEW QUESTIONS

*The correct answers are in **boldface**.*

1. **(d)** is the correct answer. The fluid overloaded patient does not need continuous fluids. (a, b, and c) all would benefit from continuous fluid administration.
2. **(b)** is the correct answer. IV medications act rapidly because they are instantly in the bloodstream. (a) Furosemide (Lasix) can be given orally. (c) IV dosing is not necessarily more accurate. (d) Oral furosemide does not have more side effects.
3. **(b)** is the correct answer. The basilic vein is the most distal vein. The nurse should always start distally and then use more proximal veins for future IV sites. (a, c, d) are all proximal and are reserved for central insertions.
4. **(c)** is the correct answer. The site must be cleaned for at least 30 seconds if alcohol is used to effectively rid the skin of bacteria. (a, b, d) are incorrect.
5. **(a)** is the correct answer. A clot could be flushed from the cannula into the circulation and lodge in a pulmonary artery, causing a pulmonary embolism. (b) Air, not a clot, causes an air embolism. (c) Arterial spasm is caused by injecting medication. (d) Extravasation is caused by infiltration of vesicant drugs.
6. **(c)** is the correct answer. Leakage of IV fluid into tissues causes puffiness. (a, b, d) indicate infection or inflammation.
7. **(c)** 125 mL per hour is the correct answer. (a, b, d) are incorrect.
8. **(c)** 50 gtt per minute is the correct answer. (a, b, d) are incorrect.
9. **(b)** is hypertonic. (a) is isotonic. (c, d) are hypotonic.
10. **(b)** is the correct answer. The date, time, IV site, type of cannula, and signature of person inserting should all be documented. (a, c, d) should all be completed before documentation.

CHAPTER 7

VOCABULARY

Antigen is a protein marker on a cell's surface that identifies the cell as self or nonself.

Asepsis is a condition free from germs, infection, and any form of life.

Bacteria are one-celled organisms that can reproduce but need a host for food and a supportive environment. Bacteria can be harmless normal flora or disease-producing pathogens.

Hand Hygiene is cleansing of the hands with hand washing or the use of alcohol-based hand rubs.

Nosocomial Infection is an infection acquired in a health-care agency.

Pathogens are microorganisms or substances capable of producing a disease.

Personal Protective Equipment are items such as gloves, gowns, masks, goggles, and face shields that help prevent the spread of infection to those wearing them.

Phagocytosis is ingestion and digestion of bacteria and particles by phagocytes that ingest and destroy particulate substances such as bacteria, protozoa, and cell debris.

Sepsis is an infection that has spread to the bloodstream.

Virulence is the ability of the organisms to produce disease.

Viruses are small intracellular parasites that can live only inside cells and may produce disease when they enter a cell.

PATHOGEN TRANSMISSION

1. **(C)**	6. **(B)**
2. **(D)**	7. **(C)**
3. **(C)**	8. **(B)**
4. **(D)**	9. **(B)**
5. **(B)**	10. **(A)**

PATHOGENS AND INFECTIOUS DISEASES

1. Staphylococci
2. Fungi
3. *Candidia albicans*
4. Epstein-Barr
5. Pneumonia (Histoplasmosis)
6. Toxoplasmosis
7. Protozoa
8. Viruses
9. Rickettsiae
10. *Clostridium difficile (C. diff)*.

CRITICAL THINKING

1. Equipment—mask, gown, gloves, a sign reading "Contact Isolation," soap and paper towels, special bags for linen and trash, wash area in the room.

2. Disposable thermometer, disposable or autoclavable blood pressure (BP) cuff, stethoscope that remains in the room and can be disinfected, grooming items, bedpan, bath basin, separate container for sharps. Intravenous (IV) equipment and any other equipment needed for the care of the patient must be able to be disinfected.

3. Visitors are limited so the patient has few social contacts and may lack a support system as a result. Environmental stimuli are limited. Activities are limited. Dependent on others for some needs due to confinement.

4. Allow visitors as appropriate and instruct them on how to implement isolation precautions. Encourage contact via telephone with family and friends who cannot visit. Maintain a cheery environment; open curtains; maintain sensory stimuli by remaining with the patient as long as possible. Encourage diversional activities, things the patient likes to do, such as TV, books, etc. Always answer call light immediately.

REVIEW QUESTIONS

*The correct answers are in **boldface.***

1. **(d)** catheter must be anchored to patient's leg per agency protocol so movement in urethra does not encourage organisms to enter the urinary tract. (a) the bag should be lower than the bladder to prevent unsterile urine return to bladder, (b) pale yellow urine indicates urine is dilute and not concentrated, keeping bacteria flushed out, (c) adequate hydration is important to reduce risk, but urine is already dilute.

2. **(c)** Washing hands before and after patient contact is considered the most important method of infection prevention. (a) Hands cannot be sterilized. (b) is a good action but it alone is not sufficient for infection control. (d) Gloves are worn only during certain procedures, when the caregiver is likely to come in contact with a moist body surface. Even when gloves are worn, hand washing before and after wearing the gloves is still essential for infection control.

3. **(a)** Surgical asepsis is aimed at the destruction of microbes before they enter the body. (b) and (d) describe medical asepsis. (c) is not related to surgical asepsis.

4. **(a, e, f)** All pathogens require moisture, food, warmth, and darkness. Some need oxygen, but others do not.

5. **(c)** The only way to obtain a sterile specimen is to catheterize the patient. (a, b, d, e) are incorrect because any voided specimen is contaminated.

6. **(a)** Urinary catheters are a cause of nosocomial infections and should be avoided if possible. (b, c, d) do not prevent infection and restricting fluids may promote infection and dehydration.

7. **(d)** A high fever indicates that the patient has developed a secondary bacterial infection. (a, b, c) are incorrect. Viral infections such as the common cold are usually associated with a low-grade fever. Symp-

toms of the common cold include stuffy nose with watery discharge, scratchy throat, dry cough, sneezing, and watery eyes.

8. (**a**) A culture identifies pathogen presence. (b) A drug level or peak and trough measures antibiotic levels. (c) A sensitivity report indicates what pathogens are sensitive to certain antibiotics. (d) is incorrect.

9. (**a**) is a sign of local infection. (b, d) are seen in shock. (c) is typical of a systemic infection.

10. (**b**) is a method of sterile technique. (a, c, d) are all medical asepsis practices.

11. (**c**) is correct. Nosocomial infections are acquired as a result of hospitalization. (a) is a chronic infection, (b) is due to a sexually transmitted disease, and (d) the infection was present prior to hospitalization.

12. (**d**) is correct. Vancomycin is the treatment of choice for methicillin-resistant *Staphylococcus aureus* (MRSA). (a, b, c) are incorrect.

13. (**b, e**) can be signs of infection in an older adult. (a, c, d) are not signs of infection.

14. (**b**) Sterile water should be used instead of tap water for an immunocompromised patient to prevent infection. (a, c, d) are appropriate actions.

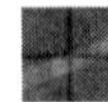 CHAPTER 8

VOCABULARY

1. acidosis
2. anaerobic
3. anaphylaxis
4. antiarrhythmics
5. coagulopathies
6. cyanosis
7. tachypnea
8. oliguria
9. tachycardia

MATCHING

1. (**C**)
2. (**A**)
3. (**B**)
4. (**B**)
5. (**B**)
6. (**C**)

CRITICAL THINKING

1. Stage: Severe/irreversible
   Category of Shock: Hypovolemic
   Initial Action: Notify physician, aid volume restoration by monitoring intravenous infusion
2. Stage: Mild/compensating
   Category of Shock: Septic
   Initial Action: Notify physician, maintain oxygen
3. Stage: Moderate/progressive
   Category of Shock: Cardiogenic
   Initial Action: Stop intravenous infusion, notify physician

REVIEW QUESTIONS

*The correct answers are in **boldface**.*

1. (**c**) Notify the physician immediately because the patient is hypovolemic and needs intravenous fluids. (a) This is not the type of intravenous fluid the patient needs; an isotonic intravenous solution such as 0.9% normal saline would be appropriate. (b) is not a priority at this time. (d) The patient requires intervention now and more frequent monitoring.
2. (**b**) Elevated creatinine indicates possible renal damage. (a, c, d) are near normal and not indicative of a problem.

SIGNS AND SYMPTOMS OF SHOCK PHASES

Signs/Symptoms	Phases		
	Mild/Compensating	Moderate/Progressive	Severe/Irreversible
Heart rate	Elevated	Tachycardia	Slowing
Pulses	Bounding	Weaker, thready	Absent
Blood pressure Systolic	Normal	<90 mm Hg *In hypertensive, 25% below baseline	<60 mm Hg
Diastolic	Normal	Decreased	Decreasing to 0
Respirations	Elevated	Tachypnea	Slowing
Depth	Deep	Shallow	Irregular, shallow
Temperature	Varies *May elevate in septic shock	Decreased	Decreasing
Level of consciousness	Anxious, restless, irritable, alert, oriented	Confused, lethargic	Unconscious, comatose
Skin/mucous membranes	Cool, pale	Cold, moist, clammy, pale	Cyanosis, mottled, cold, clammy
Urine output	Normal	Decreasing to >20 mL/hr	15 mL/hr decreasing to anuria
Bowel sounds	Normal	Decreasing	Absent

3. (**b**) The pulse elevates to compensate for decreasing cardiac output in mild shock. (a, c, d) are found in moderate shock.

4. (**a**) is correct. (b, c, d) are found in mild shock.

5. (**b**) Inform the registered nurse so the intravenous rate can be increased while the physician is being notified because the patient is hypovolemic. (a, c, d) are incorrect because the patient needs immediate intervention. (a) provides no intervention, although vital signs will be monitored continuously, and (c, d) will worsen the condition.

6. (**b**) increases blood pressure. (a, c, d) are incorrect.

7. (**b**) Decreased peripheral tissue perfusion may be seen first as slow capillary refill. (a, c, d) do not convey peripheral tissue perfusion status.

8. (**c**) Tachypnea is compensatory to maintain normal oxygen levels when cardiac output decreases. (a) If anxiety occurs, it is not the primary cause of tachypnea. (b) Decreasing retention of carbon dioxide is not the primary reason for tachypnea, although it is a benefit. (d) is incorrect.

9. (**c**) Blood pressure is dropping and peripheral vasoconstriction occurs, resulting in less blood flow to the extremities; sympathetic nervous system compensation causes sweating to cool the body for "fight or flight." (a, b, d) are incorrect.

10. (**c**) is a 25% decrease from baseline. (a, b, d) are incorrect.

11. (**b**) The goal is to increase understanding when knowledge is deficient. (a, c, d) are incorrect.

12. (**d, b, e, a, c**). Use Maslow's hierarchy as a guide: Airway is considered first (d), then oxygen. (b) Determining vital signs (e) will guide further treatment, as will urine output monitoring (a). (c) is not a priority at this time.

CHAPTER 9

VOCABULARY

1. (**D**)
2. (**C**)
3. (**F**)
4. (**A**)
5. (**I**)
6. (**H**)
7. (**J**)
8. (**E**)
9. (**B**)
10. (**G**)

CULTURAL COMPETENCE

Remember that each patient is an individual and may or may not act like others from his or her cultural group.

- Native Americans might not ask for pain medication. They may believe pain is something that must be endured.
- European Americans may be stoic and avoid taking medication even when it is necessary. They may fear addiction or dependence.
- African Americans may express pain more freely and may feel pain and suffering are inevitable.
- Hispanic Americans from Puerto Rico may moan or cry. Those from Mexico may be more stoic, especially the men, who do not want to appear weak.
- Asian Americans tend to be stoic and not express pain as freely.

CRITICAL THINKING

1. Using the WHAT'S UP? format, you would assess where her pain is, how it feels, what makes it better or worse, when it began, how severe it is on a scale of 0 to 10, related symptoms, and her perception of the pain and what will relieve it.

2. Morphine is an opioid that works by binding to opioid receptors in the central nervous system.

3. Because you can expect Miss Murphy to be in pain on her operative day, it is most beneficial to administer her analgesic every 4 hours, before pain begins to recur. This will help her walk and cough and prevent postoperative complications. Often postoperative analgesics are administered via patient-controlled anesthesia (PCA).

4. Common side effects of opioids included drowsiness, nausea, and constipation. Respiratory depression and constricted pupils are signs of overdose.

5. If the morphine has been effective, Miss Murphy will be able to ambulate and cough with minimal difficulty and will rate her pain at a level that is acceptable to her.

6. According to the equianalgesic chart, the 30 mg of oral codeine in Tylenol No. 3 would be equal to about 2 mg of intramuscular (IM) morphine, a much smaller dose than she has been receiving. The physician should be contacted for a more appropriate order.

7. Relaxation, distraction, back rubs, and imagery might all be effective in addition to the morphine. She has already been using distraction as she visits with her family.

REVIEW QUESTIONS

*The correct answers are in **boldface**.*

1. (**d**) is correct. Pain is whatever the experiencing person says it is, occurring whenever the experiencing person says it does. (a, b, c) may all be true in some situations but are not general definitions of pain.

2. (**c**) is correct. *Suffering* is the term used to describe the sense of threat that can accompany pain. (a, b, d) may all be present with pain, but they are not the same as suffering.

3. (**a**) is correct. Constipation is a common side effect. (b) is not common, (c) is not a side effect of opioids, and (d) is not common and is different than a side effect.
4. (**c**) is correct. The patient's self-assessment is the best measure of pain available. (a) Some patients may moan or cry, but others may not—this may be a cultural variation; (b) vital signs are an indirect measure, and are most reliable when assessing acute pain; and (d) the patient's request for pain medication may be unrelated to the degree of pain.
5. (**b**) is correct. Distraction can be effective when used with analgesics. (a) Some patients may deny their pain, but not most; (c) laughing and talking do not mean pain is not present; and (d) there is no evidence that laughing changes the duration of action of medications.
6. (**a**) is correct. Acute pain may be accompanied by elevated vital signs. (b, c) are incorrect because vital signs adapt to chronic pain.
7. (**d**) is correct. Meperidine has a toxic metabolite called normeperidine, which can build up and cause cerebral irritation. (a, b, c) may all be true, but the nurse must first consider the patient's safety before trying other approaches.
8. (**c**) is correct. Pain level should be assessed before giving any analgesic, and respiratory rate should be assessed before giving any medication that can depress respirations. (a) Liver and kidney function are not routinely assessed, (b) blood glucose is not routinely assessed, and (d) the physical cause of pain may not always be known.
9. (**a**) is correct. Naloxone is a narcotic antagonist. (b, c, d) are not narcotic antagonists.
10. (**c**) is correct. There is no research to justify the use of placebos to treat pain. (a, b, d) all imply that the placebo will be given. Placebos should be given only in research settings with patient consent.
11. (**c**) is correct. Most patients who are too drowsy to push the button are not in pain. Further assessment is needed to determine if he is in pain and how to proceed. (a, b) No one but the patient should ever push the button. (d) The medication should be increased only as ordered after a complete assessment and assurance that Mr. Brown is safe.
12. (**b**) is correct. The patient should always be believed. (a, c, d) may all be true, but if the nurse makes a wrong assumption, a patient in pain may go without treatment. Injuries sustained in a motorcycle accident are likely to be painful.

◼ CHAPTER 10

VOCABULARY

1. alopecia
2. anorexia
3. leukopenia
4. xerostomia
5. palliative
6. Chemotherapy
7. cytotoxic
8. Neoplasm
9. metastasizes
10. benign

CELLS

1. True
2. False—for one protein
3. False—to the ribosomes
4. True
5. False—on the messenger RNA
6. True
7. False—only those needed for its specific functions are active
8. False—46
9. False—each cell has a full 46 chromosomes
10. False—it is also necessary for repair of tissues

BENIGN VERSUS MALIGNANT TUMORS

Benign tumors typically grow slowly, cause minor tissue damage, remain localized, and seldom recur after treatment. Cells resemble tissue of origin. Malignant tumors often grow quickly, cause damage to surrounding tissue, spread to other parts of the body (metastasize), and recur after treatment. Cells are altered to be less like their tissue of origin.

CRITICAL THINKING

1. Leukopenia: Use careful handwashing; teach Delmae and her family the importance of doing the same. Teach her to avoid crowds, people with infections, and bird, cat, or dog excreta. Instruct her to avoid fresh fruits or vegetables that cannot be peeled. Teach her signs and symptoms of infection to report.
2. Thrombocytopenia: Teach Delmae the importance of avoiding injury to prevent bleeding. Avoid IM injections. Teach her to watch for and report symptoms of bleeding, such as bruising, petechiae, or blood in urine, stool, or emesis.
3. Anemia: Provide a balanced diet, with supplements as prescribed. Administer oxygen as ordered for dyspnea. Provide opportunities to rest. Administer or teach self-administration of epoetin alfa as ordered.
4. Stomatitis: Offer soft, mild foods. Offer frequent sips of water. Provide a mouthwash such as diphenhydramine diluted in water or saline. Teach her to avoid hot, cold, spicy, and acidic foods.
5. Nausea and vomiting: Give antiemetics as ordered. Use prophylactically, not just when nausea is present. Provide mouth care before meals. Provide small, frequent meals and room-temperature or cool foods. Serve

meals in a clean, pleasant environment that is free from odors and unpleasant sights. Offer hard candy. Use music or relaxation as distractions.

6. Alopecia: Offer an accepting attitude. Help the patient locate a wig or other head covering if she wishes. Tell her that her hair will grow back.

REVIEW QUESTIONS

*The correct answers are in **boldface**.*

1. (**b**) is correct.
2. (**c**) is correct.
3. (**b**) is correct. High-fat foods may increase the risk of some cancers. (a) Broccoli and cauliflower help reduce cancer risk. (c) Chicken and fish are low-fat meats that are healthy choices. (d) Cakes and breads are not problems unless they are high in fat or other high-risk ingredients.
4. (**c**) is correct. A biopsy enables the pathologist to examine and positively identify the cancer. (a) Cultures diagnose infection. (b) X-ray can help locate a tumor but cannot determine whether it is benign or malignant. (d) A bronchoscopy may be done, but a biopsy is necessary to positively identify the cancer.
5. (**a**) is correct. Frequent mouth care will help prevent the discomfort and dryness that accompany mucositis. (b) Cold liquids may worsen mucositis. (c) High-carbohydrate foods will not help. (d) Juices are acidic and may irritate the mucous membranes.
6. (**b**) is correct. Remember the importance of time, distance, and shielding. (a) Leaving the patient alone for 24 hours is inappropriate. (c) Body fluids should not be touched, but it is not feasible to care for the patient and avoid touching altogether. (d) A "contaminated" sign will make the patient feel isolated and afraid.
7. (**b**) is correct. Petechiae are small hemorrhages into the skin. (a) Fever is a sign of infection. (c) Pain is not usually a sign of bleeding. (d) Vomiting is not a sign of bleeding unless it is bloody.
8. (**a**) is correct. Washing hands frequently is an excellent way to help prevent infection in the patient at risk. (b) Avoiding injections will help prevent bleeding but will do little to prevent infection. (c) Visitors with infections should be discouraged, but the patient needs the support of family at this time. (d) Fresh fruits and vegetables can transmit infection.
9. (**d**) is correct. Alternative methods for pain control can be helpful but should never be expected to substitute for analgesics in the patient with cancer. (a) Distraction should be used with, not instead of, medication. (b) The nurse must believe the patient's report of pain. (c) Distraction can be effective when used with medication and in no way indicates that the patient's pain is not real.
10. (**c**) is correct. The goal of hospice is to help patients achieve a comfortable death. (a, b, d) are all aimed at curing the patient's cancer. If cure is the goal, a referral to hospice is inappropriate.

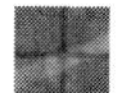 # CHAPTER 11

VOCABULARY

1. surgeons
2. perioperative
3. postoperative
4. induction
5. preoperative
6. intraoperative
7. adjunct
8. dehiscence
9. anesthesiologists
10. anesthesia
11. atelectasis
12. debridement
13. hypothermia
14. evisceration

SURGERY URGENCY LEVELS

1. (**D**)	6. (**A**)
2. (**C**)	7. (**B**)
3. (**C**)	8. (**A**)
4. (**D**)	9. (**C**)
5. (**B**)	10. (**A**)

NOURISHING THE SURGICAL PATIENT

*Corrections are in **boldface**.*

Healing requires increased vitamin **A and D** for collagen formation, vitamin **K** for blood clotting, and **zinc** for tissue growth, skin integrity, and cell-mediated immunity. **Proteins** are essential for controlling fluid balance and manufacturing antibodies and white blood cells. Hypoalbuminemia, a low **serum** albumin, impedes the return of interstitial fluid to the venous return system, **increasing** the risk of shock. A serum **albumin** level is a useful measure of protein status.

MEDICATIONS

1. True
2. False—the surgeon determines if the anticoagulant therapy is stopped several days before surgery, which it often is.
3. False—the patient may be told by the physician to either take no insulin, the normal dose of insulin, or half of the normal dose.
4. True
5. True
6. False—surgery is a great stressor for the body.
7. True

8. False—circulatory collapse can develop if steroids are stopped abruptly.

INTRAOPERATIVE NURSING DIAGNOSES AND OUTCOMES

1. Free from injury
2. Maintains skin integrity
3. Maintains blood pressure, pulse, and urine output within normal limits
4. Is free of symptoms of infection
5. Reports pain is relieved to satisfactory level

WOUND HEALING PHASES

Phase	Time Frame	Wound Healing	Patient Effect
Phase I	Incision to second postoperative day	Inflammatory response	Fever, malaise
Phase II	Third to fourteenth postop day	Granulation tissue forms	Feeling better
Phase III	Third to sixth postop week	Collagen deposited	Raised scar formed
Phase IV	Months to 1 year	Wound contracts and shrinks	Flat, thin scar

CRITICAL THINKING

1. For nursing interview, diagnostic testing, anesthesia interview, and preoperative teaching to ensure patient is in the best possible condition for surgery.
2. Laboratory tests: blood glucose, creatinine, blood urea nitrogen (BUN), electrolytes, complete blood count (CBC), prothrombin time (PT), partial thromboplastin time (PTT), bleeding time, type and screen, and urinalysis, are some common tests; oxygen saturation, electrocardiogram (ECG), chest x-ray.
3. Explain what is to be done in preadmission testing; explain preadmission prep: bathing, scrubs, preps, medications, nil per os (NPO) time, no nail polish or make-up; admission procedures the day of surgery: registration, nursing unit, emotional support, consent signed, preoperative checklist completion; intravenous (IV) line insertion, medications, surgery, postanesthesia care unit and family waiting locations, surgery time frames; postoperative care: pain control, deep breathing and coughing, leg exercises, activity, leg abduction, drains.
4. Explain admission procedures; get consent signed, preoperative checklist completion; IV insertion; give medications.
5. Greeting the patient; verifying patient's name, age, and allergies; surgeon performing the surgery; consent; surgical procedure, especially right or left when applicable, and medical history; answering questions; and alleviating anxiety. Explain what to expect in surgery: "The room may feel cool, but you can request extra blankets."

"There is a lot of equipment, including a table and large bright overhead lights." "Several health-care team members will introduce themselves to you." "The physician will greet you."

6. Licensed practical nurses/licensed vocational nurses (LPN/LVNs) may scrub in surgery to hand instruments to the surgeon. The LPN/LVN must know sterile technique, surgical instruments, and medications placed in the sterile field for use during surgery.
7. Maintaining the patient's airway and safety.
8. Pain control is essential to prevent physiological harm to the patient and to ensure that the patient can participate in recovery activities such as deep breathing and coughing and activity. Deep breathing and coughing prevents atelectasis and pneumonia. Leg exercises and activity prevent thrombophlebitis. Drains are inserted to prevent fluid accumulation and infection.

REVIEW QUESTIONS

*The correct answers are in **boldface**.*

1. (**c**) The LPN/LVN can offer emotional support as needed to patients. (a) is the role of the registered nurse (RN). (b, d) are roles of the physician.
2. (**b**) The registered nurse must be informed so the surgeon can be notified. (a, c, d) are not appropriate interventions, and if the patient is extremely scared, the surgeon must be told because surgery may need to be canceled.
3. (**a**) Higher steroid levels are needed during stress to the body, which surgery produces. (b, c, d) are not complications of steroid withdrawal; circulatory collapse is.
4. (**d**) Eliminate background noise because the elderly cannot filter out noise. (a) This increases glare, which will interfere with vision. (b) Large black-on-white print should be used. (c) A low tone should be used.
5. (**d**) The nurse's signature verifies that it was the patient who signed the consent after informed consent was provided by the surgeon. (a, b, c) are not the role of the nurse and are not indicated by the witnessing of the consent.
6. (**b**) Skin integrity is maintained during surgery with proper positioning and avoidance of pressure points. (a, c, d) are preoperative goals.
7. (**a**) Oxygen saturation must be above 90%. (b) is incorrect. (c) Patients do not have to void before postanesthesia care unit (PACU) discharge. (d) IV narcotics cannot have been given less than 30 minutes ago.
8. (**c**) Patients and a responsible adult must understand discharge instructions before discharge. (a) Patients cannot drive home. (b) Patient does not have to have home telephone but must be able to be contacted in some way for follow-up. (d) IV narcotics cannot have been given less than 30 minutes ago.

9. (**c**) Pneumonia can be prevented with lung expansion promoted by ambulation. (a, b, d) are not prevented with ambulation.
10. (**b**) Use two people to assist patient for first time in case patient is light-headed. (a) One person may not be enough to support patient if fainting occurs. (c) Patient should not self-dangle for safety. (d) Narcotics should be given about 1 hour before ambulation so patient is comfortable but hypotension is less likely.
11. (**c**) Presence of flatus occurs with normal bowel function. (a, d) indicate the bowel is not functioning. (b) is not related to bowel function.
12. (**c**) Have patient lie down to reduce pressure on the incisional area to help prevent evisceration. (a) Having patient sit upright promotes evisceration. (b) Intravenous fluids should be maintained at ordered rate and increased fluid needs anticipated because of large fluid loss occurring with dehiscence and evisceration. (d) This would not be the nurse's first action, and the patient would likely be prepared for surgery.
13. (**d**) Exhaling deeply to reach target is incorrect and would indicate need for teaching. (a, b, c) are incorrect because they are the appropriate way to use the spirometer.
14. (**a**) Sympathetic nervous system saves fluid in response to stress of surgery, which reduces urine output initially. (b, c, d) are incorrect.
15. (**b, e**) A fever occurring shortly after surgery is often due to atelectasis because infection takes longer to develop, so encouraging coughing and deep breathing and ambulating to expand lungs can help prevent pneumonia. (a) An infection is not usually the cause of a fever in this time frame. (c) Tylenol is not necessary for a low-grade fever and will not help the cause. (d) Fluid intake should be maintained to help thin lung secretions.

CHAPTER 12

VOCABULARY

1. (**C**)
2. (**B**)
3. (**A**)
4. (**E**)
5. (**D**)
6. (**G**)
7. (**F**)
8. (**H**)
9. (**I**)
10. (**J**)

PRINCIPLES FOR TREATING SHOCK

1. True
2. False—direct pressure
3. False—Apply blanket to keep patient warm.
4. True
5. False—Take frequent vital signs.
6. False—Do not give the patient oral fluids.
7. True

SIGNS AND SYMPTOMS OF INCREASED INTRACRANIAL PRESSURE

1. (**B**)
2. (**A**)
3. (**A**)
4. (**B**)
5. (**A**)
6. (**B**)
7. (**B**)
8. (**A**)
9. (**A**)
10. (**A**)
11. (**B**)
12. (**B**)

ASSESSMENT OF MOTOR FUNCTION

If the patient is unable to	The lesion is above the level of
Extend and flex arms	C-5 to C-7
Extend and flex legs	L-2 to L-4
Flex foot, extend toes	L-4 to L-5
Tighten anus	S-3 to S-5

HYPERTHERMIA

1. (**A**)
2. (**A**)
3. (**B**)
4. (**B**)
5. (**A**)
6. (**B**)
7. (**A**)
8. (**B**)
9. (**B**)
10. (**A**)

PRINCIPLES FOR DISASTER OR BIOTERRORISM RESPONSE

1. Overwhelms
2. disaster plans
3. called in, discharged
4. triage, stabilization
5. seriously, full
6. drills
7. familiar, role
8. natural

CRITICAL THINKING

1. Unresolved grieving of his wife's death.
2. Withdrawn, rarely leaves home, has not bathed, wearing soiled clothing, refrigerator is empty, curtains drawn, paces, says "I want to die." He is exhibiting cognitive, emotional, and behavioral disorganization.
3. He no longer possesses coping skills necessary to maintain usual level of functioning. His moods, thoughts, and actions are so disordered that they have the potential to lead to suicide if the situation is not quickly controlled.
4. Dysfunctional grieving related to spouse's unexpected death; risk for injury related to impaired judgment; ineffective health maintenance related to disturbed thought processes.
5. Establish an atmosphere of trust. Use active listening. Make environment safe. Reduce external sources of stimulation. Speak directly and truthfully to patient. Include supportive members of patient's family. Patient

is prepared for each new development as circumstances evolve. Threatening, challenging, or arguing with disturbed patient is not done.

REVIEW QUESTIONS

*The correct answers are in **boldface**.*

1. (**c**) Respiratory distress may be experienced in anaphylactic shock because of fluid in the air passages and constricted bronchi. (a, b, c) are not common with anaphylactic shock.
2. (**a**) Arterial blood flow is assessed with capillary refill. (b, c, d) are not assessed with capillary refill.
3. (**b**) Activated charcoal would be given to help absorb the medication. (a, b, d) would not be appropriate for a semiconscious patient.
4. (**b**) Patient is alert and oriented. (a, c, d) are incorrect. Core body temperature should be within normal range. Skin should be warm and dry.
5. (**c**) (3 mg/5 mg) $\times$ 1 mL = 3/5 = 0.6 mL. (a, b, d) are incorrect.
6. (**c**) A rapid, thready pulse indicates compensation (rapid) and loss of blood volume (thready). (a, b, d) are incorrect.
7. (**c, b, a, d**) Airway is the first priority, then breathing, circulation, disability.
8. (**b**) The brachial artery is the proximal artery to the radial artery. (a, c, d) are not the most proximal arteries to the radial artery.
9. (**b, c, d**) are needed for the unvaccinated nurse when caring for a patient with smallpox. (a) is for the vaccinated nurse and (e) is not required.
10. (**a**) Morbidity and mortality are usually from pulmonary aspiration secondary to loss of the gag reflex. (b, c, d) are neurological signs that would occur later with complications. The nurse's priority is monitoring that will prevent complications from occurring.

 # CHAPTER 13

VOCABULARY

1. respite care
2. powerlessness
3. chronic
4. spirituality
5. hopelessness
6. developmental stage

CHRONIC ILLNESS AND THE OLDER ADULT

*Corrections are in **boldface**.*

Older adults constitute one of the **largest** age groups living with chronic illness. Older adult spouses or older family members are **increasingly being called on** to care for a chronically ill family member. Children of older adults who themselves are reaching their **60s** are being expected to care for their parents. These older adult caregivers **may also be** experiencing chronic illness. For older adult spouses, it is usually the less ill spouse who provides care to the other spouse. The older adult family unit is at great risk for ineffective coping or further development of health problems. Nurses should assess **all** members of the older adult family to ensure that their health needs are being met.

Older adults are **very** concerned about becoming dependent and a burden to others. They may become depressed and give up hope if they feel that they are a burden to others. Establishing **short-term** goals or self-care activities that allow them to participate or have small successes are important nursing actions that can **increase** their self-esteem.

CRITICAL THINKING

1. The nurse should explore Mrs. Martin's spiritual needs: Is she hopeful? What makes her feel at peace? How does she usually meet her spiritual needs? Does she have certain religious customs?
2. Spiritual distress; potential for enhanced spiritual well-being; hopelessness; powerlessness.
3. Interventions may include using the meditation room for quiet reflection or prayer, chaplain visits, or worship services; assisting Mrs. Martin with transportation to the meditation room or worship services; and providing desired reading material such as a Bible or prayer book.
4. If Mrs. Martin expresses a feeling of peace or hopefulness.

REVIEW QUESTIONS

*The correct answers are in **boldface**.*

1. (**d**) Integrity versus despair. (a, b, c) are earlier developmental stages.
2. (**a**) stress management directly influences how a patient ages. (b, c, d) do not directly influence a patient's aging.
3. (**d**) This empowers the patient to control her own health care. (a, b, c) take control away from the patient.
4. (**b**) Home care nurses can strengthen a patient's self-care capacity by saying, "Let me assist you" instead of "Let me do this for you." (a) Being a caretaker instead of a partner is not helpful in improving self-esteem. (c) Empowering the patient instead of doing it all for the patient would be helpful. (d) Doing everything for the patient instead of assisting makes the patient feel dependent and useless.
5. (**a**) Offering praise for small patient efforts shows interest in the patient and motivates the patient to try other tasks. (b) If praise is offered only for major patient efforts, opportunities to praise small tasks are lost; if the patient never accomplishes major tasks, no praise is ever given. (c) If ADLs are done for the patient, no opportunity for independence and success is allowed

for the patient. (d) Assisting patient at first sign of difficulty with ADLs allows the patient no opportunity to succeed at a difficult task.

6. (**b**) Using humor can be helpful, and this is one method of using humor. (a) Avoiding the use of humor is not beneficial because humor has been shown to enhance health. (c) A serious manner may not be as helpful in improving a patient's mood. (d) Limiting conversation to a minimum further isolates the patient.

7. (**d**) Stress decreases when the caregiver is given personal time away from the patient, which everyone needs. (a) Personal time increases. (b) Rest time increases. (c) There is no cost for most volunteer respite services.

8. (**d**) Allowing the patient to make informed decisions should foster health promotion. (a, b, c) Making the choices for the patient and family may not result in implementation of those choices because input was not obtained from them.

9. (**a**) Providing educational information empowers the patient to make informed choices. (b) Limiting visiting hours for family members isolates the patient and does not allow patient free choice. (c) Asking family members to provide care makes the patient dependent if some independence is possible. (d) Setting the goals for the patient and family takes the decision-making process away from the patient.

10. (**a**) Peripheral vascular disease is a chronic illness. (b, c, d) are acute illnesses.

11. (**a**) Being willing and able to carry out the medical regimen is important in dealing positively with the illness. (b, c, d) would be unhelpful behaviors in adapting to a chronic illness.

12. (**b**) Malabsorption syndrome is a congenital disorder. (a, c, d) are acquired illnesses.

13. (**a**) is correct. (b, c) are incorrect.

CHAPTER 14

VOCABULARY

1. activities of daily living
2. arrhythmia
3. cataract
4. attitude
5. aspiration
6. edema
7. glaucoma
8. expectoration
9. constipation
10. homeostasis
11. contracture
12. pressure ulcer
13. nocturia
14. extrinsic factors
15. macular degeneration
16. osteoporosis
17. sensory deprivation
18. optimal functioning
19. reality orientation
20. sensory overload

AGING CHANGES

1. (**A**)		14. (**L**)
2. (**C**)		15. (**O**)
3. (**E**)		16. (**P**)
4. (**F**)		17. (**Q**)
5. (**B**)		18. (**R**)
6. (**H**)		19. (**T**)
7. (**D**)		20. (**U**)
8. (**G**)		21. (**S**)
9. (**K**)		22. (**V**)
10. (**N**)		23. (**W**)
11. (**M**)		24. (**Z**)
12. (**J**)		25. (**X**)
13. (**I**)		26. (**Y**)

COMMUNICATING WITH THE HEARING IMPAIRED

1. True
2. False—face patient so the speaker's face is visible to patient
3. False—speak toward patient's best side of hearing
4. True
5. True
6. False—recognize that high-frequency tones and consonant sounds are lost first, *z*, *sh*, *ch*, *d*, *g*
7. True

MEDICATIONS

*Corrections are in **boldface**.*

Older patients are **more** susceptible to drug-induced illness and adverse medication side effects for various reasons. They take **many** medicines for the **more than** one chronic illness that they have. Different medications interact and produce side effects that can be dangerous. Over-the-counter medicines older patients take, as well as the self-prescribed extracts, elixirs, herbal teas, cultural healing substances, and other home remedies commonly used by individuals of their age cohort, **do** influence other medications.

If an older patient crushes a large enteric-coated pill so that it can be taken in food and is easily swallowed, it **destroys** the enteric protection and can inadvertently cause damage to the stomach and intestinal system. Some patients **intentionally** skip prescribed doses in an effort to save money. When prescribed doses are not being taken as expected, problems do not clear up as quickly and new problems may result. The nurse should educate the older patient and the patient's family. Patients need to know what each prescribed pill is for, when it is prescribed to be taken, and how it should be taken.

CRITICAL THINKING

This is a values clarification exercise, so answers are your own individualized answers that should be based on guiding principles.

1. An individual response
2. Your values and beliefs (what are they)
3. Be tactful and provide privacy during situation resolution.
4. Consider professionalism issues, agency policy, patient safety.
5. Consider professionalism, respect for others' values.

REVIEW QUESTIONS

*The correct answers are **in boldface.***

1. (**c**) is the only symptom for glaucoma. (a, b, d) are incorrect.
2. (**d**) There is a decreased taste sensitivity for salt and sweet flavors. (a, b, c) are not aging changes.
3. (**b**) Peripheral vascular resistance increases with age, contributing to hypertension development. (a, c, d) decrease with aging.
4. (**b**) Circulatory status is the reason for slow, deliberate movements because gravity shifts body fluids with position change. (a, c, d) are incorrect.
5. (**a**) The older circulatory system is very sensitive to fluid-overload situations, and intravenous therapy increases the risk potential. (b, c, d) are incorrect.
6. (**c**) Whispering lowers the pitch of the sounds, making your words easier to hear for someone who has lost only high-pitched frequencies. (a, b, d) are incorrect for high-pitched hearing loss.
7. (**b**) Wax can obstruct the conduction pathway, causing a bone-conduction problem. (a, c) are not related to a bone-conduction problem, but a nerve problem.
8. (**b**) Psychological factors are the primary source of sexual dysfunction, as documented in the literature. (a, c, d) are not the primary source.
9. (**a**) This puts the patient's needs ahead of the nurse's needs. (b, c, d) do not show respect for the patient's needs.
10. (**b**) Weight-bearing exercise helps fight the degeneration of bone in osteoporosis. (a) Calcium intake should be increased. (c, d) do not have any influence on osteoporosis.

CHAPTER 15

VOCABULARY

1. (**F**)   6. (**B**)
2. (**D**)   7. (**H**)
3. (**E**)   8. (**J**)
4. (**C**)   9. (**A**)
5. (**G**)   10. (**I**)

HOME HEALTH SERVICES

1. (**D**)   4. (**B**)
2. (**E**)   5. (**A**)
3. (**C**)

CRITICAL THINKING

1. Four times per week for 4 weeks.
2. Dressing changes, reinforcement of medication teaching including blood glucose monitoring, vital sign monitoring, O_2 therapy precautions, and management.
3. "No smoking" signs need to be posted because Mrs. Thompson is receiving O_2 therapy. Environment needs to be assessed for potential safety hazards including long O_2 tubing, scatter rugs, inadequate lighting, need for assistive devices, and need for monitoring system.
4. Yes, social services for meals on wheels, OT/PT for strength training, and identification and instruction of assistive devices, and a home health aide.

REVIEW QUESTIONS

*The correct answers are in **boldface**.*

1. (**c**) is correct. (a, b, d) are incorrect as they were involved in nursing in other ways.
2. (**a**) is correct as it shows caring, understanding and insight into the patient's needs. (a, b, d) are incorrect. (b) is part of the process for making a visit but does not influence trust. (c) should be done as needed as part of providing nursing care but does not influence trust. (d) reflects confidentiality requirements but others may be included with patient's permission such as family members as well as other health care team members involved in the patient's care.
3. (**d, e, f**) are correct and are general safety measures for any person who is ambulating. (a, b) are incorrect as the patient may need to get out of bed or ambulate when others are not there— the means to do so safely should be provided. (c) is not a skilled nursing function. If there are concerns with housekeeping, it can be discussed with family and possibly addressed with other services.
4. (**d**) is correct as the spouse is the caregiver. (a, b, c) are incorrect as they do not relate to the caregiver.
5. (**b**) is correct. (a, c, d) are incorrect as they promote the risk of infection.
6. **0.8 mL** is correct.
7. (**b, c, d, e**) are correct to promote learning. (a) is incorrect as information should be provided in brief, organized concepts to allow learning and retention.
8. (**d**) is correct. (a, b, c) are incorrect as the patient is in control in the home environment.
9. (**a**) is correct so that the RN can perform an assessment and determine an appropriate plan of action. (b, d) are not correct as it is inappropriate to direct the patient as to what to do in the patient's own home and washing the dishes is not the LPN's function. (c) is not correct as this is an assumption that may not be true and requires assessment by the RN.

10. (**a, c, e**) are correct. (b) is not usually possible, so a time range should be given. (d) is not done for safety but so that the nurse's car is not blocked in.

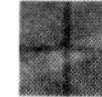

CHAPTER 16

VOCABULARY

Fill in the blank.

1. living wills
2. durable power of attorney
3. hospice
4. postmortem care
5. advocate

TRUE OR FALSE?

1. False, they usually lose weight.
2. False, most companies provide a hospice benefit.
3. True
4. True
5. False, they will only be discharged if they are no longer terminal.
6. True
7. False, CPR must be started within 3 to 5 minutes.
8. True
9. True
10. False, weight loss and functional decline are two common indicators.

CRITICAL THINKING

Dyspnea: *Administer morphine, administer oxygen, elevate head of bed, place a fan in the room, provide massage and muscle relaxation.*

Bowel and bladder incontinence: *Keep perineal area clean, change diapers often.*

Copious oral secretions: *Adjust patient's head so secretions go down throat, place humidifier in room, administer hyoscyamine or scopolamine, administer low-dose morphine, suction.*

Body temperature changes: *Administer Tylenol, change clothing as needed, provide warm blankets, change bedclothes and bed linens as needed.*

Restlessness: *Assess for discomfort, assess for urinary retention or fecal impaction, assess for medication toxicity, reposition in bed, administer oxygen.*

REVIEW QUESTIONS

*The correct answers are in **boldface**.*

1. (**b**) is correct. (a and d) are not associated with tube feeding. (c) could occur, but was not shown with research.
2. (**b**) is correct. (a and d) are also effects of morphine, but are not the reason it is given to a dying patient. (c) morphine will not affect temperature.

3. (**b**) is correct. (a, c, and d) may also be necessary steps, but allowing the family time to spend with the patient (and having the patient look presentable) is the most important.
4. (**c**) is correct. (a) redirecting a patient is appropriate if he is expected to improve; (b) the medications may play a part but this statement does not help the family; (d) oxygen may be used for comfort, but may not improve the thought processes of a dying patient.
5. (**a**) is correct, and is a therapeutic response. (b, c, and d) help the staff or other patients, but do not help the family.
6. (**d**) is correct, and validates the wife's feelings. This may help her make a decision. (a) may be appropriate if she needs clarification, but is not the best response while she is upset. (b and c) may be true, but do not address her feelings of upset.
7. (**d**) is correct. (a, b, and c) are important, but do not address the specific circumstance of home resuscitation.
8. (**c**) is correct. (a, b, and d) are good questions, but do not assess the patient's understanding.
9. (**b**) is correct. Cultural traditions should be supported if at all possible. (a, c, and d) are incorrect—they ignore the importance of the family's cultural tradition.

CHAPTER 17

STRUCTURES OF THE IMMUNE SYSTEM

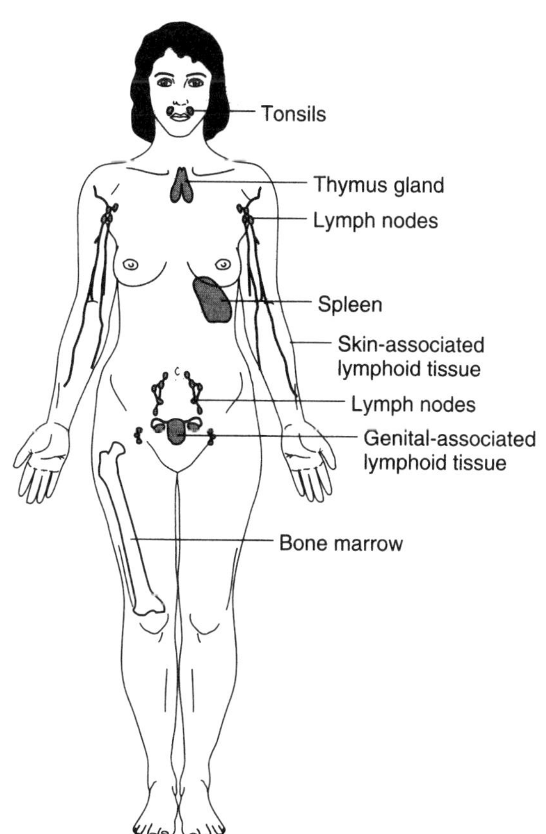

IMMUNE SYSTEM CELLS

1. (D)   5. (C)
2. (G)   6. (A)
3. (E)   7. (F)
4. (B)

ANTIBODIES

1. IgA
2. IgG
3. IgD
4. IgE
5. IgG
6. IgA
7. IgM

VOCABULARY

1. Antigens
2. Immunity
3. Natural killer cells, T cells, B cells
4. T cells (or T lymphocytes)
5. Immunoglobulins
6. Cell mediated
7. Naturally acquired active
8. IgG
9. Inflammation
10. Neutrophils

IMMUNE SYSTEM

1. (G)   5. (B)
2. (D)   6. (H)
3. (E)   7. (C)
4. (A)   8. (F)

NURSING ASSESSMENT—SUBJECTIVE (HISTORY)

*Corrections are in **boldface.***

Demographic Data

The patient's age, gender, race, and ethnic background are important. Systemic lupus erythematosus affects **women** eight times more frequently than **men.** The patient's place of birth gives insight to ethnic ties. Where the patient has lived and does live may shed light on the current illness. The patient's occupation, such as that of a coal miner, may contribute to **respiratory** symptoms.

Common signs and symptoms found with immune system disorders include fever, fatigue, joint pain, swollen glands, **weight loss,** and skin rash.

History

Food, medication, and environmental allergies should include those that the patient experiences and those present in the family history. With a family history a previous exposure to a substance is **not** required before a severe reaction occurs. Conditions such as systemic lupus erythematosus, ankylosing spondylitis, and asthma are thought to be either familial or have a **genetic** predisposition. If the patient's thymus gland has been removed (thymectomy), **T**-cell production may be altered. Corticosteroids and immunosuppressants **alter** the immune response. The patient's lifestyle may place the patient at **high** risk for contracting the human immunodeficiency virus. The patient's diet and usage of vitamins give insight into the **reserve** of the immune system. Stress (environmental, physical, and psychological) can **depress** immune system function.

CRITICAL THINKING

1. Demographic data (age, gender, race and ethnic background, place of birth, place of residence, occupation [past and present]); patient history (blood transfusions, high-risk behaviors, allergies [drug, food, environmental], surgeries, diagnosed medical conditions [past, present]); physical (general appearance, cardiovascular, skin, mucous membranes, respiratory, gastrointestinal, renal, musculoskeletal, nervous).
2. Normal lymph nodes are not palpable. Nodes that are nontender, hard, fixed, and enlarged are frequently associated with cancer.
3. If cancer is suspected: recent weight loss, occupational exposures, any high-risk lifestyle behaviors such as smoking, sexual patterns, previous medical history, and family history.

REVIEW QUESTIONS

*The correct answers are in **boldface.***

1. (a)   7. (d)
2. (b)   8. (c)
3. (b)   9. (c)
4. (a)   10. (a)
5. (b)   11. (b)
6. (b)   12. (c)

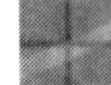 ## CHAPTER 18

VOCABULARY

1. (J)   9. (B)
2. (K)   10. (D)
3. (H)   11. (F)
4. (M)   12. (G)
5. (C)   13. (O)
6. (I)   14. (A)
7. (P)   15. (E)
8. (N)   16. (L)

IMMUNE DISORDERS

1. Type I, type II, type III, type IV
2. Hay fever
3. Sinusitis, nasal polyps, asthma, chronic bronchitis
4. Infection
5. Epinephrine
6. Hives
7. is less pruritic, has more diffuse edema, may last longer
8. Coombs' test
9. Shock, renal failure
10. Penicillins, sulfonamides
11. MSG, bisulfates
12. Poison ivy (or oak)
13. Vitamin B_{12}
14. Erythrocytopheresis
15. Sacroiliac, costovertebral, large peripheral

IMMUNE WORD SEARCH SOLUTION

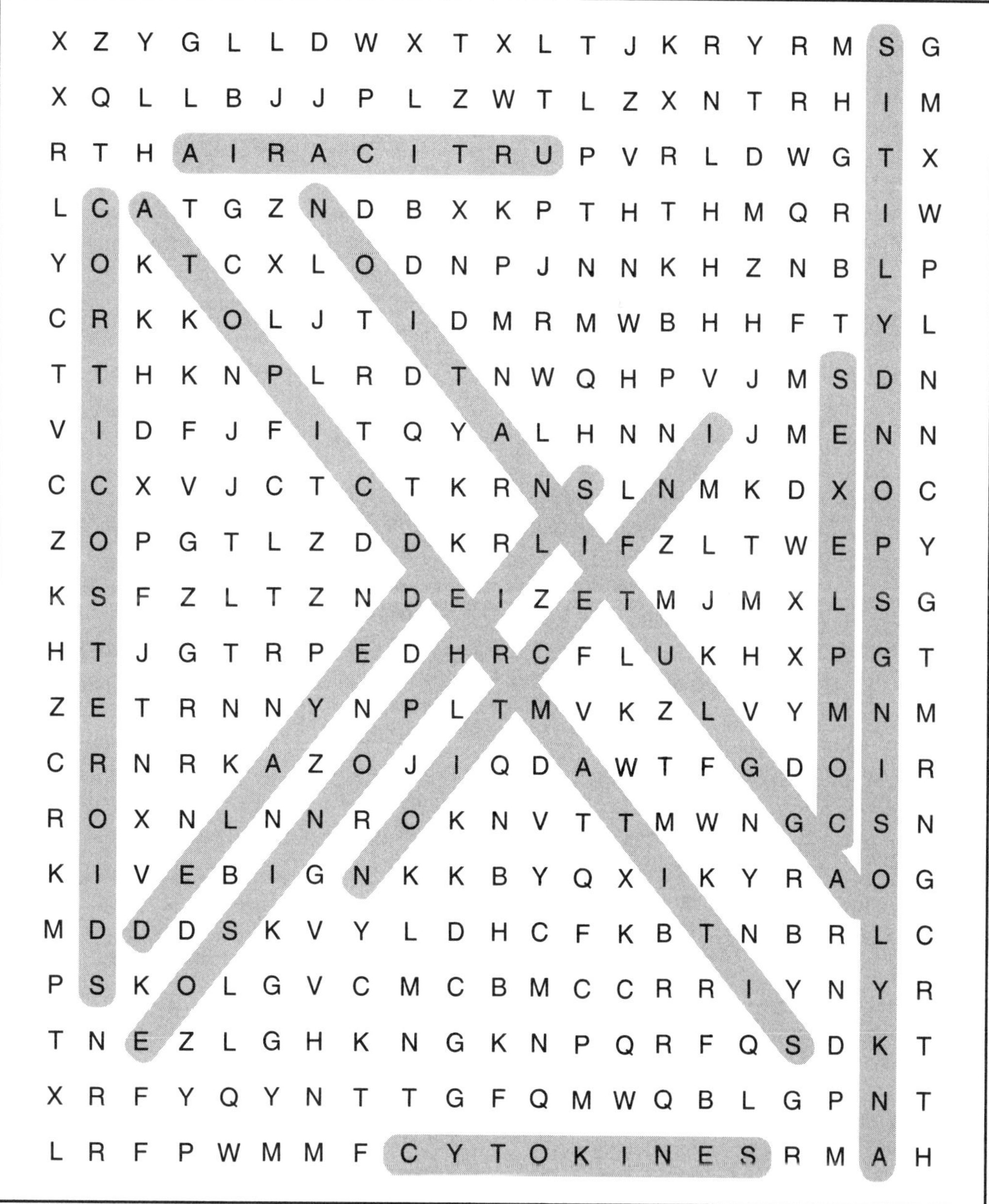

IMMUNE DISORDERS PUZZLE SOLUTION

Across	Down
1. Pernicious	1. Penicillins
3. Fifteen	2. Obstruction
6. Anaphylaxis	4. Epinephrine
8. Humoral	5. Fatique
9. Monocytes	7. Hypogammaglobulinemia
13. Hypothyroidism	10. Sacroiliac
15. Nasal polyps	11. Mast cells
17. Angioedema	12. Latex allergy
19. Intrinsic factor	14. Autoimmunity
20. Steroids	16. Allergen
21. Butterfly	18. Stress
22. Discoid	

REVIEW QUESTIONS

*The correct answers are in **boldface**.*

1. (**a**) An infection can develop if treatment is not followed. (b, c, d) are incorrect.
2. (**c**) The physician must be informed to determine if the medication should be given. It is not within the nurse's scope of practice to make that decision. (a, b, d) are incorrect.
3. (**d**) The antibiotic, which is the cause of the problem, should be stopped immediately so that no more medication enters patient. (a, b) would be done next or as the antibiotic is stopped if assistance is available. (c) is incorrect.
4. (**d**) Respiratory distress with wheezing occurs in anaphylaxis. (a, b, c) are incorrect.
5. (**a**) Epinephrine is the initial treatment for anaphylaxis. (b, c, d) are incorrect.
6. (**a**) Red blood cells are destroyed by this condition, so red cell fragments would be present. (b, c, d) are incorrect.
7. (**b**) When a portion of the stomach is removed, intrinsic factor, which is necessary for the absorption of vitamin B_{12}, is reduced. Patients must have lifelong vitamin B_{12} to prevent pernicious anemia from developing.
8. (**b**) is correct. (a, c, d) are incorrect.
9. (**d**) is correct. (a, b, c) are incorrect.
10. (**c, e, f**) Respiratory distress with stridor, dyspnea occurs in anaphylaxis. Tachycardia occurs as a compensatory mechanism. (a, b, d) are incorrect.
11. (**b**) Opening windows will allow pollen to enter the car. (a, c, d) will control the allergy.
12. (**d**) is correct. (a, b, c) are incorrect.
13. (**a**) is correct. (b, c, d) are incorrect.
14. (**b**) is correct. (a, c, d) are incorrect.

CHAPTER 19

VOCABULARY

1. Acquired immune deficiency syndrome (AIDS)
2. $CD4^+$ cell
3. Enzyme-linked immunosorbent assay (ELISA)
4. Opportunistic infections
5. Human immunodeficiency virus (HIV) wasting syndrome
6. Viral load

DIAGNOSTIC TESTS

1. ELISA test: the typical HIV diagnostic tests and testing pattern include the following:
   A. ELISA test is done to detect antibodies to HIV antigen on test plates.
   B. If positive, the ELISA test is repeated.
   C. If the ELISA test is again positive, another test, often the Western blot, is done for confirmation.
   D. If all test results are positive, the patient is HIV-antibody positive.
   E. Other tests can be used, especially if initial test results are not conclusive. It is important that the patient be counseled before and after the ELISA test is done. Patients need to be instructed on safe-sex practices, resources, and support systems.
2. Viral load: measures the amount of HIV RNA in plasma and is extremely important for determining prognosis and monitoring the response to antiretroviral therapy. Viral loads should be preformed at diagnosis, 1 month after initiation of new treatments, and at 3–4-month intervals thereafter.
3. $CD4^+$ cell count: is essential for evaluating the status of the immune system. In healthy adults, levels average approximately 600 to $1400/mm^3$. It is recommended that $CD4^+$ cell counts be performed at 4-month intervals for most patients.

HIV

1. Blood, semen, vaginal secretions, and breast milk
2. Many
3. Early
4. Women

HIV AND AIDS

1. True
2. False—end stage of HIV infection is AIDS
3. False—anyone may contract HIV if exposure occurs
4. True

5. False—an incubation period occurs following exposure, so testing 1 to 2 days later would be inconclusive; antigens are detectable 2 weeks after infection with the virus
6. False—standard precautions are used with all patients, so isolation is not routinely necessary for patients with AIDS unless ordered for special reasons

CRITICAL THINKING

1. The patient is told that he is HIV positive but does not have AIDS at this time. With treatment, HIV is considered a chronic condition that may not develop into AIDS for many years. If AIDS develops, there is currently no cure, but it is treatable in most cases.
2. CD4$^+$ T-cell count of less than 200/mL and/or the presence of 1 of 25 clinical conditions. These conditions are often opportunistic infections or cancers.
3. To prevent *Pneumocystis carnii* pneumonia (PCP) and toxoplasmosis opportunistic infections from developing.
4. (a) Candidiasis, medications, and peripheral and central nervous system disease tend to decrease the senses of taste and smell. This, along with discomfort, anorexia, and fatigue, predisposes the patient with AIDS to nutritional deficiencies. (b) Medicated swish and swallows, topical anesthetic sprays, and flavor enhancers may promote an increased food intake.
5. It occurs from encephalopathy caused by direct infection of brain tissue by HIV.

6. Bodily secretions of infected person coming in contact with recipient's blood through a break in the skin.
7. The recommended disinfectant is household bleach in a 1:10 dilution mixture. This needs to be prepared within 24 hours of use. Use it to (a) clean toilet seats and bathroom fixtures; (b) clean inside the refrigerator to avoid growth of mold; and (c) wash clothing separately that is soiled with blood, urine, feces, or semen. Dishes are washed normally in hot soapy water and rinsed thoroughly after use.

REVIEW QUESTIONS

*The correct answers are in **boldface.***

1. (**c, d, e**) are correct. (a, b) are incorrect.
2. (**d**) is correct. (a, b, c) are incorrect.
3. (**a**) is correct. (b, c, d) are incorrect.
4. (**d**) is correct. (a, b, c) are incorrect.
5. (**c**) is correct. (a, b, d) are incorrect.
6. (**b**) is correct. Fruits and vegetables increase bowel function. (a, c, d) are incorrect.
7. (**a**) is correct. (b, c, d) are incorrect.
8. (**d**) is correct. (a, b, c) are incorrect.
9. (**b**) is correct. Cooked vegetables are safer. (a, c, d) are incorrect because they contain raw foods, which are riskier for infection.
10. (**b**) is correct. Standard precautions are used for all patients. (a, c, d) are incorrect.

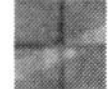

CHAPTER 20

STRUCTURES OF THE CARDIOVASCULAR SYSTEM

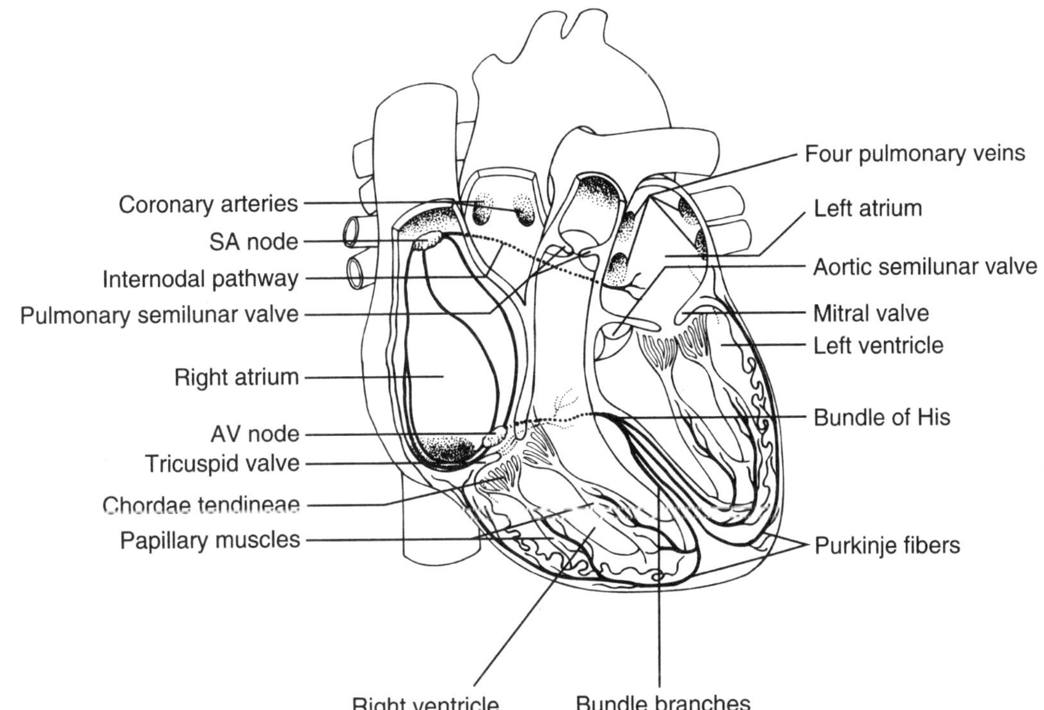

CARDIAC BLOOD FLOW

A. 14	H. 7
B. 10	I. 12
C. 1	J. 8
D. 3	K. 9
E. 13	L. 11
F. 6	M. 2
G. 5	N. 4

AGING AND THE CARDIOVASCULAR SYSTEM

*Corrections are in **boldface**.*

It is believed that the "aging" of blood vessels, especially arteries, begins in **childhood.** Average resting blood pressure tends to **increase** with age and may contribute to stroke or **left**-sided heart failure. The **thinner**-walled veins, especially those of the legs, may also weaken and stretch, making their valves incompetent. With age, the heart **muscle** becomes less efficient, and there is a **decrease** in both maximum cardiac output and heart rate. The health of the myocardium depends on **its** blood supply. Hypertension causes the **left** ventricle to work harder, so it may **hypertro-phy.** The heart valves may become **thickened by** fibrosis, leading to heart murmurs. Dysrhythmias become more common in the elderly as the cells of the conduction pathway become **less** efficient.

CARDIOVASCULAR SYSTEM

1. cardiovascular system
2. heart's
3. vascular system, capillaries
4. stiffen
5. lubb, diastole
6. absent, normal
7. cardiac, catheterization
8. peripheral, pain, poikilothermia
9. vascular, venography

ACUTE CARDIOVASCULAR NURSING ASSESSMENT

1. Allergies
2. Smoking
3. Pain
4. Weight gain
5. Crackles
6. Dizziness
7. Fatigue
8. Pink-tinged sputum

CRITICAL THINKING: SUGGESTED ANSWERS

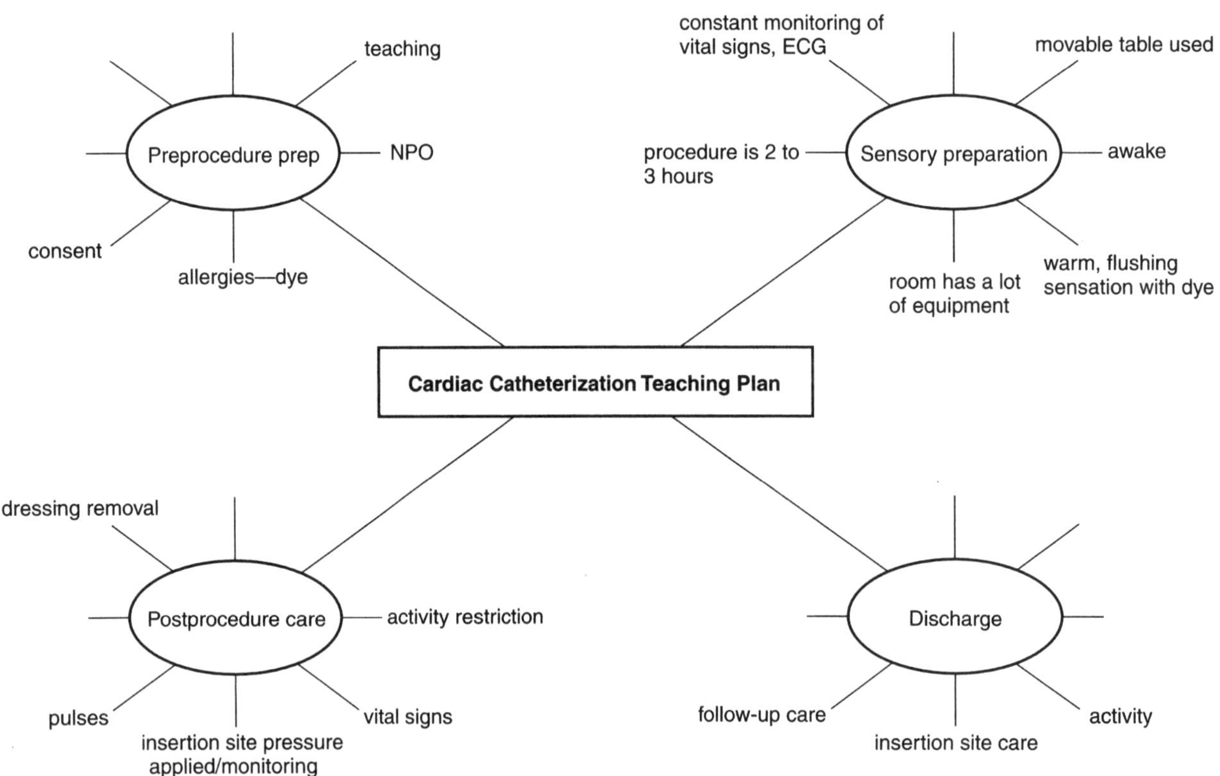

REVIEW QUESTIONS

*The correct answers are in **boldface**.*

1. **(a)**
2. **(b)**
3. **(c)**
4. **(d)**
5. **(a)**
6. **(d)**
7. **(a)** The leg reading is 10 mm Hg higher. (b, c, d) are incorrect.
8. **(b)** is the arm with the higher reading, which is what should be used. (a) The reading is lower. (c) It is not as practical to use the leg because the higher reading arm is available, although the leg could be used. (d) The arm with the lower reading should not be used.
9. **(a)** is correct. (b, c, d) are incorrect.
10. **(c)** It normally increases to compensate for the position change. (a, b) It does not drop. (d) This indicates orthostatic hypotension.
11. **(b)** Reduced blood supply results in a lack of oxygen and nutrients that contribute to the signs seen. (a, c, d) are incorrect.
12. **(b)** Medication is used in lieu of exercise when the patient cannot tolerate exercise to simulate the increased blood flow that would occur with exercise. (a, c, d) are incorrect.
13. **(d, e)** Third-degree heart block that interferes with normal heart rate and symptomatic bradycardia can be treated with a pacemaker. (a, b, c) are not usually treated with a permanent pacemaker.

CHAPTER 21

VOCABULARY

1. **(A)**
2. **(G)**
3. **(F)**
4. **(E)**
5. **(D)**
6. **(C)**
7. **(B)**
8. **(K)**
9. **(J)**
10. **(I)**
11. **(H)**

DIURETICS

1. **(C)**
2. **(B)**
3. **(A)**
4. **(C)**
5. **(B)**
6. **(C)**
7. **(A)**
8. **(A)**
9. **(B)**

HYPERTENSION RISK FACTORS

1. False
2. True
3. False
4. True
5. False

STAGES OF HYPERTENSION AND RECOMMENDATIONS FOR FOLLOW-UP

1. False—1 year
2. True
3. True
4. False—1 month
5. True
6. False—2 months
7. True
8. False—1 month
9. True
10. True

CRITICAL THINKING

1. Weight, smoking history, diet and salt intake, alcohol use, exercise patterns, life roles, finances, knowledge base. Feedback: 5 feet 4 inches, 156 lb; does not smoke or use alcohol; salts food liberally, eats three meals and snacks, moderate fat intake; walks when time permits; deals with issues as they come, which is often in her roles as wife and mother to three children; has no prescription insurance coverage; knows very little about hypertension.
2. Individualized teaching plan for Mrs. Martin's needs should include addressing knowledge deficits through teaching according to protocols for weight management, diet and salt intake, exercise importance and medications.
3. Provide information regarding the importance of controlling her hypertension; financial assessment to ensure that she has a funding source to buy medication because she may need lifelong medication.
4. Blood pressure readings on follow-up visits are within normal limits with medication.

REVIEW QUESTIONS

*The correct answers are in **boldface**.*

1. **(b, c, d)** are modifiable risk factors for hypertension. (a, e) Race and age are nonmodifiable risk factors.
2. **(c)** Isolated systolic hypertension has been found in the elderly population when the systolic blood pressure is 140 mm Hg or more but the diastolic blood pressure is less than 90 mm Hg. (a) Primary hypertension is the result of unknown causes. (b) Secondary hypertension has an identifiable cause. (d) Hypertension emergency is blood pressure >180 mm Hg systolic or >120 mm Hg diastolic complicated by risk for or progression of target organ dysfunction.
3. **(b)** *Hypertension* is defined as a blood pressure of more than 140/90 on two separate occasions. (a) Blood pressure measurement is the heart contracting or systolic, as well as relaxing, or diastolic. (c) Stress, activity, and emotions may temporarily raise blood pressure. (d) Peripheral vascular resistance may help

determine blood pressure, but it does not define hypertension.

4. (**a**) Smoking is associated with a high incidence of stages 1 and 2 hypertension. (b, c) Patients who smoke may show an increase in blood pressure because nicotine vasoconstricts the blood vessels. (d) Smoking is a major risk factor for cardiovascular disease but has not been shown to cause hypertension.

5. (**d**) is correct. (a, b, c) do not have headache as a common side effect.

6. (**c**) Stage II hypertension is classified as a systolic blood pressure of ≥160 and a diastolic blood pressure of ≥100. (a) Prehypertension is systolic blood pressure 120 to 139 and/or diastolic blood pressure 80 to 89. (b) Stage I is 140 to 159/90 to 99.

7. (**c**) Medications for hypertension should be taken daily as directed. (a) Sunbathing may increase dehydration, a side effect of the drug. (b) Lifestyle modifications are to be continued with antihypertensive therapy. (d) The medication is keeping the blood pressure lowered and will have to be taken daily.

8. (**b**) Thiazide diuretics reduce the reabsorption of potassium, so patients should be monitored for signs of hypokalemia or muscle weakness. (a, c, d) Numb hands, gastrointestinal distress, and nightmares are not common side effects of metolazone.

9. (**a**) Enalapril maleate (Vasotec) inhibits the conversion of angiotensin I to angiotensin II, thereby decreasing the levels of angiotensin II, which decreases vasopressor activity and aldosterone secretion. (b, c, d) The actions of enalapril maleate (Vasotec) achieve antihypertensive effects by suppression of the renin-angiotensin-aldosterone system, but not by adjusting the fluid volume, dilating vessels, or decreasing cardiac output.

10. (**c**) Cough is the common side effect of enalapril maleate. (a, b, d) Acne, heartburn, and diarrhea are not common side effects of enalapril maleate.

11. (**b**) Propanolol (Inderal) blocks the effects of beta-adrenergic stimulation, decreasing blood pressure, cardiac output, and cardiac contractility. (a, c, d) Propanolol (Inderal) does not increase heart rate, affect fluid volume, or increase cardiac contractility.

12. (**c**) Stopping propanolol (Inderal) abruptly may cause withdrawal syndrome. (a) Propanolol (Inderal) does not affect fluid volume or electrolytes unless combined with a diuretic. (b) Gastrointestinal side effects are not common. (d) Patients are instructed to avoid prolonged standing and to make position changes slowly because they may experience hypotension.

13. (**d**) Knowledge is needed to control this chronic condition. (a) Defining characteristics of activity intolerance include abnormal electrocardiographic readings and vital signs and reports of dyspnea or fatigue. (b) Ineffective airway clearance is the state in which an individual is unable to clear secretions. (c) Impaired physical mobility is a temporary limitation of the ability to move freely, which is not the focus of care for hypertension.

14. (**c**) Although a patient may feel better after taking medication, the hypertension is well controlled but not cured. (a, b, d) Hypertension can damage the target organs if it is not controlled. Accurate statements by patients regarding complications of hypertension and lifestyle modifications may indicate that patients are well informed.

15. (**a**) The Joint National Committee (JNC) recommends regular aerobic exercise to prevent and control hypertension. (b) Smoking, even low-tar cigarettes, is a risk factor for heart disease. (c) Alcohol intake is limited to 1 oz/day by the JNC. (d) A daily multivitamin supplement has not been shown to prevent or control hypertension.

CHAPTER 22

VOCABULARY

1. chorea
2. pericarditis
3. myocarditis
4. petechiae
5. pericardiocentesis
6. cardiac tamponade
7. cardiomyopathy
8. cardiomegaly
9. myectomy
10. thrombophlebitis

INFLAMMATORY AND INFECTIOUS CARDIOVASCULAR DISORDERS

1. (**B**)
2. (**E**)
3. (**A**)
4. (**C**)
5. (**D**)

RHEUMATIC FEVER AND RHEUMATIC HEART DISEASE

*Corrections are in **boldface**.*

Rheumatic fever **is a complication of** a streptococcal infection such as a sore throat. Rheumatic fever signs and symptoms include polyarthritis, subcutaneous nodules, **chorea** with rapid, **uncontrolled** movements, carditis, fever, arthralgia, and **pneumonitis.** A throat culture diagnoses **a streptococcal infection at the time of the infection.** Rheumatic carditis can be a complication of rheumatic fever. The heart valves and their structures can be scarred and damaged. Rheumatic fever can be prevented by detecting and treating streptococcal infections promptly with **penicillin.** The signs and symptoms of a pharynx streptococcal infection include sudden sore throat, fever **of 101°F to 104°F,** chills, throat redness with exudate, sinus or ear infection, and lymph node enlargement. Nursing care focuses on relieving the patient's pain and anxiety, maintaining normal cardiac function, and educating the patient about rheumatic heart disease.

THROMBOPHLEBITIS

NURSING DIAGNOSIS
Acute Pain Related to Infection of Vein

Interventions	Rationale	Evaluation
Assess pain using rating scale such as 0 to 10.	Self-report is the most reliable indicator of pain	Does patient report pain using scale?
Provide analgesics and non-steroidal anti-inflammatory drugs (NSAIDs) as ordered.	Pain is reduced when inflammation is decreased.	Is patient's rating of pain lower after medication?
Apply warm, moist soaks.	Heat relieves pain and vasodilates, which increases circulation to reduce swelling. Moist heat penetrates more deeply.	Does patient report increased comfort with warm, moist soaks?
Maintain bed rest with leg elevation above heart level.	Elevation decreases swelling, which reduces pain.	Is swelling reduced?

NURSING DIAGNOSIS
Deficient Knowledge Related to Lack of Knowledge About Disorder and Treatment

Interventions	Rationale	Evaluation
Explain condition, symptoms, and complications.	Patient must have basic knowledge to comply with therapy.	Is patient able to verbalize knowledge taught?
Explain medications, therapies ordered, monthly lab test monitoring, and need for Medic Alert identification.	Compliance and safe use of medications are promoted with an adequate knowledge base.	Can patient explain medications, therapies, lab tests, purpose of Medic Alert identification?
Teach patient not to massage extremity.	Massage can dislodge an embolus.	Does patient avoid massaging extremity?

DIAGNOSTIC TESTS FOR INFECTIVE ENDOCARDITIS

1. (G) 5. (B)
2. (E) 6. (D)
3. (C) 7. (H)
4. (F) 8. (A)

CRITICAL THINKING

1. Enlargement of heart muscle, especially along the septum without dilation of the ventricle, which does not relax or fill easily.

2. Smaller, reduced because of decreased relaxation and size.
3. Chest x-ray.
4. It would increase contractility in a heart that does not relax easily, so filling would be decreased with even less relaxation.
5. (a) Because cardiac output is reduced, dehydration must be avoided to prevent a further decrease in cardiac output. (b) Exertion is avoided so that an increase in cardiac output, which the compromised heart is unable to provide, is not required.
6. The family will feel useful and included in the patient's care if they are taught cardiopulmonary resuscitation

(CPR). They will feel a sense of control and purpose in the event that CPR is required.

REVIEW QUESTIONS

*The correct answers are in **boldface**.*

1. (**b**) A throat culture must be done to rule out a streptococcal infection, which can lead to complications. (a, c, d) are not as essential to prevent complications.
2. (**d**) is a bacterial infection that can precede rheumatic fever. (a, b, c) are incorrect.
3. (**a**) To prevent endocarditis from recurring because of increased risk from previous heart damage. (b) is not the reason they are given. (c, d) are not prevented by antibiotics.
4. (**c**) They can cause the clot to dislodge and become an embolus. (a) They do not prevent calf swelling. (b) Preventing a life-threatening complication is the priority. (d) They do not cause a clot to form.
5. (**c**) is monitored for heparin. (a, b, d) are not monitored for heparin; b and d are monitored for warfarin (Coumadin) therapy.
6. (**a**) Vitamin K is the antidote. (b, c, d) are incorrect; d is the antidote for heparin.
7. (**b**) The desired outcome for pain is that it is satisfactorily relieved according to patient. (a) is the outcome for anxiety. (c, d) would not be appropriate for a patient with acute thrombophlebitis because bedrest is ordered.
8. (**b**) The next dose of warfarin (Coumadin) should be held until the physician is informed because prothrombin time (PT) monitors Coumadin effects and it is over high end of therapeutic range. (a) is incorrect because the PT is elevated and could cause bleeding. (c, d) are incorrect because PT does not monitor heparin.
9. (**a, e, f**) Bedrest is essential to prevent emboli development. It is OK to apply stocking to nonaffected leg to prevent venous stasis. Heat provides pain relief and increases circulation. (b, c, d) would encourage emboli development if the affected leg is involved.
10. (**b**) is above therapeutic range. (c) measures for heparin. (a) does not measure warfarin. (d) is normal.
11. (**d**) The patient is experiencing paroxysmal nocturnal dyspnea, which occurs from increased fluid returning to the heart from reclining; the fluid then builds up in the lungs. (a, b, c) are incorrect.
12. (**b**) Anorexia is a side effect of digoxin (Lanoxin). (a, c, d) are incorrect.
13. (**b**) 45 mg/60 mg × 2 mL = 90/60 = 1.5 mL. (a, c, d) are incorrect.
14. (**d**) Friction of inflamed pericardial and epicardial layers rubbing together. (a, b, c) are incorrect.

15. (**c**) Chest pain is the most common symptom, especially with deep inspiration. (a, b, d) are incorrect.

CHAPTER 23

VOCABULARY

1. (**D**)	11. (**C**)
2. (**I**)	12. (**A**)
3. (**M**)	13. (**H**)
4. (**J**)	14. (**K**)
5. (**R**)	15. (**N**)
6. (**P**)	16. (**S**)
7. (**L**)	17. (**O**)
8. (**B**)	18. (**Q**)
9. (**E**)	19. (**T**)
10. (**G**)	20. (**F**)

ATHEROSCLEROSIS

1. A fatty streak appears on the lining of an artery. This build-up of fatty deposits is known as *plaque*. Plaque has irregular, jagged edges that allow blood cells and other material to adhere to the wall of the artery. With time, this build-up can cause stenosis of the vessel, which leads to partial or total occlusion of the artery. When this occurs, the area distal to it can become ischemic due to lack of blood flow. This build-up will become calcified and harden, leading to damage of the vessel with loss of elasticity and compliance.
2. Cigarette smoking, hypertension, elevated serum cholesterol, diabetes mellitus, obesity, stress, and sedentary lifestyle.
3. Assess readiness to learn. Example for smoking: Explain what occurs when one smokes, including changes to vessels and effect on blood flow. Determine when patient craves cigarettes most, and teach patient to try a different activity to distract from smoking. Teach patient to avoid caffeine products—chocolate, cocoa, and caffeinated soft drinks. Avoid stimulants. Increasing fluid intake, especially during the first 3 days of quitting smoking, will help wash nicotine out of the system. Have patients read books instead of magazines; magazines have many cigarette ads.

MYOCARDIAL INFARCTION

*Corrections are in **boldface**.*

Myocardial infarction (MI) is the death of a portion of the **heart muscle** caused by a blockage or spasm of a coronary artery. When the patient has an MI, the affected part of the muscle becomes damaged and can no longer function properly. Ischemic injury takes **several hours** before complete necrosis and infarction take place. The ischemic process affects the subendocardial layer, which is **most** sensitive to hypoxia. Myocardial contractility is depressed, so the body attempts to compensate by triggering the **autonomic** nervous system. This causes an **increase** in myocardial oxygen demand, which further depresses the myocardium. After necrosis, the contractility function of the muscle is **permanently** lost. If treatment is initiated at the **first sign** of an MI, the area of damage can be minimized. If prolonged ischemia is allowed to take place, the size of the infarction can be quite **large.**

The area that is affected by an MI depends on which coronary artery is involved. The left anterior descending (LAD) branch of the left main coronary artery is the area that feeds the **anterior** wall. The right coronary artery (RCA) feeds the **inferior** wall and parts of the atrioventricular node and the sinoatrial node. An occlusion of the RCA leads to abnormalities of impulse conduction and formation. The left circumflex coronary artery feeds the **lateral** wall and part of the posterior wall of the heart.

Pain is the **most** common complaint. The pain **may radiate to one or both arms and shoulders, the neck, and the jaw.** The patient usually **denies** that an MI is occurring. Other symptoms may include restlessness, a feeling of impending doom, nausea, diaphoresis, and cold, clammy, ashen skin. The only symptom that might be present in the elderly patient may be a **sudden onset of shortness of breath.**

The three strong indicators of an MI are patient history, abnormal electrocardiographic (ECG) readings, and **troponin I** levels.

Initially, patients are kept on bedrest to **decrease** myocardial oxygen demand. Patients are medicated promptly when complaining of chest pain. **Morphine sulfate** is the most widely used narcotic. It helps decrease anxiety, **slows** respirations, and has a **vasodilation** effect on coronary arteries. Oxygen is given usually at **2 L/min** via nasal cannula. Nitroglycerin sublingual, topical, or by intravenous drip can also be administered. Thrombolytic therapy is a frequent option of **lysing** a clot that is occluding a coronary artery.

A nursing care plan should include factors that may contribute to **increased** cardiac workload. Changes in diet, stress reduction, regular exercise program, cessation of smoking, and following a medication schedule require extensive patient and family teaching.

PHARMACOLOGICAL TREATMENT

1. **(D)**
2. **(C)**
3. **(A)**
4. **(G)**
5. **(B)**
6. **(F)**
7. **(I)**
8. **(E)**
9. **(H)**

CRITICAL THINKING

1. **(a)** is correct.
2. Associated with arterial occlusive disease. This is pain in the calves of the lower extremities associated with activity or exercise. With poor blood supply to the muscles, they are unable to receive increased oxygen to meet the demand of increased activity. As ischemia increases, a cramping-type pain develops.
3. When activity stops, the muscle does not have the increased oxygen demand, so the pain begins to subside with rest.
4. Smoking contributes to loss of high-density lipoproteins, which are the best type to have present to decrease the risk of cardiovascular disorders. The rate of progressive damage to vessels is increased with smoking. Smoking also contributes to vasoconstriction, which leads to angina and cardiac dysrhythmias.

REVIEW QUESTIONS

*The correct answers are in **boldface.***

1. **(d)** A stress ECG demonstrates the extent to which the heart tolerates and responds to the additional demands placed on it during exercise. The heart's ability to continue adapting is related to the adequacy of blood supplied to the myocardium through the coronary arteries. If the patient develops chest pain, dangerous cardiac rhythm changes, or significantly elevated blood pressure, the diagnostic testing is stopped. (a, b, c) are incorrect.
2. **(d)** When a patient is apprehensive and afraid, the nurse should listen and encourage the patient to express his or her feelings. This can ease the mental burden and help the patient feel less overwhelmed, alone, and helpless. Listening is an active process even if the patient does most of the talking. (a) Learning is impaired during times of anxiety. (b) Avoiding the subject may indicate to the patient that the nurse does not care. (c) How others have done ignores the fact that for this person, the experience is unique.
3. **(c)** Iodine is the base for the radiopaque dye used for the arteriogram. Notify the physician if the patient is allergic to it. The physician may cancel the procedure or take other precautions, such as the administration of an antihistamine or other emergency medication. (a, b, d) are not related to the test dyes used.
4. **(a)** If nitroglycerin tablets are fresh, the patient should feel a tingling or fizzing in the mouth. Tablets usually need to be replaced about every 3 months. (b, d) Nitroglycerin tablets do not disintegrate or change color when old. (c) Aspirin smells like vinegar when it becomes old.
5. **(b)** Fresh vegetables without added salt are low in sodium. (a, c, d) are high in sodium.
6. **(c)** Pulmonary edema. These symptoms are classic signs of pulmonary edema. (a, b, d) Respiratory distress may be observed, but the frothy sputum is symptomatic of pulmonary edema.
7. **(b)** Capillary refill is normally less than 3 seconds. (a, c, d) are all symptomatic of atherosclerosis.

8. (**c**) 30%. (a, b, d) are incorrect.
9. (**c**) Lack of sufficient oxygen to the myocardium is the cause of chest pain. (a) causes wasting of heart muscle. (b) causes dysrhythmias. (d) will not cause chest pain unless oxygen supply is insufficient to meet the workload.
10. (**a, e, f**) Hypertension and diabetes can be controlled with proper diet, exercise, and medications. Smoking can be stopped. (b, c, d) cannot be changed.
11. (**b**) Coconut oil is saturated. (a, c, d) are examples of unsaturated fats.
12. (**a, b, d**) are all found with venous insufficiency. (**c**) Edema, moderate to severe, is a manifestation of venous insufficiency. (e) is not a sign of venous insufficiency but may indicate thrombophlebitis.
13. (**b**) Pain is the outstanding symptom. (c) Cramping is also a feature to a lesser extent. (a, d) Numbness and swelling are not characteristic.
14. (**b**) Arteriolar vasoconstriction. (a, c, d) are not descriptive of Raynaud's disease.

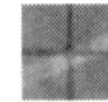 # CHAPTER 24

VOCABULARY

1. annuloplasty
2. commissurotomy
3. insufficiency
4. regurgitation
5. stenosed
6. valvuloplasty

MITRAL VALVE PROLAPSE

*Corrections are in **boldface**.*

During ventricular **systole,** when pressures in the left ventricle rise, the leaflets of the mitral valve normally remain **closed.** In mitral valve prolapse (MVP), however, the leaflets bulge backward into the left **atrium** during systole. Often there are **no** functional problems seen with MVP. However, if the leaflets do not fit together, mitral **regurgitation** can occur with varying degrees of severity.

MVP tends to be hereditary, and the cause is **unknown.** Infections that damage the mitral valve may be a contributing factor. It is the most common form of valvular heart disease and typically occurs in **women** age 20 to 55. Most patients with MVP have **no** symptoms. Symptoms that may occur include chest pain, dysrhythmias, palpitations, dizziness, and syncope.

No treatment is needed unless symptoms are present. Stimulants and caffeine should be avoided to prevent symptoms. Information on endocarditis prevention is essential.

VALVULAR DISORDERS

1. False—narrowing
2. True
3. True
4. False—allows
5. True
6. False—mitral, aortic
7. True
8. False—late
9. True
10. True
11. True
12. True
13. False—enlarges
14. True
15. False—new protocols consider antibiotics for some invasive procedures per protocols

CRITICAL THINKING

1. Aging.
2. Ask if there is a history of rheumatic fever.
3. The left ventricle increases atrial kick; the left ventricle hypertrophies to increase contractility.
4. Left ventricular failure.
5. Decreased coronary artery blood flow results from the reduced cardiac output at the same time that the left ventricular workload is increased. This imbalance in oxygen supply and demand results in angina.
6. Prophylactic antibiotics.
7. Hypertrophy is a compensatory mechanism.
8. Sudden death may occur from aortic stenosis, so the valve is replaced.

REVIEW QUESTIONS

*The correct answers are in **boldface**.*

1. (**b**) Impaired emptying of blood from the left ventricle occurs because the blood cannot easily leave the left ventricle through the narrowed aortic valve. (a) The aortic valve is narrowed. (c) Backflow of blood into the left atrium occurs with mitral regurgitation. (d) Impaired emptying of the left atrium occurs with mitral stenosis.
2. (**a**) Backflow of blood into the left atrium occurs through the mitral valve, which does not close tightly. (b, c, d) are incorrect.
3. (**c**) Ventricular hypertrophy occurs to help maintain cardiac output. (a, b, d) are incorrect.
4. (**b**) Left ventricular failure results in decreased cardiac output, which reduces oxygen to the tissues and causes fatigue. (a, c, d) are incorrect.
5. (**a**) Furosemide helps prevent pulmonary edema, a complication of decreased cardiac output and heart failure. (b, c, d) help prevent complications not related to

decreased cardiac output. (e) Potassium supplement is needed with furosemide, a potassium-wasting diuretic.

6. (**d**) Cardiac catheterization measures chamber pressures. (a, b, c) do not.

7. (**c**) The patient's goal would be to be able to verbalize knowledge of disorder. (a, b, d) are incorrect.

8. (**a**) Assessing the patient's learning priorities helps ensure that he is motivated to learn because his needs and not the nurses' needs are being met. (b, d) do not promote learning and may hinder it. (c) is not correct.

9. (**a**) Wearing Medic Alert identification is essential in case of a bleeding problem or loss of consciousness. (b) An increased intake of green leafy vegetables can counteract the effects of warfarin (Coumadin) because they contain vitamin K, the antidote for Coumadin. (c) Blood test appointments are monthly. (d) An electric razor is to be used when shaving.

10. (**a**) If the patient understands to breathe normally when moving, Valsalva's maneuver will not occur. (b, c) are incorrect. (d) results in Valsalva's maneuver.

11. (**d**) Dyspnea and coughing are indicators of heart failure because of fluid congestion in the lungs, so you would listen to lung sounds to see if crackles are present. (a, b, c) are incorrect.

CHAPTER 25

VOCABULARY

1. (**S**)	12. (**J**)
2. (**I**)	13. (**P**)
3. (**E**)	14. (**A**)
4. (**O**)	15. (**G**)
5. (**H**)	16. (**N**)
6. (**D**)	17. (**C**)
7. (**L**)	18. (**Q**)
8. (**K**)	19. (**T**)
9. (**U**)	20. (**R**)

10. (**B**)   21. (**F**)
11. (**M**)

COMPONENTS OF A CARDIAC CYCLE

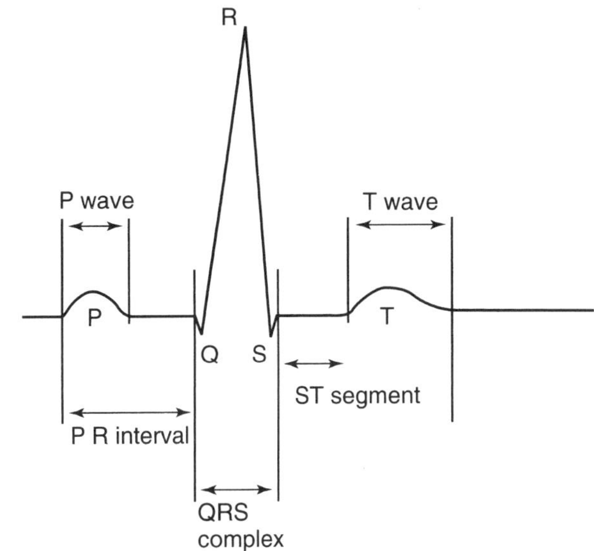

HEART RATE

1. 100
2. 110
3. 80

CARDIAC CONDUCTION

1. (**E**)	13. (**V**)
2. (**I**)	14. (**T**)
3. (**L**)	15. (**N**)
4. (**R**)	16. (**C**)
5. (**X**)	17. (**S**)
6. (**U**)	18. (**P**)
7. (**Q**)	19. (**D**)
8. (**A**)	20. (**G**)
9. (**W**)	21. (**J**)
10. (**M**)	22. (**K**)
11. (**H**)	23. (**F**)
12. (**O**)	24. (**B**)

ELECTROCARDIOGRAM INTERPRETATION

A.

1. Rhythm: Regular

2. Heart rate: 100 beats per minute

3. P waves: Smoothly rounded and upright in lead II, precede each QRS complex, alike

4. PR interval: 0.14 seconds

5. QRS interval: 0.06 seconds

6. Electrocardiogram (ECG) interpretation: Normal sinus rhythm

B.

1. Rhythm: Regular
2. Heart rate: 56 beats per minute
3. P waves: Smoothly rounded and upright, precede each QRS complex, alike
4. PR interval: 0.20 seconds
5. QRS interval: 0.08 seconds
6. ECG interpretation: Sinus bradycardia

CRITICAL THINKING

1. Assess patient: vital signs, heart sounds, note symptoms, place on heart monitor per agency protocol.
2. Report the patient findings to the registered nurse or physician. Elevate head of bed (HOB) for comfort, monitor vital signs, maintain oxygen per nasal cannula at 2 L/min per agency protocol, remain with patient to help alleviate anxiety.
3. Hypokalemia or ischemia causing irritability of the heart.
4. Lightheadedness, feel heart skipping, chest pain, or fatigue.
5. ECG, oxygen, administration of potassium, electrolyte levels, may consider antidysrhythmic agent if symptomatic.

REVIEW QUESTIONS

*The correct answers are in **boldface**.*

1. (**c**) The complete heartbeat consisting of contraction, or systole, and relaxation, or diastole, of the atria and ventricles. (a, b) The circulation of the blood is a result of the action of the cardiac cycle. (d) is the contraction portion of the cardiac cycle.
2. (**b**) Assess patient. Monitored rhythms can be deceptive. Always "treat the patient, not the monitor." (a, c, d) may be appropriate actions *after* the patient is assessed, if indicated.
3. (**c**) The superior and inferior venae cavae. (a) delivers the blood back to the left side of the heart after oxygenation in the lungs. (b) receives the blood pumped from the left ventricle into the systemic circulation. (d) is a part of the heart's own circulation.
4. (**d**) is correct. (a) controls the flow of blood from one heart chamber to another and into the pulmonary and systemic circulations. (b) is the sac covering the heart. (c) collects blood to then be pumped out of the heart into the circulation.
5. (**a**) The left ventricle is the largest chamber. (b) The right ventricle is smaller. (c, d) Both the right and the left atria are smaller than either ventricle.
6. (**d**) The T wave represents ventricular *repolarization,* or the resting state of the heart. The U wave is frequently seen in patients with hypokalemia. (b) represents ventricular depolarization. (c) represents atrial *depolarization.*

7. (**b**) 40 to 60 beats per minute is the inherent rate for the atrioventricular node. (a) is the inherent rate for the ventricles. (c) is the normal rate for the sinoatrial node. (d) is not a normal heart rate.
8. (**c**) Sinus rhythms identify the impulse as having originated in the sinoatrial node. (a) Escape beats are late beats occurring when a more rapid focus fails to initiate a beat. (b) A block occurs when the normal conduction pathway of the heart is disturbed. (d) Ectopic rhythms are abnormal beats.
9. (**b**) Digoxin (Lanoxin) slows the heart rate and increases the force of contraction. (a) To decrease ectopic beats, you would give an antiarrhythmic such as procainamide or lidocaine intravenously, or quinidine orally. (c) To relieve chest pain, you would give nitroglycerin sublingually or intravenously. (d) To raise blood pressure, you would give a vasopressor such as dopamine or dobutamine.
10. (**a**) Atrial fibrillation can cause interruptions in the movement of blood through the heart and the formation of a thrombus, with serious consequences. (b) Swelling of hands and feet, often an early sign of heart failure, could be a less serious result of atrial fibrillation. (c, d) are not the result of atrial fibrillation.
11. (**d, e**) Both are appropriate treatments for atrial fibrillation. (a) Lidocaine is not an appropriate treatment, and oxygen only for the symptoms of extremely fast or slow atrial fibrillation while correcting the dysrhythmia. (b) Nitroglycerin is not an appropriate treatment, and bedrest only to conserve energy while correcting the dysrhythmia. (c) Isuprel is not a treatment for atrial fibrillation.
12. (**a**) Three or more premature ventricular contractions (PVCs) in a row constitute ventricular tachycardia. (b) Bigeminy is a PVC every second beat. (c) Trigeminy is a PVC every three beats. (d) Multifocal PVCs are PVCs arising from different foci in the ventricle and therefore vary in appearance.
13. (**d**) In a hemodynamically stable patient, treatment with medication is the first choice. (a) Cardioversion would be tried only if other measures did not work. (b) Pacing is seldom an option for this. (c) Defibrillation is not appropriate treatment.
14. (**c**) is the correct answer. (a) is the name of the rhythm

of a dying heart with wide QRS complex and slowing irregular rate. (b) is a pattern with no ventricular activity. (d) is the absence of a firing mechanism in the sinus node.

15. (**c**) Elevate the head of the bed and start oxygen by nasal cannula to improve oxygenation because oxygen hunger is a common cause of heart irritability per agency policy. (a) An ECG is next after the previously stated actions. (b) Call the physician next. (d) is not an appropriate action; in fact, it would likely cause harm by compromising breathing by pressure of the diaphragm on the heart and lungs.

 CHAPTER 26

VOCABULARY

1. Pulmonary edema (acute heart failure)
2. Cor pulmonale
3. splenomegaly, hepatomegaly
4. peripheral vascular resistance
5. Paroxysmal nocturnal dyspnea
6. preload
7. afterload
8. Orthopnea

FLUID ACCUMULATION PATTERNS

Left-sided Heart Failure

Left ventricle → left atrium → pulmonary veins → lungs

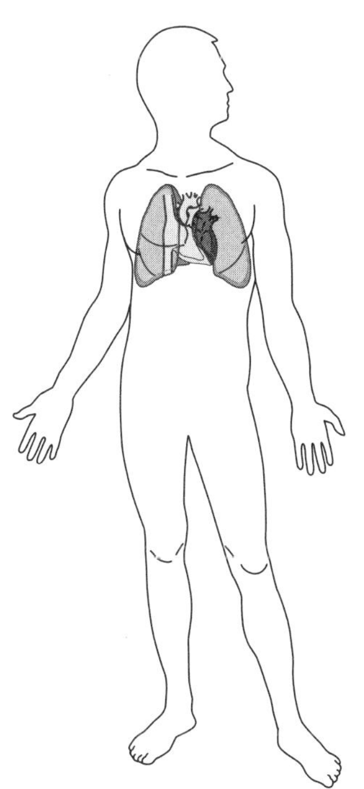

Right-sided Heart Failure

Right ventricle → right atrium → vena cavae → jugular vein distention → hepatomegaly → splenomegaly → peripheral edema

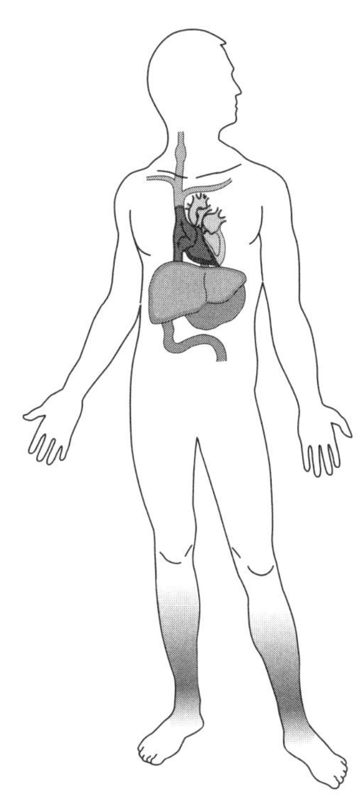

SIGNS AND SYMPTOMS OF HEART FAILURE

1. (**L**)
2. (**R**)
3. (**L**)
4. (**R**)
5. (**R**)
6. (**L**)
7. (**R**)
8. (**L**)

CRITICAL THINKING

1. Left-sided heart failure leading to backward fluid accumulation in lung tissues and decreased cardiac output.
2. Left: dyspnea, cough, crackles, orthopnea. Right: jugular vein distention, peripheral edema.
3. (a) Potent diuretic to reduce fluid congestion and fluid returning to the heart (preload) to improve cardiac output. (b) Positive inotropic agent to strengthen heart's contraction. It also slows the heart rate, allowing better emptying of the ventricle. Cardiac output is increased. (c) Restricting sodium may reduce fluid volume and aid in reducing edema. (d) Provides greater availability of oxygen to the tissues by increasing the percentage of oxygen in inhaled air.
4. Mr. Donner is experiencing acute heart failure—pulmonary edema. Fluid accumulation in his lungs is severe and requires immediate treatment.
5. (a) Decreases fluid returning to the heart (preload) to ease the heart's workload and improve cardiac output. (b) Provides greater availability of oxygen in inhaled

air. (c) Potent diuretic; when given intravenously (IV) has a quicker onset of action to reduce the amount of fluid congestion and fluid returning to the heart to improve cardiac output. (d) Positive inotropic agent given to strengthen the heart's contraction. (e) Sedative action reduces anxiety, and given IV, it has a quicker onset of action.

6. Excess fluid volume related to (r/t) pump failure; clear breath sounds and free of edema. Activity intolerance r/t fatigue; tolerates activity with appropriate increases in heart rate, blood pressure, and respirations. Sleep pattern disturbance r/t nocturnal dyspnea; awakens refreshed and is less fatigued during day. Impaired gas exchange r/t pump failure; maintains clear lung fields. Anxiety r/t dyspnea; verbalizes decrease in anxiety. Self-care deficits (total) r/t fatigue and dyspnea; activities of daily living (ADLs) completed with assistance. Ineffective management of therapeutic regimen r/t lack of knowledge; states understanding of treatment plan and willingness to follow it.

7. Signs and symptoms of heart failure; medications; purpose, monitoring (heart rate, potassium), side effects; diet; energy conservation; daily weights.

REVIEW QUESTIONS

*The correct answers are in **boldface**.*

1. (**b**) Decreased cardiac output occurs with heart failure, leading to reduced oxygenation of the tissues and therefore fatigue. (a, c, d) all result from heart failure, as does fatigue. They do not cause the fatigue.

2. (**d**) The heart is failing as a pump to move blood forward. (a) occurs in cardiac arrest, (b) occurs in a myocardial infarction, (c) is the opposite of what occurs with heart failure.

3. (**c**) Fluid in the lungs is heard as crackles. (a, b, d) are related to right-sided heart failure.

4. (**a**) If fluid accumulates from heart failure, weight will increase and is detectable by daily weights. (b) would be monitored for problems with an adequate caloric intake, not a fluid problem. (c) would be monitored for the effects of digitalis toxicity. (d) would be monitored for ascites development.

5. (**c**) 0.25 mg by mouth (PO) is the usual adult daily dose of digoxin (Lanoxin). (a, b) are less than the usual daily dose of Lanoxin. (d) is greater than the usual daily dose of Lanoxin.

6. (**b**) Lanoxin increases the strength of the heart's contraction. This allows better emptying of the ventricle, which improves cardiac output and increases blood flow to the kidneys, so increased urine output occurs. (a) If urine output decreases, the Lanoxin has not improved cardiac output to increase blood flow to the kidneys. (c) Lanoxin slows the heart rate. A rapid heart rate occurs to compensate for reduced cardiac output. (d) A slow heart rate is expected with Lanoxin, but below 50 is slower than desired for effectiveness.

7. (**a**) Hypokalemia may predispose to Lanoxin toxicity. (b, c, d) do not predispose to Lanoxin toxicity.

8. (**a**) Poor appetite is a common sign of Lanoxin toxicity. (b) Diarrhea is a side effect of Lanoxin. (c) Yellow lights, not halos, are a sign of toxicity. (d) Bradycardia occurs with toxicity.

9. (**d**) Furosemide is a loop diuretic that may deplete electrolytes, especially potassium, so ongoing monitoring of potassium is necessary. (a, b, c) are not affected directly by furosemide (Lasix) and are not monitored for this therapy.

10. (**a, e**) Morphine sulfate is given to relieve the patient's anxiety caused by the dyspnea of pulmonary edema. It also reduces preload and afterload to decrease the workload of the failing heart. (b) Chest pain is usually associated with a myocardial infarction, not pulmonary edema. (c) It does not strengthen the heart's contraction. (d) It may decrease blood pressure.

11. (**d**) The right ventricle enlarges from the extra workload that occurs from the increased pulmonary pressures while ejecting blood into the pulmonary artery. (a, b, c) are not directly affected by pulmonary pressures.

12. (**c**) is a common sign of pulmonary edema. (a, b) are associated with right-sided heart failure. (d) Tachycardia occurs in pulmonary edema as a compensatory mechanism.

13. (**d**) Inotropic agents strengthen the heart's contractions. (a) An agent that slows the heart rate is a chronotropic agent. (b) An inotropic agent does not increase heart rate. (c) Conduction time is not affected by the inotropic property of a medication.

14. (**a**) Furosemide is a potent diuretic that works quickly when given IV to increase urine output. (b, c, d) are not the reasons a diuretic is given.

15. (**b**) An anxious patient is comforted by the presence of the nurse and does not want to be left alone. (a) would increase oxygen needs and increase dyspnea and anxiety. (c, d) could make the dyspneic patient feel more confined, increasing dyspnea and anxiety.

CHAPTER 27

VOCABULARY

1. Ecchymosis
2. Lymphedema
3. petechiae
4. Purpura
5. thrombocytopenia

LYMPHATIC SYSTEM

1. (**B**)   4. (**A**)
2. (**D**)   5. (**C**)
3. (**E**)

STRUCTURES OF THE LYMPHATIC SYSTEM

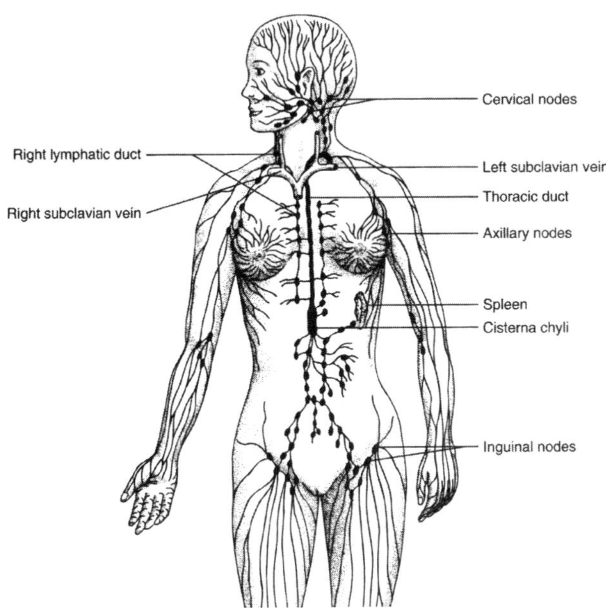

HEMATOPOIETIC SYSTEM

1. **(J)**	6. **(C)**
2. **(F)**	7. **(D)**
3. **(B)**	8. **(A)**
4. **(G)**	9. **(H)**
5. **(I)**	10. **(E)**

CRITICAL THINKING

1. Fever may indicate a febrile or hemolytic reaction. Back pain is an early symptom of hemolytic reaction. Respiratory distress may signal circulatory overload or anaphylaxis. Crackles are a symptom of circulatory overload. Hives indicate an urticarial reaction.
2. Even though 20 breaths per minute may be normal, it is an increase for Mr. Foster. A thorough assessment should be done and the registered nurse notified in case this is an early sign of a reaction.
3. The maximum time blood can hang is 4 hours from the time it is picked up from the blood bank.

REVIEW QUESTIONS

*The correct answers are in **boldface**.*

1. **(b, c, d)**
2. **(d)**
3. **(d)**
4. **(b)**
5. **(c)** is correct. The partial thromboplastin time (PTT) is monitored for heparin therapy. (a, b) are used to monitor warfarin therapy. (d) indicates platelet function.
6. **(d)** is correct. Cryoprecipitate contains clotting factors. (a, b, c) do not contain clotting factors.
7. **(b)** is correct. The international normalized ratio (INR) should be between 2 and 3; 1.6 is low. (a) The patient

is unlikely to bleed with a low INR. (c) The dose should be altered only by the physician. (d) Vitamin K might be given if the INR is prolonged.

8. **(a)** is correct. Blood flows more easily through a larger gauge needle. (b, c, d) are too small and may damage red blood cells (RBCs).
9. **(c)** is correct. The transfusion must be stopped immediately because these are symptoms of a possible deadly hemolytic reaction. (a) A physical assessment would be nice, but this is an emergency and there is not time. (b) There is no time for a pain assessment. (d) An analgesic can be administered after emergency care has stabilized the patient.
10. **(b)** is correct. A bone marrow biopsy is painful. (a) Explaining the procedure to the family should be done, but it is not as important as pain control for the patient. (c) The patient is observed for bleeding after, not before, the procedure. (d) The physician can drape the site.

CHAPTER 28

VOCABULARY

1. False	7. False
2. True	8. False
3. True	9. True
4. True	10. False
5. False	11. True
6. True	12. True

CRITICAL THINKING: LEUKEMIA

1. Mr. Frantzis is in the final stage of his disease, and he has opted for no treatment. Rehabilitation is no longer a goal. On days when he is feeling especially tired, it would be appropriate to bring him his breakfast in bed. A liquid supplement that is easy to drink might also be helpful.
2. Do a complete pain assessment using the WHAT'S UP? format. The pain might be sternal or rib tenderness from crowding of bone marrow. Administer analgesics as ordered.
3. Not all runny noses are infectious. Find out if the nursing assistant has a cold. If so, reassign Mr. Frantzis' care to another assistant because he is at risk of infection.
4. Mr. Frantzis may be developing confusion if the leukemia has invaded the central nervous system. Clarify with him who Jennifer is, and assess him for confusion (keep in mind that you may look like someone named Jennifer, and he may not be confused at all). If he is becoming confused, assess for other causes, such as medication use or oxygen saturation, and institute measures to keep him safe.
5. Provide good mouth care after each meal and as required. Use a soft toothbrush or a swab if irritation is severe. Avoid giving him foods that are irritating, acidic,

or extremely hot or cold. Remove his dentures for cleaning and at bedtime. Inspect his mouth carefully while dentures are out.

CRITICAL THINKING: HODGKIN'S DISEASE

*Corrections are in **boldface.***

Joe is a 28-year-old construction worker diagnosed with stage I Hodgkin's disease. He initially went to his physician because of a **painless** lump in his neck. He is also experiencing **low-grade fevers** and weight loss. The diagnosis was confirmed by the presence of Reed-**Sternberg** cells by the laboratory. He expresses his fears to his nurse, who tells him that **although Hodgkin's disease is a cancer,** it is often curable. Joe takes a leave from work and begins **curative** radiation therapy. (At age 28, it would be very unusual for Joe to choose palliative therapy.)

SICKLE CELL ANEMIA

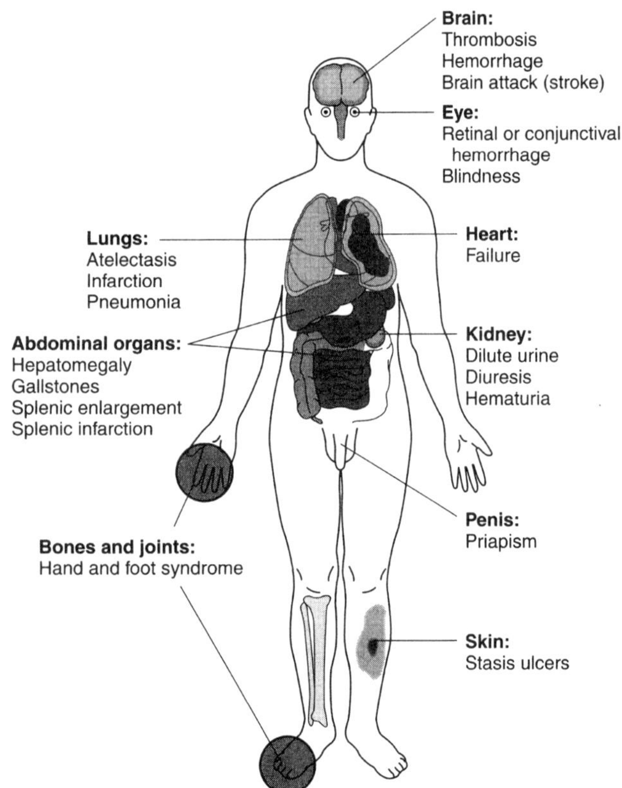

REVIEW QUESTIONS

*The correct answers are in **boldface.***

1. (**b**) is correct. Red meat is high in iron. (a, c, d) are not as high in iron.
2. (**b**) is correct. Hemoglobin carries oxygen to tissues; hemoglobin level is reduced in anemia. (a) Oxygen transport to tissues is the problem. (c) Oxygen, not nutrients, is the problem. (d) Anemia does not cause lung damage.
3. (**d**) is correct. The conjunctivae are pale in a patient with anemia. (a, b, c) are not necessarily pale in anemia, especially in a dark-skinned patient.
4. (**a**) is correct. The patient with anemia may experience palpitations as an early compensatory mechanism. (b, c, d) are later signs.
5. (**b**) is correct. Chilling and exercise may both contribute to hypoxemia and a crisis. (a, c, d) do not cause hypoxemia.
6. (**a**) is correct. Infarction of small bones in the fingers and toes causes unequal growth. (b, c, d) are not symptoms of hand-foot syndrome.
7. (**c**) is correct. The best measure of effective teaching is actual change in behavior, as evidenced by the patient using an electric razor. (a, b, d) are all good measures of learning, but they are not as convincing as the actual change in behavior.
8. (**b**) is correct. Often the patient knows best when bleeding is occurring, and treatment should be initiated as soon as possible. (a) Deep palpation may injure tissue and worsen bleeding. (c) An x-ray will waste valuable time when the patient could be receiving treatment. (d) Heat is a vasodilator and could increase bleeding. Also, waiting before beginning treatment is not recommended.
9. (**d**) is correct. Multiple myeloma attacks bone, making it prone to fractures. (a, b, c) are not directly related to multiple myeloma.
10. (**a**) is correct. Fluids help minimize complications of hypercalcemia. (b) Respiratory problems are not related to hypercalcemia. (c) Activity should be encouraged to keep calcium in the bones. (d) Heat will not affect calcium levels.
11. (**d**) is correct. Fatigue is subjective and is best described by the patient. (a, b, c) may be indirectly related to fatigue, but they rely on the nurse's interpretation.
12. (**a**) is correct. Going to church will place the patient in a crowd of people, which will increase risk of exposure to infection. (b, c, d) do not expose the patient to infection.
13. (**c**) is correct. This can assist her to identify support systems that can help her cope. (a, b) offer false reassurance. (d) is inappropriate because there is no evidence that she is terminal at this time, and it will not help her cope. It may be addressed at a time when she is coping better.
14. (**a**) is correct. Vitamin K can help correct clotting problems and prevent bleeding during surgery. (b, c, d) are not affected by vitamin K.
15. (**b**) is correct. A high incision often discourages deep breathing and coughing because of the resulting pain. This can result in infection. (a) platelet count does not increase risk of infection; (c, d) early ambulation and discharge may help prevent infection.
16. (**d**) is correct. Fever is a sign of infection. (a, b, c) are not signs of infection.
17. (**c**) is correct. Vaccines will help guard against infection. (a, b) do not help prevent infection; (d) is unnecessary.

CHAPTER 29

VOCABULARY

1. dyspnea
2. Crepitus
3. thoracentesis
4. barrel chest
5. respiratory excursion
6. adventitious
7. tracheotomy
8. tidaling
9. Apnea
10. tracheostomy

ANATOMY

1, 6, 8, 5, 2, 4, 10, 3, 7, 9, 11

VENTILATION

1, 4, 3, 6, 2, 5, 7

THE RESPIRATORY SYSTEM

ADVENTITIOUS LUNG SOUNDS

1. **(E)**   3. **(F)**   5. **(C)**
2. **(A)**   4. **(D)**   6. **(B)**

CHEST DRAINAGE

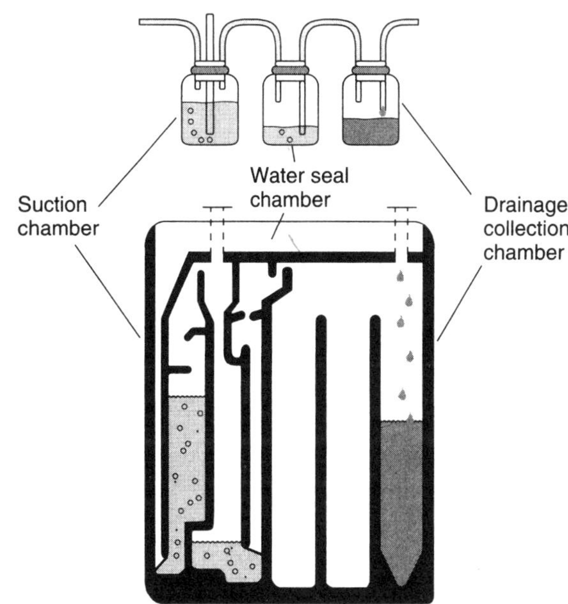

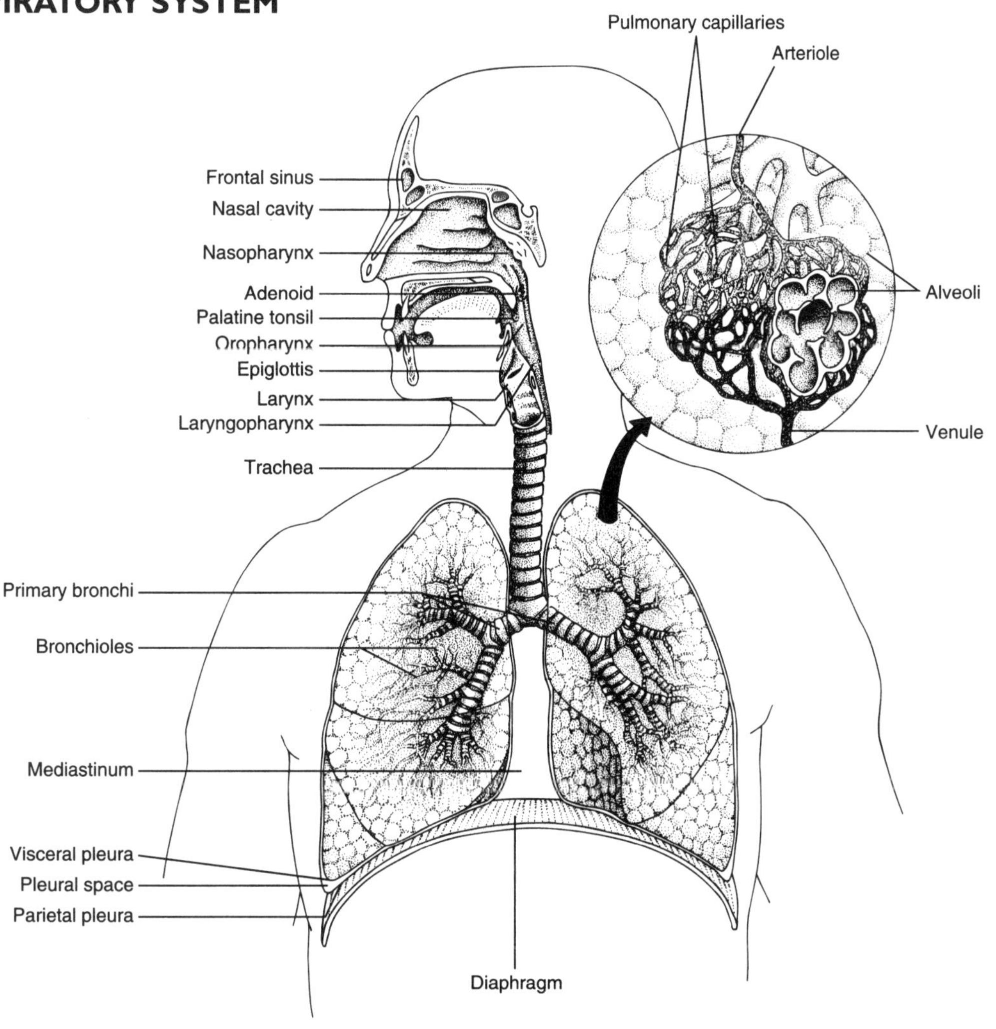

CRITICAL THINKING

1. Mr. Howe's cough should be assessed using the WHAT'S UP? technique. He should be asked how it feels, how bad it is, what makes it better or worse, and when it started. In addition, he should be asked about amount, color, odor, and consistency of sputum.
2. Night sweats, cough, and weight loss are typical symptoms of tuberculosis (TB). Bloody sputum is also common. These symptoms should alert the nurse to ask the physician about the likelihood of TB and the need for isolation to protect staff and other patients.
3. A chest x-ray and sputum culture and sensitivity will be ordered. Additional tests for TB are discussed in Chapter 31.
4. Mr. Howe should be kept NPO (nothing by mouth) according to institution policy before the bronchoscopy. An injection of atropine may be ordered to dry secretions. After the test, Mr. Howe's vital signs and respiratory status should be closely monitored. Mr. Howe will remain NPO until his gag reflex returns. The nurse should consult the physician's orders for additional postprocedure instructions.

REVIEW QUESTIONS

*The correct answers are in **boldface.***

1. (**d**) is correct.
2. (**b**) is correct.
3. (**d**) is correct.
4. (**b**) is correct.
5. (**c**) is correct.
6. (**c**) is correct. Cilia help remove potential pathogens. (a, b, d) are not affected by changes in cilia.
7. (**b**) is correct. Wheezes sound like a violin. (a) crackles sound like Velcro being pulled apart. (c) A friction rub sounds like leather rubbing together. (d) Crepitus is not an adventitious sound.
8. (**b**) is correct. The first concern is increasing oxygenation, and replacing the oxygen will help. (a, c) may be appropriate, but oxygen should be tried first. (d) 72% is not normal.
9. (**a**) is correct. Pursed-lip breathing helps excrete carbon dioxide. (b, c, d) are not promoted by pursed-lip breathing.
10. (**d**) is correct. "Good lung down" has been shown to increase oxygenation. (a, b, c) do not increase oxygenation.
11. (**a**) is correct. Assistance with cleaning the catheter two to three times a day should be provided. (b) Transtracheal oxygen usually prevents the need for another oxygen source. (c) Removal of the catheter for this length of time may cause the tract into the trachea to close. Also, if removed, another oxygen source would be needed. (d) A transtracheal catheter is not hooked to humidification.
12. (**d**) is correct. Chest physiotherapy (CPT) helps mobilize secretions. (a) CPT does not affect chest muscles. (b) CPT does not use humidification. (c) CPT does not promote expansion.
13. (**c**) is correct. Reducing the level of wall suction will reduce the bubbling. (a) Bubbling in the water-seal chamber, not the suction chamber, indicates a system leak. (b) There is no need to replace the system. (d) Increasing the water level will increase the level of suction.

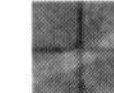 **CHAPTER 30**

VOCABULARY

1. laryngectomee
2. epistaxis
3. Exudate
4. rhinoplasty
5. dysphagia
6. Rhinitis

CRITICAL THINKING: NASAL SURGERY

1. Wake Mr. Jones and examine his throat. He may be swallowing blood. Vital signs should also be checked for signs of blood loss. Make sure that he is in semi-Fowler's position to help prevent aspiration and reduce swelling.
2. "You may need to ask your physician for an antihistamine or cough suppressant. If you must sneeze, be sure to do so with your mouth open. A stool softener and plenty of liquids and fiber can help keep your stools soft."
3. "Aspirin and related drugs such as ibuprofen can increase your risk for bleeding and should be avoided." Check with his physician to see if acetaminophen can be recommended.

CRITICAL THINKING: INFLUENZA

1. Influenza is caused by a virus. Antibiotics will not be effective. Antibiotics must be used with discretion to prevent the development of resistant strains of bacteria.
2. Fever and illness can lead to dehydration. Fluids will also help thin respiratory secretions so that they are more easily expectorated.
3. Fever may be beneficial if it is not too high. Ask the physician at what temperature she or he recommends acetaminophen. Some sources say to give it only if fever reaches above 103°F (39.4°C) or if discomfort is severe.
4. Influenza is contagious, so if symptoms are the same, it would be reasonable to provide the same care as was recommended for your son. (If any medications were

prescribed, they should not be shared.) It is probably not necessary to take her to the doctor unless additional symptoms develop or symptoms persist. A call to the physician can always be placed to be sure a visit is not recommended.

5. The elderly are more at risk for complications of influenza, especially pneumonia. She should see her physician. Tamiflu might be helpful if given within 48 hours of exposure.

REVIEW QUESTIONS

*The correct answers are in **boldface**.*

1. (**a**) is correct. Facial tenderness is a symptom of a sinus infection. (b, c, d) are not symptoms of sinus infection.
2. (**c, d, and f**) are correct. Hot moist packs can help reduce inflammation, humidity will help loosen secretions, and semi-Fowler's position helps reduce pressure. (**e**) is effective for pulmonary, not sinus, secretions; (b) is not a nursing intervention.
3. (**d**) is correct. Interventions were aimed at comfort. (a, b, c) do not evaluate effectiveness of comfort measures.
4. (**d**) is correct. Dysphagia and hoarseness are common symptoms of cancer of the larynx. (a, b, c) may possibly develop later or as complications, but they are not early symptoms.
5. (**c, d, a, b**) A patent airway is always a priority. Remember your ABCs (airway, breathing, circulation). Pain is second, because it is physiological. Physiological needs are priorities according to Maslow. Ambulation is third, because it promotes recovery. A visit from a laryngectomee is important, but acceptance of the laryngectomy would come after physiological needs.
6. (**a**) is correct. If a patient places a finger over his laryngectomy, he will cut off his air supply. (b, c, d) are all options for communication for a patient with a laryngectomy.
7. (**a**) is correct. Narcotics depress the respiratory rate and cough reflex, which would increase risk for postoperative complications. (b) Narcotics do not increase secretions; (c) they do not cause stomal edema; and (d) narcotics can be addicting, but not when they are taken for legitimate pain.
8. (**c**) is correct. Pollutants in the tracheostomy can cause infection and irritation. (a) He will be taught to suction his tracheostomy as needed. (b) This is not a therapeutic statement. (d) He, not his physician, will need to do routine tracheostomy care.
9. (**d**) is correct. A sitting position will help reduce bleeding. Leaning forward will allow the blood to drain out of the nose so that bleeding can be monitored. (a, c) Lying down increases pressure in the nose and may increase bleeding, and (b) extending the neck will allow blood to drain down the back of the throat and be swallowed, making it impossible to monitor the severity of the bleeding.
10. (**d**) is correct. Epinephrine is a vasoconstrictor. (a) Raising the blood pressure (BP) can increase bleeding. (b) It may dilate bronchioles, but this will not help bleeding. (c) Epinephrine does not enhance clotting.

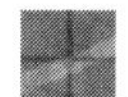 # CHAPTER 31

VOCABULARY

Across

3. ARDS (acute respiratory distress syndrome)
4. Paradoxical
7. Hemoptysis
9. MDI (metered dose inhaler)
10. Mucous
13. Thoracotomy
18. NMT (nebulized mist treatment)
20. Pleurodesis
21. Bleb
22. TB

Down

1. AP (anteroposterior)
2. Ectopic
3. Antitussive
5. Adjuvant
6. ABG (arterial blood gases)
8. Anergy
11. Status
12. Exudate
14. Hemothorax
15. Tachypnea
16. Induration
17. Risk
19. SOB (shortness of breadth)

RESPIRATORY MEDICATIONS

1. (**B**)   5. (**A**)
2. (**D**)   6. (**C**)
3. (**E**)   7. (**G**)
4. (**F**)

CRITICAL THINKING

1. A complete respiratory assessment should be completed. Edith's respiratory symptoms can be assessed using the WHAT'S UP? format. Rate degree of dyspnea on a scale of 0 to 10. Auscultate lung sounds and assess activity tolerance. Note skin color and ask about cough and sputum.

2. A 48–pack-year history can mean two packs a day for 24 years, or three packs a day for 16 years, and so on. Multiply packs per day by number of years for pack-years.
3. Emphysema causes destruction of alveolar membranes and adjacent capillaries, reducing the surface area available for gas exchange. Reduced gas exchange results in hypoxia, which causes dyspnea.
4. Edith's lung sounds will most likely sound diminished.
5. Edith probably has a chronically high P_{CO_2}, making a low P_{O_2} her stimulus to breathe. If a high flow rate of oxygen is administered, it will reduce her stimulus to breathe.
6. Emphysema increases the risk for occurrence of bullae and blebs. Rupture of these can cause pneumothorax.
7. Fowler's, semi-Fowler's, or orthopneic (leaning over bedside table) position increases room for lung expansion and helps reduce dyspnea. Sitting in a chair may also help if it is not too tiring.
8. Edith has probably had many lectures on the evils of smoking. Assess her desire to quit, and her knowledge of the relationship between her illness and her smoking. If she is willing, ask her physician for an order for nicotine patches and medication, and she can be referred to a local stop-smoking program (check yellow pages). Assist her to identify a friend who has quit smoking for support.

REVIEW QUESTIONS

*The correct answers are in **boldface**.*

1. (**a**) is correct; 86% is low, and the patient would benefit from supplemental oxygen. (b) 86% is not normal. (c) 86% does not warrant emergency treatment unless additional symptoms are present. (d) Walking in the hall will further reduce his S_{aO_2}.
2. (**a**) is correct. A bronchoscopy is an endoscopic procedure. (b, c, d) A bronchoscopy does not involve dyes or x-rays.
3. (**d**) is correct. The patient's throat will have been numbed and irritated by the scope. A gag reflex must be present before he can safely eat. (a) Breakfast should be held until the gag reflex returns. (b) There is no dye. (c) The patient did not receive a general anesthesia. Any sedation given should be gone before he returns to his room.
4. (**b, c, d, f**) are correct; all have been shown to increase risk. (a, e) do not increase cancer risk.
5. (**b**) is correct. Radiation for lung cancer is palliative. (a) Surgery is the treatment for cure. (c) He will probably require oxygen eventually. (d) Treatment may slow the spread but will probably not totally prevent it.
6. (**a**) is correct. Airways are inflamed and spastic in asthma. (b) Asthma does not cause fluid collection. (c) Asthma constricts rather than stretches airways.

(d) Asthma is not caused by infection, although infection may exacerbate it.
7. (**b**) is correct. Emphysema destroys alveoli, causing loss of elasticity and air trapping. (a) Inflammation and secretions are more characteristic of bronchitis. (c) Capillaries are damaged in emphysema, but the entire blood supply is not destroyed. (d) Large sacs of sputum are not present in emphysema.
8. (**d**) is correct. Corticosteroids have potent anti-inflammatory action. (a, b, c) are not affected by corticosteroids.
9. (**a**) is correct; 2 L/min is the maximum rate for patients with chronic respiratory disease. (b, c, d) are too high and may reduce respiratory drive.
10. (**c**) is correct. Intravenous morphine can reduce acute dyspnea. (a) Cortisone is slower acting. (b) Meperidine (Demerol) will not help. (d) A beta blocker may worsen dyspnea.
11. (**b**) is correct. It is the only placement that keeps the system below the patient's chest. (a, c, d) all risk having the system above the patient's chest, which can cause return of drainage to the chest.
12. (**a**) is correct. Bubbling in the water-seal chamber indicates an air leak. (b) will reduce bubbling in the suction-control chamber. (c) Vigorous bubbling is not expected in the water-seal chamber. (d) Asking the patient to cough will not correct the problem.
13. (**b**) is correct. Auscultating lung sounds will help determine whether the lung is re-expanding. (a, c, d) may all be appropriate, but they do not monitor whether the chest-drainage system is effectively reducing the pneumothorax.
14. (**a**) is correct. Smoking is a major risk factor for many kinds of lung disease. (b, c, d) are risk factors for a variety of problems, but they are not as significant as smoking in causing lung disease.

CHAPTER 32

FUNCTIONS OF THE GASTROINTESTINAL SYSTEM

1. lower esophageal
2. ileocecal
3. pyloric
4. small
5. stomach
6. large
7. small
8. esophagus
9. external anal
10. salivary
11. teeth, tongue
12. villi
13. rectum

STRUCTURES OF THE GASTROINTESTINAL SYSTEM

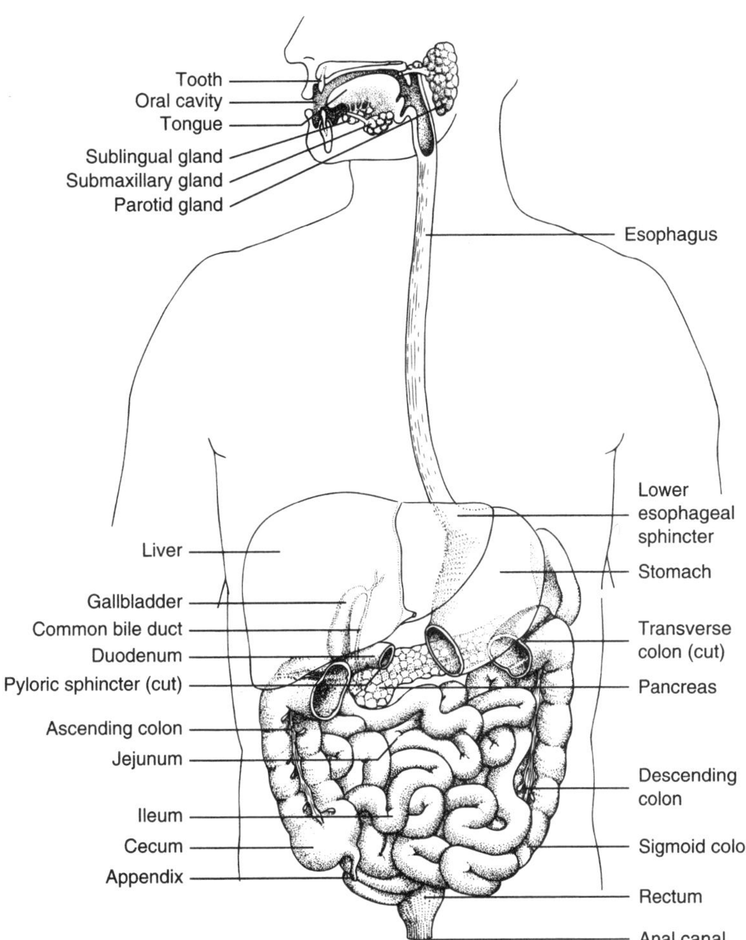

VOCABULARY

1. endoscope
2. bowel sounds
3. colonoscopy
4. gavage
5. impaction
6. guaiac
7. fluoroscope
8. steatorrhea
9. gastric analysis
10. gastroscopy

LABORATORY TESTS

1. (**E**)   4. (**A**)
2. (**D**)   5. (**C**)
3. (**B**)

BOWEL PREPARATION

Corrections are in **boldface.**

A **bowel** preparation is required for several procedures that visualize the lower bowel. This preparation is important for effective test results. An incomplete bowel preparation may prevent the test from being done or cause the need for it to be repeated. This can result in the patient's **delayed** discharge and **increased costs.** The patient usually receives a **clear liquid** diet 24 hours before the test. A bowel preparation medication (liquid or pill) may be given. A **warm** tap-water enema or Fleet enema may be given **until returns are clear.** Elderly or debilitated patients should be carefully assessed during the administration of multiple enemas, which can fatigue the patient and **decrease** electrolytes. In patients with bleeding or **severe diarrhea,** the bowel preparation may not be ordered by the physician.

PANCREAS

1. Trypsin
2. Lipase
3. Amylase

CRITICAL THINKING

1. The total parenteral nutrition (TPN) rate should be started at a lower rate and gradually increased until the ordered rate is reached. This allows body systems and

the pancreas time to adjust to the high dextrose concentration.

2. The high dextrose percentage can cause the patient to be hyperglycemic, so it is necessary to monitor serum glucose levels to detect this and treat it with insulin. If the patient becomes hyperglycemic, it does not indicate that he or she is diabetic. When the high dextrose percentage is stopped, the patient's blood glucose returns to baseline levels. If insulin is given, it is used only temporarily to control the hyperglycemia.

3. (a) Dextrose of 12% or less may be given in peripheral veins; (b) dextrose greater than 12% must be given in a central vein such as the subclavian or jugular vein because the high glucose concentration is irritating to veins.

4. It is important to run TPN on an infusion pump to carefully control the rate. It is important not to allow the TPN to go in too quickly, or hyperglycemia and then dehydration from the high blood sugar can result. Dehydration occurs from the body's attempt to dilute and eliminate the high levels of blood sugar.

5. Maintain the ordered rate. TPN should never be increased to catch it up if it is behind schedule because the patient would become hyperglycemic and dehydrated.

6. When TPN is discontinued, the infusion usually is slowly weaned off to prevent hypoglycemia from occurring if the dextrose was abruptly stopped. This weaning can take several hours.

7. When TPN is ordered to be stopped, the patient is fed, if not contraindicated, to prevent hypoglycemia from occurring when the dextrose is stopped.

8. *Possible nursing diagnosis:* Imbalanced nutrition: less than body requirements.
   Outcome: Patient will maintain ideal body weight or gain weight toward goal weight.
   Interventions:
   Obtain baseline patient weight and identify ideal body weight.
   Identify barriers to nutrient ingestion.
   Weigh patient weekly and report changes to physician.
   Administer and monitor TPN as ordered according to TPN protocols.
   Monitor lab values such as albumin and absolute lymphocyte levels.
   If patient is receiving TPN, monitor blood glucose levels.
   Teach patient about TPN and necessary management of it if it is used in the home setting.

REVIEW QUESTIONS

*The correct answers are in **boldface.***

1. **(b)**
2. **(b)**
3. **(a)**
4. **(c)**
5. **(d)**

6. **(c)** Hypoactive bowel sounds occur less than 5 to 30 per minute. (a) There are some bowel sounds, so they are not absent. (b) Hyperactive bowel sounds occur at a rate greater than 30 per minute. (d) The rate of 4 per minute is less than normal.

7. **(c)** Stool cultures must be collected using sterile technique so as not to introduce any pathogens into the specimen that would alter the test results. (a, b, d) can be done using clean technique.

8. **(b)** A flat plate x-ray can be done with food in the stomach or feces in the bowel, which does not impair visibility of the structures and has no risk for aspiration. (a, c, d) all require clear visibility or may have a risk of aspiration.

9. **(a)** Barium can produce constipation if it is not diluted. (b) is incorrect because there is no pain during or after a barium swallow; (c) is incorrect because nutritional intake is not excessive as a result of the barium ingestion; (d) is incorrect because the barium can produce constipation, not diarrhea, if it is not diluted.

10. **(c)** The chalky barium will cause the patient's stool to look white for 1 to 3 days after the procedure. (a) Stools usually gradually return to a brown color; (b, d) are not associated with the color of barium and are not normal stool colors.

11. **(b)** The gag reflex must return before the patient eats or drinks to prevent aspiration. (a) Keeping the patient nil per os (NPO) does not rest the vocal cords. (c) There is no reason to keep the throat dry after an esophagogastroduodenoscopy (EGD). (d) An absent gag reflex does not stimulate vomiting.

12. **(d)** The patient sits upright to facilitate the tube moving down into the stomach by gravity. (a, b, c) do not facilitate insertion of the nasogastric (NG) tube by gravity and would inhibit the tube insertion.

13. **(c)** Disturbed body image is expressed by how patients see themselves and the pride they take in their appearance. (a, b, d) do not address the embarrassment the patient expresses.

14. **(b)** Swallowing helps insertion by closing the epiglottis, thus preventing the NG tube from slipping into the trachea, which could obstruct the airway and be dangerous to the patient. (a, c) close the throat, preventing passage of the tube into the esophagus. (d) has no effect on the insertion of the NG tube.

CHAPTER 33

VOCABULARY

1. *Helicobacter pylori*
2. anorexia
3. gastritis
4. aphthous stomatitis
5. bulimia nervosa
6. dumping syndrome

7. gastrectomy
8. obesity
9. hiatal hernia
10. gastrojejunostomy

GASTRITIS

1. (**A**)   5. (**B**)
2. (**B**)   6. (**A**)
3. (**A**)   7. (**C**)
4. (**C**)   8. (**A**)

GASTRECTOMY

PEPTIC ULCER DISEASE

*Corrections are in **boldface**.*

Most peptic ulcers are caused by the **bacterium *Helicobacter pylori.*** Peptic ulcers are commonly found in the **duodenum.** Symptoms of peptic ulcers include burning and a gnawing pain in the **epigastric region.** With a duodenal ulcer, there is pain and discomfort on an **empty** stomach, which may be relieved by **ingesting** food. Peptic ulcers **can** be cured. Medication treatment for most peptic ulcers should include **antibiotics** as indicated.

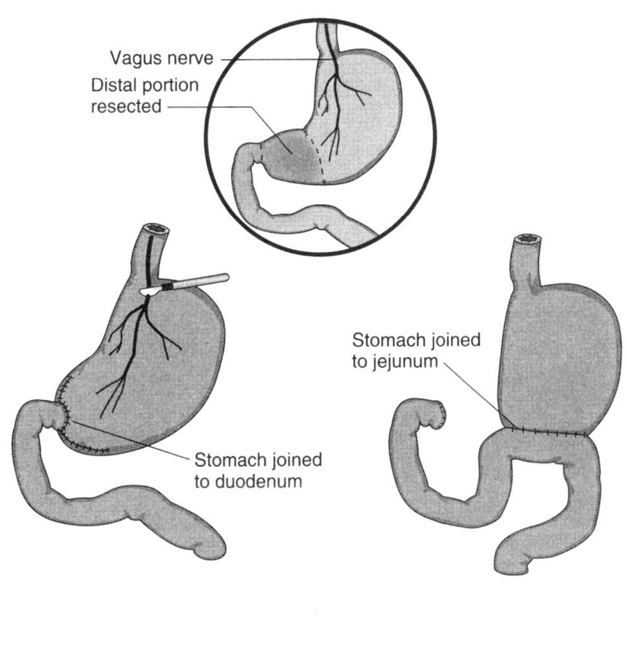

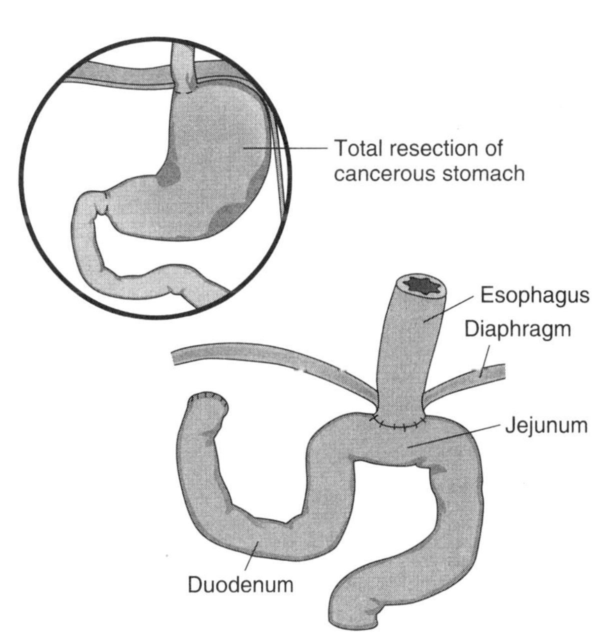

CRITICAL THINKING

1. Your first action is to prevent Mrs. Sheffield from aspirating. You maintain her side-lying position and remind her to remain in this position, propping her with pillows so she does not aspirate.
2. Your next action is to take her vital signs.
3. You determine that Mrs. Sheffield is in the early stages of hypovolemic shock (increased pulse and respirations, decreased temperature and blood pressure, and diaphoresis), and her gastric bleeding needs to be stopped immediately. You maintain her intermittent low-wall suction to aspirate the gastric output, thus preventing further gastric distention. You also maintain her intravenous (IV) setting to compensate for her fluid loss.
4. You notify the physician of Mrs. Sheffield's condition.
5. Current vital signs; signs and symptoms—diaphoresis, nausea, slightly distended abdomen; intake and output—vomitus (amount and color), nasogastric output (amount and color), IV (solution and rate), urine output since return to your unit; other data: the time Mrs. Sheffield returned from the postanesthesia care unit, her

vital signs, and your general assessment of her on return to your unit.

6. Apply oxygen at 2 L via nasal cannula and reassure the patient that her condition is being closely monitored and that her physician is taking her back to surgery to repair her abdomen. Request the laboratory work. Gather the equipment necessary to transport Mrs. Sheffield with oxygen, an emesis basin, and some extra blankets.

REVIEW QUESTIONS

*The correct answers are in **boldface**.*

1. (**a**) Confusion is a common side effect of cimetidine, especially in the elderly. (b, c, d) are not side effects of cimetidine.
2. (**a**) Anorexia is a symptom of chronic gastritis type B. (b) Dysphagia is seen in gastroesophageal reflux disease. (c) Diarrhea is not a sign of chronic gastritis type B. (d) A feeling of fullness can occur in patients with dumping syndrome.
3. (**d**) Gastrectomy is the only effective treatment for gastric cancer. (a) Gastroplasty reduces the size of the stomach to treat morbid obesity. (b) Gastrorrhaphy is suturing of the stomach wall. (c) Gastric stapling is a surgical treatment for obese patients.
4. (**b, e**) Diaphoresis and hypotension are common signs of hypovolemic shock. (a) Hypotension, not hypertension, is a sign of hypovolemic shock. (c) The pulse would be weak and thready, not bounding. (d) There would not be edema associated with hypovolemic shock.
5. (**c**) A low-fat diet is advised to decrease the fat content in the stool. (a) A bland diet may decrease irritation of the bowel, but the patient's problem stems from inadequate mixing of food with pancreatic and biliary secretions to digest fats, and a low-fat diet would be more helpful for this. (b) A high-carbohydrate diet does not prevent fat from being introduced in the diet. (d) A pureed diet would not be helpful because it could contain fat.
6. (**d**) Diet management and exercise are the first interventions used to promote weight loss in the obese patient because they are noninvasive. Also, monitoring the patient in a diet and exercise program gives the health-care provider information about the patient's metabolism, food preferences, food habits, rate of weight loss, and activity tolerances. (a) is a surgical procedure that would be considered if noninvasive interventions were not successful. (b, c) are not surgical procedures used for treating obesity; they are used for diseases such as cancer.
7. (**a**) Eating small, frequent meals that can pass easily through the esophagus prevents the rapid filling of the stomach and thus heartburn and regurgitation. (b) The patient should avoid reclining for 1 hour after eating because reclining would promote reflux, not prevent it. (c) The patient should sleep in an elevated position to prevent reflux by raising the head of the bed on 6-inch blocks and using pillows. (d) Eating before bedtime should be avoided so the stomach is empty, to prevent reflux.
8. (**d**) Start the oxygen first. Use Maslow's hierarchy to help prioritize interventions. Oxygen administration will increase the amount of oxygen in the vascular system, thus increasing the oxygen to the tissues. (a) The IV should be hung next to help restore and maintain volume. (b) The laboratory can be called to draw blood for a complete blood cell count while other interventions are occurring, which will give you a hemoglobin level that will indicate oxygen-carrying capacity. (c) While his blood is being drawn and processed, insert the nasogastric tube, which will decompress his stomach, and keep the head of his bed up 30 to 45 degrees to prevent aspiration of any emesis.
9. (**a**) A painless ulcer is common early in oral cancer. (b) White painful ulcers describe aphthous stomatitis (canker sore). (c) Feeling of fullness occurs with hiatal hernia or esophageal cancer. (d) Heartburn occurs with hiatal hernia.
10. (**b**) Esophageal dilation is performed to enlarge the esophagus and allow food to pass the obstruction caused by the tumor. (a) Gastrectomy is done for stomach cancer. (c, d) Radical or modified neck dissection is performed for oral cancer that has metastasized to cervical lymph nodes.
11. (**d**) Foods that cause discomfort need to be identified so they can be avoided. (a) Large meals promote reflux, so small meals should be eaten. (b) Sleeping flat without pillows promotes reflux, so the patient should be elevated. (c) Lying down after each meal would promote reflux, so the patient should sit up for 2 hours after a meal.

CHAPTER 34

VOCABULARY

1. (**L**)		7. (**H**)
2. (**J**)		8. (**I**)
3. (**B**)		9. (**C**)
4. (**K**)		10. (**E**)
5. (**A**)		11. (**G**)
6. (**D**)		12. (**F**)

OSTOMIES

*Corrections are in **boldface**.*

1. Michelle Braun is a 16-year-old with ulcerative colitis. She is taking cortisone and **sulfasalazine (Azulfidine) or another aminosalicylate.** She is on a **low**-residue diet. She is now admitted to the hospital for a colectomy and **permanent end ileostomy.** You monitor her intake and output (I&O), daily weights, and elec-

trolytes. You also monitor for signs of inflammation in her joints, skin, and other parts of her body. You teach her to **increase** fluids following surgery, **but it is not feasible** to limit the number of stools she has daily.

2. James Key is a 46-year-old with a new sigmoid colostomy. Following surgery you monitor his stoma every shift for 3 days to ensure that it remains **pink** and moist. You explain that the stool will be **formed** and that **irrigation is optional to establish regularity.** You contact the dietitian to provide a list of the high-fiber foods that he should eat.

CRITICAL THINKING

1. Assess Mrs. Hendricks' abdomen for normal bowel sounds, distention, tenderness, and other signs of problems. Assess her diet, exercise, fluid intake, and other possible factors that may have caused constipation.

2. Because Mrs. Hendricks has arthritis, she may not be getting much exercise. Lack of teeth probably prevents her from eating many fresh fruits or vegetables. Poor fluid intake and certain medications may also be factors. Chronic laxative abuse can be a factor, but Mrs. Hendricks only takes milk of magnesia occasionally.

3. Mrs. Hendricks is only 1 day behind her normal bowel movement schedule. This is not a major concern. However, you should intervene to prevent the problem from becoming worse. Unrelieved constipation can lead to fecal impaction, megacolon, and complications related to use of Valsalva's maneuver.

4. Before giving Mrs. Hendricks more milk of magnesia, you can try giving her some prune juice, walk her in the halls if she is able, and have her sit on the toilet or bedside commode (avoid use of bedpan) to attempt to have a bowel movement. Placing her feet on a footstool while sitting on the toilet may also help.

5. Prevention is the best treatment for constipation. Place Mrs. Hendricks on a regimen of 2 g bran with her cereal each morning. Include pureed fresh fruits and vegetables as much as possible in her diet. Encourage fluids and assist her to walk in the halls several times each day. Establish a regular time each day (or two) for Mrs. Hendricks to have the bathroom to herself for a bowel movement. Offer a warm drink such as a cup of coffee or tea or warm water before this time. If these measures do not work, add Metamucil to her daily regimen. Avoid the milk of magnesia, senna (Sennakot), and enema as much as possible.

REVIEW QUESTIONS

*The correct answers are in **boldface**.*

1. (**b**) is correct. Ulcerative colitis affects the colon and rectum. (a) is a better description of diverticulitis; (c) describes Crohn's disease; and (d) is not true of ulcerative colitis.

2. (**d, e**) are correct. Complete blood count (CBC) should be monitored because ulcerative colitis can cause bleeding; electrolytes are monitored because of loss with diarrhea. (a) monitors liver problems, (b) monitors muscle damage, and (c, f) monitors pancreas function.

3. (**d**) is correct. Fresh fruits and vegetables can exacerbate diarrhea. (a, b, c) can all exacerbate diarrhea symptoms.

4. (**c**) is correct. Total parenteral nutrition (TPN) is the only way to adequately feed a person for an extended period without using the gut. (a, b) both require a functional bowel; (d) provides inadequate nutrition for an extended period.

5. (**a**) is correct. A low-fiber diet increases risk of diverticulosis. (b, c, d) do not increase risk for diverticulosis.

6. (**a**) is correct. Foods with seeds may need to be avoided. (b, c, d) do not exacerbate diverticulosis.

7. (**c**) is correct. A bowel obstruction can cause nausea and vomiting. (a, b) are not related to diverticulitis. There is no evidence that (d) is correct.

8. (**d**) is correct. The loop can be replaced after the resected area of bowel has healed. (a) transverse ostomies do not usually drain constant liquid stool, (b) there is no such thing as a looped bag, and (c) the ostomy will drain stool.

9. (**a**) is correct. Fluids are needed to replace those lost in liquid stools. (b, c, d) can all increase liquid stools and fluid loss.

10. (**b**) is correct. Pouches are made of odor proof plastic. (a) nothing will absorb all odor, (c) effluent does have an odor, and (d) daily pouch changes are hard on skin and not recommended.

CHAPTER 35

VOCABULARY

1. (**D**)		7. (**L**)
2. (**C**)		8. (**A**)
3. (**J**)		9. (**I**)
4. (**E**)		10. (**B**)
5. (**G**)		11. (**H**)
6. (**K**)		12. (**F**)

LIVER

Across	Down
2. HBV	1. Encephalopathy
6. Caput medusae	2. Hepatorenal
9. TIPS	3. Portal
10. Asterixes	4. Hepatitis
11. HAV	5. RUQ
	6. Cirrhosis
	7. Ascites
	8. Varices

GALLBLADDER

1. (**D**)	6. (**H**)
2. (**F**)	7. (**I**)
3. (**G**)	8. (**J**)
4. (**E**)	9. (**B**)
5. (**A**)	10. (**C**)

PANCREAS

1. (**A**) Serum glucose may elevate because damage to the islets of Langerhans causes decreased insulin production.
2. (**A**) The digestive enzyme amylase is released in large quantities by an inflamed pancreas.
3. (**N**)
4. (**A**) Pleural effusion is caused by a local inflammatory reaction to the irritation from pancreatic enzymes.
5. (**N**)
6. (**A**) Serum albumin is decreased, usually from decreased protein metabolism.
7. (**A**) A positive Cullen's sign indicates hemorrhage from pancreatic destruction.
8. (**A**) Urinary output of less than 30 mL/hr can indicate hepatorenal syndrome or shock from circulatory collapse.
9. (**A**) Indicates neuromuscular irritability from decreased serum calcium levels.
10. (**A**) Indicates malabsorption of dietary fats from decreased lipase.

CRITICAL THINKING

1. The data collected about Ms. Smith that support the diagnosis of chronic liver failure are a grossly distended abdomen, jaundiced sclerae and skin, multiple bruises, and 2+ pitting edema of the lower extremities. Ms. Smith also scratches her arms and legs frequently, indicating itching. Her laboratory data indicate that her serum bilirubin, ammonia, and prothrombin time are elevated and that her serum albumin, total protein, and potassium are below normal.
2. You note that Ms. Smith is irritable, has difficulty answering questions, and appears to doze off often during the interview. Other observations you might make include asterixis, increasing difficulty in arousing the patient, muscle twitching, and fetor hepaticus.
3. The 2+ pitting edema and abdominal distention are due to the decreased amount of serum albumin produced by the failing liver permits fluid to seep into the abdominal cavity and other body tissues.
4. You expect the physician to order a severely protein-restricted diet for the hepatic encephalopathy. In addition, the patient may be ordered saline or magnesium sulfate enemas, neomycin, or lactulose to rid the body of excess ammonia.
5. You can anticipate that the physician will order a vasoconstrictor drug such as vasopressin for Ms. Smith. If the vasoconstrictor does not stop the bleeding from the esophageal varices, a Senstaken-Blakemore tube may be ordered. In addition, the physician may decide to do injection sclerotherapy in an attempt to prevent further episodes of bleeding.
6. Observe for aspiration or suffocation, such as increased respiratory rate and effort, increased confusion and irritability, noisy breathing, pallor, or cyanosis. Also carefully monitor the inflation pressure of the esophageal balloon to ensure that the pressure remains under 25 mm Hg to prevent erosion of the esophagus.
7. Monitor the patient's emesis, stool, and urine at least every 8 hours for blood. Observe for any increase in bruising or bleeding from the gums. Monitor blood clotting laboratory studies such as the prothrombin time, as well as the CBC for excess blood loss.
8. Measure Ms. Smith's abdomen and weigh her daily; document results. Report any weight gain or increase in circumference promptly. Because Ms. Smith will usually be ordered a low-sodium diet and will have fluids restricted, carefully monitor and record intake and output. Assess Ms. Smith's vital signs and mental status every 4 hours and report changes promptly. Administer diuretics as ordered.
9. Teach Ms. Smith that acetaminophen (Tylenol) is to be avoided because it is toxic to the liver and may cause further damage.

REVIEW QUESTIONS

*The correct answers are in **boldface**.*

1. (**c**) is correct. This is a low-sodium meal. (a, b, d) are all high in sodium.
2. (**d**) is correct. The gastric balloon helps keep the tube in place. (a, b, c) are all appropriate interventions.
3. (**b**) is correct. Straining will further increase pressure and may cause bleeding. (a, c, d) are not appropriate. Coughing could rupture a varix, and increasing fluid intake can further increase pressure.
4. (**b**) is correct. Standard precautions protect the nurse from exposure to disease. (a) reverse isolation protects the patient, not the nurse; (c, d) do not protect from blood exposure.
5. (**d**) is correct. Hepatitis B virus (HBV) is the most common cause. (a, b, c) are not the most common causes.
6. (**a**) is correct. These are symptoms of hepatic encephalopathy. They are not symptoms of (b, c, d).
7. (**b**) is correct; 20% to 60% of patients rebleed.
8. (**b, c, d, e**) are correct. Females are more at risk for gallbladder disease, so (a) is not a risk.
9. (**d**) is correct. Meperidine (Demerol) is most helpful. (a, b, c) morphine may cause painful spasms.
10. (**d**) is correct. Pro-Banthine is an antispasmotic agent that may help relieve biliary colic. (a) will worsen gallbladder spasms, (b) will not help, and (c) is used to dissolve stones.

11. **(c)** is correct. Excessive alcohol intake is associated with pancreatitis. (a, b, d) are not associated with pancreatitis.

12. **(a)** is correct. Patients describe their pain as dull, boring, and beginning in the mid-epigastrium and radiating to the back. (b, c, d) are not characteristic of pancreatitis.

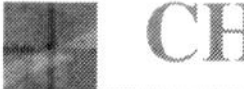

CHAPTER 36

VOCABULARY

1. **(C)**   5. **(H)**
2. **(A)**   6. **(F)**
3. **(D)**   7. **(E)**
4. **(B)**   8. **(G)**

ANATOMY

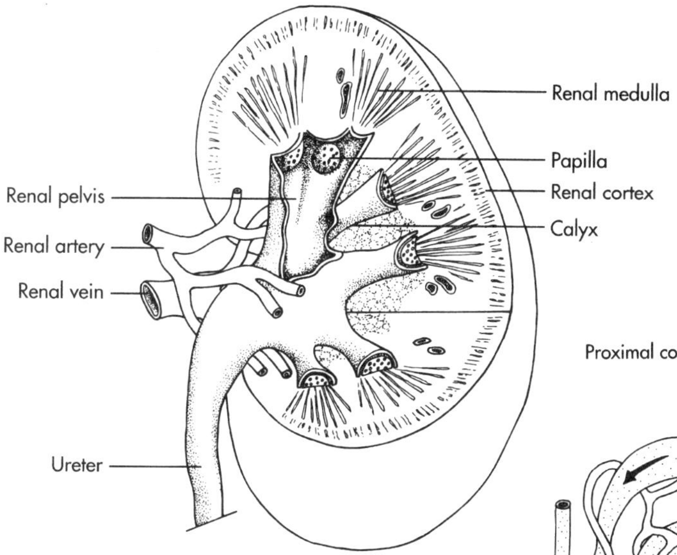

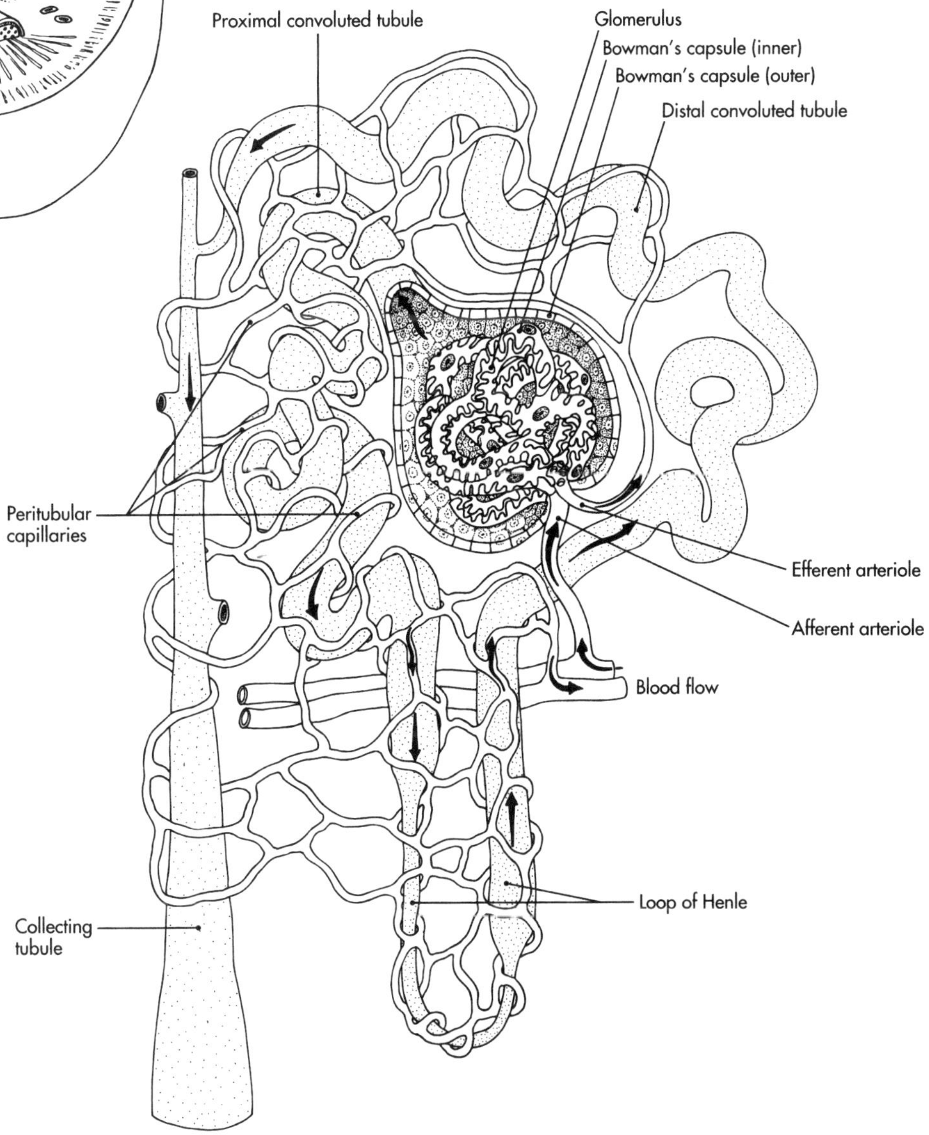

SAMPLE URINALYSIS RESULTS

Patient A: urinary tract infection
Patient B: dehydration, deficient fluid volume
Patient C: liver disease

RENAL DIAGNOSTIC TESTS

1. False—intravenous pyelogram
2. False—renal ultrasound
3. False—urine culture and sensitivity
4. True
5. False—allergic reactions are possible; can be nephrotoxic

CRITICAL THINKING

1. These are classic symptoms of stress incontinence.
2. She should be taught how to perform Kegel's exercise. She also should be referred to a urologist or gynecologist who specializes in incontinence. She may benefit from medications or surgery.
3. Functional incontinence. She would have been continent if she had been able to call the nurse for assistance in time.
4. The patient should receive a call light that she can feel and that is pinned to the front of her gown. It would also be helpful if she had a roommate who could turn on the call light for her if needed.
5. Fluids should not be restricted. Fluid restriction can result in concentrated urine, which is more irritating to the urinary tract, and cause incontinence. Some people become continent only by increasing their fluid intake and setting up a regular pattern of voiding.

REVIEW QUESTIONS

*The correct answers are in **boldface.***

1. (**a**)
2. (**b**)
3. (**c**)
4. (**b**)
5. (**d**)
6. (**a**) is correct. The perineum should be washed before collecting a urine sample from a female to decrease contamination of the specimen. (b, c, d) are not necessary for a routine urine specimen.
7. (**a**) is correct. The elevated specific gravity is seen with dehydration because the urine is more concentrated. When a patient is dehydrated, the amount of urine that the patient makes is decreased, which makes the urine more concentrated. A small amount of bacteria is normally found in the urinalysis. (b, c) A small amount of bacteria does not indicate infection. (d) No blood was noted on the results.
8. (**d, e**) are correct. The elevated creatinine level and BUN reflects reduced kidney function. (a, b, c) are incorrect.
9. (**b**) is correct. The patient should be nil per os (NPO) before undergoing an intravenous pyelogram (IVP) so the dye is more concentrated for better visualization of renal structures. After the IVP, the nurse should force fluids to clear the dye from the kidneys. (a, c, d) are not restricted.
10. (**a**) is correct. It is important that the nurse determine whether the patient is able to urinate. There may be edema of the urethra after a cystoscopy, which can result in urinary retention. (b, c, d) are not necessary.
11. (**a**) is correct. Urge incontinence is associated with difficulty retaining urine once the urge to urinate is sensed. (b) is stress incontinence. (c) is not a specific type of incontinence. (d) is total incontinence.
12. (**c**) is correct. It is important to keep the catheter taped to prevent movement of the catheter, which increases the chance of introducing bacteria into the urine and trauma to the urethra. (a) increases risk of infection. (b) is not necessary. (d) A full bag increases risk of backflow and contamination.
13. (**d**) is correct. With total incontinence, the patient is unable to control urination and an adult incontinence brief is appropriate. (a) Cranberry juice would be helpful to decrease onset of a urinary tract infection, but the patient would still be incontinent of urine. (b) A urinal will not help if the patient cannot tell when he or she has to go. (c) Kegel's exercises will not help total incontinence.

CHAPTER 37

VOCABULARY

1. Urethritis
2. Cystitis
3. Pyelonephritis
4. urethroplasty
5. calculi
6. Nephrolithotomy
7. hydronephrosis
8. nephrostomy
9. nephrectomy
10. nephrosclerosis

URINARY TRACT INFECTIONS

1. The usual cause of urinary tract infections (UTIs) in women is contamination in the area from the close proximity of the rectum to the urinary meatus. Women who void infrequently are predisposed to UTIs.
2. The usual cause of UTIs in men is the presence of prostatic hypertrophy leading to obstruction of urinary flow predisposing to infection.

3. The patient should be advised to drink large amounts of water and a glass of cranberry juice daily. If the patient cannot void frequently, he or she should drink less water.
4. The single most important thing a patient with a history of UTIs should do is void frequently to prevent stasis of urine and then infection.

5.

	Cystitis	**Pyelonephritis**
Symptoms	Dysuria; frequency; urgency; cloudy, foul-smelling urine; sometimes hematuria	Dysuria; frequency; urgency; cloudy, foul-smelling urine; sometimes hematuria; also chills and fever, flank pain, and general malaise
Urinalysis results	Increased bacteria, white blood cells (WBCs); positive nitrites; positive leukocyte esterase	Increased bacteria, WBCs; positive nitrites, positive leukocyte esterase; may also have casts in the urine
Prognosis	Good with treatment; can become chronic condition with repeat infections	Acute pyelonephritis has a good prognosis; with repeat infections the patient can develop chronic pyelonephritis with scarring and eventual destruction of the kidneys

URINARY TRACT OBSTRUCTIONS

1. The most common symptom of cancer of the bladder is hematuria because cancerous tissue readily bleeds.
2. The most common risk factor for cancer of the bladder is smoking because of continual exposure of the bladder mucosa to the carcinogenic by products of smoking.
3. The most common symptom of cancer of the kidney is bleeding, again because cancerous tissue bleeds readily, just as in cancer of the bladder.
4. The urine of a patient with an ileal conduit is cloudy due to the presence of mucus because a portion of the small intestine is used and it continues to secrete mucus.
5. To care for a patient with an ileal conduit, an appliance is kept on at all times that either holds urine or drains into a Foley bag. When the appliance needs changing, it is necessary to use a wick to catch urine until the appliance can be applied. See text for how to apply an appliance to a patient with an ileal conduit.
6. The most important care of a patient with a kidney stone is to strain all urine to catch the stone. Pain relief measures are also very important.
7. The patient with a calcium oxalate kidney stone should avoid foods high in calcium, such as large quantities of milk, and sources of oxalate, such as colas and beer. It can also be helpful to keep the urine acidic. The patient with a uric acid kidney stone should avoid foods that are high in purines, such as organ meats and sardines.

CRITICAL THINKING

1. Mrs. Zins is having incidences of hypoglycemia because she is developing renal failure. The kidney helps degrade insulin and excrete it from the body. As the kidneys fail, smaller amounts of insulin are needed because it is not removed from the body.
2. It is important that Mrs. Zins not receive orange juice as would normally be given for a hypoglycemic patient because her potassium level is already high. Instead, cranberry juice or another low-potassium carbohydrate source should be given.
3. Diabetes causes atherosclerotic changes in the kidney vessels. In addition, diabetes causes an abnormal thickening of the glomerulus, which damages the glomerulus. The diabetic patient is predisposed to frequent pyelonephritis (kidney infections), which can damage the kidney. Also, the diabetic patient can develop a neurogenic bladder, which predisposes the patient to both infection and obstruction of the urinary system.
4. Good control of diabetes, keeping blood sugars within a defined range, can decrease the development of diabetic complications including development of renal failure.
5. Nursing diagnoses that would be relevant for Mrs. Zins include excess fluid volume (she has edema, weight gain, and jugular vein distention) and fatigue (she states she feels exhausted and also has a hemoglobin level of 7.2).
6. The serum creatinine of 5.4 is most diagnostic of renal failure. A 24-hour creatinine clearance is more diagnostic, but this laboratory test is not available in this case study.
7. Mrs. Zins is anemic because her kidneys have decreased or stopped production of a substance called erythropoietin, which stimulates the bone marrow to make red blood cells. It is also possible that she has slowly been bleeding through her gastrointestinal tract, a common occurrence in renal patients.
8. The three most important assessments when caring for a patient with renal failure are daily weight, intake and output (with fluid restriction if prescribed), and monitoring laboratory test for dangerous levels of electrolytes.
9. Mrs. Zins would probably be on a defined diabetic diet that was also low sodium, low potassium, decreased protein, and fluid restricted. If her phosphorus level was elevated, she would also be put on a low-phosphorus diet. This is one of the most restrictive diets possible and is very difficult to follow.

RENAL FAILURE

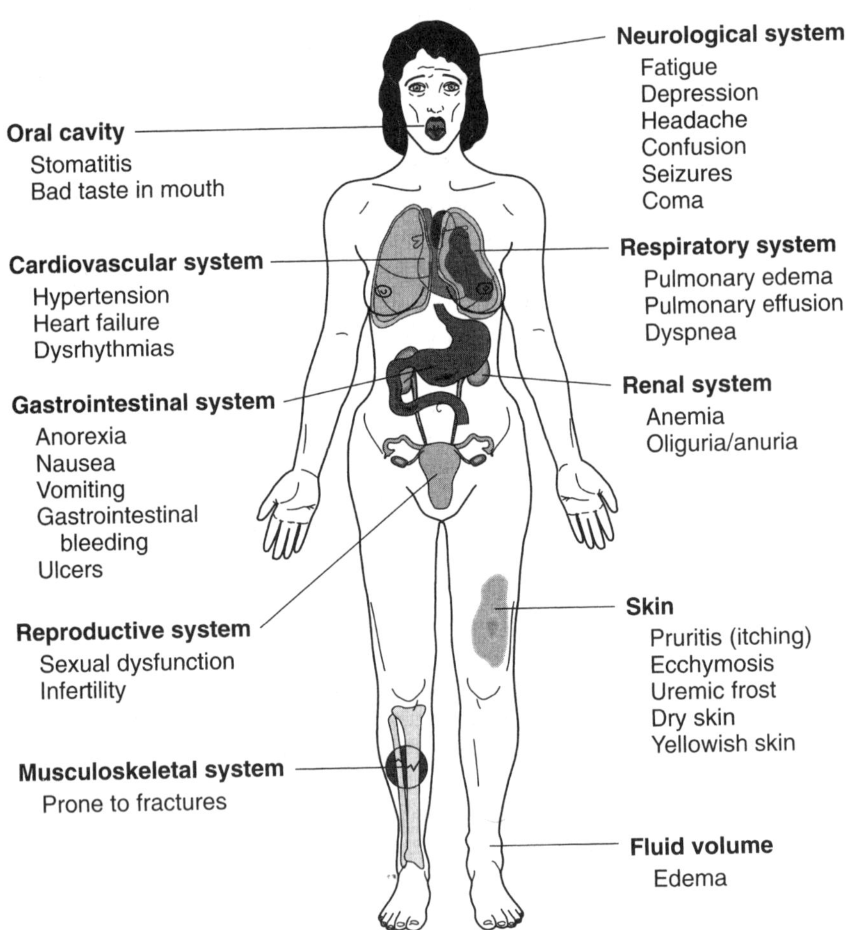

REVIEW QUESTIONS

The correct answers are in **boldface.**

1. (**d**) is correct. Hematuria is the most common symptom of cancer of the bladder. (a) nocturia or (b) dysuria may occur related to a resulting infection, or (c) retention may occur because of obstruction, but these are not the most common symptoms.

2. (**d**) is correct because the mucus is normally found in the urine of a patient with an ileal conduit. This is because a portion of the small bowel is used to make the conduit, and that portion of bowel continues to secrete mucus. (a, b, c) are not necessary.

3. (**c**) is correct because often the first and most obvious sign of acute renal failure is a decrease in urine output. (a) the blood pressure may elevate later as the patient continues into renal failure, but the urine output is most significant. (b, d) may occur in some patients, but they are not the most common.

4. (**b**) is correct because a 24-hour creatinine clearance is most diagnostic of renal failure; a result of 5 mL per hour means that the patient has approximately 5% of normal kidney function. (a, c, d) would be elevated in the patient with renal failure, but the creatinine clearance is most diagnostic.

5. (**d, e**) are correct because they are the only foods listed that do not contain significant potassium. (a, b, c) are all high in potassium.

6. (**d**) is correct because there is a sudden decrease in urine output, and the patient has symptoms of urinary retention, which are distention and pain in the suprapubic area. (a) Decreased renal perfusion would be an appropriate answer if the patient had not had symptoms of urinary retention; (b, c) would not cause the symptoms of urinary retention.

7. (**b**) is correct. Beer is high in oxalate, which predisposes the patient to calcium oxalate kidney stones. (a, c, d) are not especially high in oxalate or calcium.

8. (**c**) is the correct answer because the patient should collect the specimen partway through urination. (a, b, d) are all relevant to other diagnostic tests of the urine but not relevant to a midstream culture.

9. (**b**) is the correct answer because the most serious complication of a high potassium level is cardiac dysrhythmias. (a, c, d) may be present in renal failure but are not associated with high potassium levels.

10. (**c**) is the correct answer because the daily weight is the single best determinant of fluid balance in the body. (a, b, d) are also important, but daily weight remains most significant.

11. (**b**) is the correct answer because orange juice is high in potassium, and the patient's potassium level is already high. (a, c) would still give the patient too much potassium; (d) it would be important to check the kind of diet later, but the first priority is to protect the patient from a dangerously high potassium level.

12. (**a**) is the correct answer because there is a larger blood flow, and dialysis is more efficient. (b) All blood access sites can clot. (c) It is harder to access a graft than a two-tailed subclavian. (d) Either site can be damaged by trauma.

13. (**b**) is the correct answer because the patient must be weighed following dialysis to determine fluid balance. (a, c, d) are not relevant.

14. (**b**) is correct because this is the mechanism by which dialysis works. (a, c, d) do not describe how dialysis works.

15. (**c**) is correct because these are symptoms that are seen with fluid retention related to untreated renal failure.

(a, b, d) are not symptoms of fluid excess and renal failure.

16. (**d**) is correct because hematuria is the most common symptom of trauma to the kidney because the kidney has a very large blood supply. (a, b, c) are not symptoms of trauma.

17. (**b**) is correct because the patient has symptoms of too much fluid in the body, which is fluid volume excess. (a, c, d) are not relevant. In certain situations, a nursing diagnosis of noncompliance may have caused the symptoms, but there is not enough information in the question to make this diagnosis.

CHAPTER 38

VOCABULARY

1. glycogen
2. hyperglycemia
3. affect
4. exophthalmos
5. feedback

ENDOCRINE GLANDS AND HORMONES

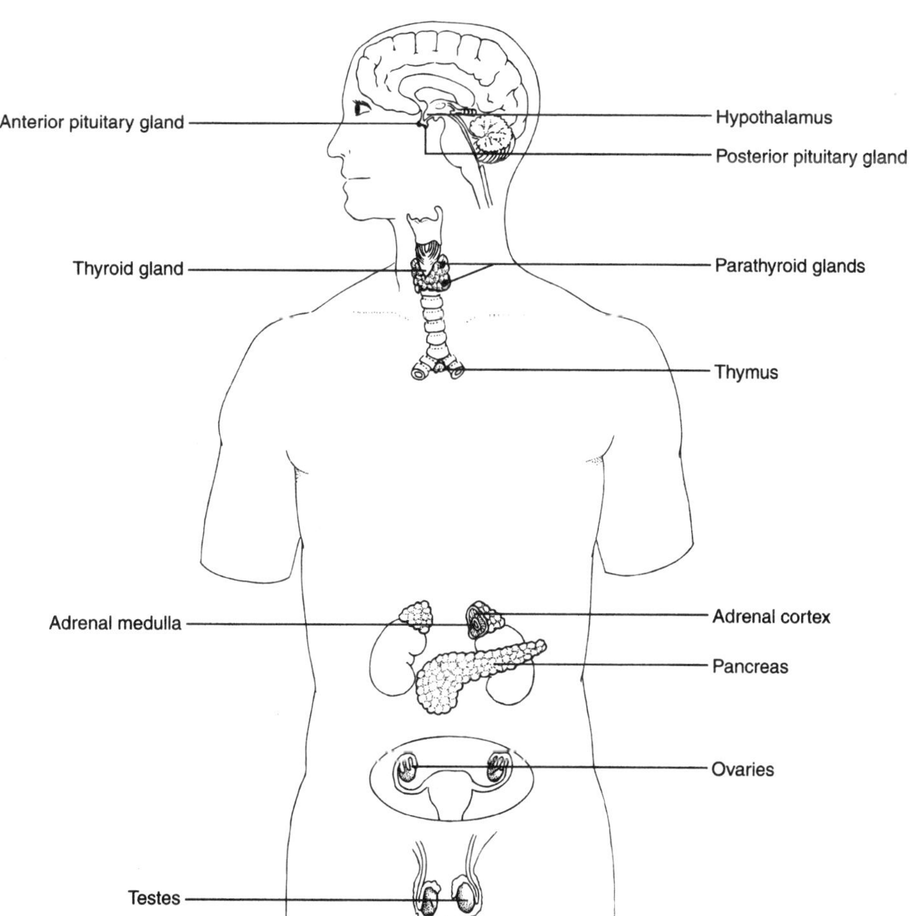

HORMONES

1. **(J)**	10. **(C)**
2. **(Q)**	11. **(N)**
3. **(A)**	12. **(F)**
4. **(H)**	13. **(G)**
5. **(E)**	14. **(D)**
6. **(M)**	15. **(O)**
7. **(P)**	16. **(B)**
8. **(K)**	17. **(L)**
9. **(I)**	

REVIEW QUESTIONS

*The correct answers are in **boldface.***

1. **(b)** is correct.
2. **(d)** is correct.
3. **(a)** is correct.
4. **(c)** is correct.
5. **(b)** is correct.
6. **(c)** is correct. The final urine voided at 24 hours must be added to the specimen. (a) The first, not the last, urine voided is discarded. (b) A separate container is not necessary. (d) All urine produced in 24 hours is necessary for the test.
7. **(a)** is correct. A history is appropriate. (b) could cause release of hormone and exacerbate symptoms. (c) evaluates diabetes, not thyroid function. (d) A buffalo hump is present when there is too much cortisol, not thyroid hormone.
8. **(c)** is correct. This answers her question. Further testing must be done to determine a definite diagnosis. (a) She may have cancer of the thyroid, but she needs further testing; also, the nurse does not make a medical diagnosis. (b) is not true. (d) A cold spot is not normal.

CHAPTER 39

VOCABULARY

1. euthyroid	6. dysphagia
2. goiter	7. myxedema
3. polydipsia	8. nocturia
4. polyuria	9. amenorrhea
5. pheochromocytoma	10. ectopic

HORMONES

Disorder	Hormone Problem	Signs and Symptoms
Diabetes insipidus	Antidiuretic hormone (ADH) deficiency	Polyuria
Syndrome of inappropriate ADH (SIADH)	ADH excess	Water retention
Cushing's syndrome	Steroid excess	Moon face
Addison's disease	Deficient steroids	Hypotension
Graves' disease	High T_3 and T_4	Exophthalmos
Hypothyroidism	Low T_3 and T_4	Weight gain and fatigue
Pheochromocytoma	Epinephrine excess	Labile hypertension
Hyperparathyroidism	High calcium	Muscle weakness, brittle bones
Dwarfism	Growth hormone (GH) deficiency	Short stature
Acromegaly	GH excess	Growing feet
Hypoparathyroidism	Low calcium	Tetany

CRITICAL THINKING

1. Because Sam has too much ADH, he will be retaining water. An appropriate nursing diagnosis would be excess fluid volume.
2. The best way to monitor fluid balance is by daily weights, at the same time each day, on the same scale, and in about the same clothes. In addition to daily weights, intake and output, vital signs, urine specific gravity, lung sounds, and skin turgor can be monitored.
3. Sam will retain water, which will reduce the osmolality of his blood. This in turn can cause cerebral edema, increased intracranial pressure, and seizures.
4. Sam's side rails should be padded. If a seizure occurs, he should be protected from harming himself.
5. Sam's urine will be very concentrated because he is not excreting much water.
6. When Sam is effectively treated, his urine will look more dilute because he will be excreting more water.
7. A head injury can directly or indirectly damage the pituitary gland, placing the patient at risk for reduced ADH secretion and DI.
8. Polyuria and polydipsia are symptoms of both DI and DM.
9. Judy's urine specific gravity will be low because she is excreting too much water.

10. Judy's serum osmolality will be high because she is losing water and becoming dehydrated.
11. Judy is at risk for deficient fluid volume.
12. Judy should watch for signs of fluid overload, such as increasing weight and concentrated urine.

THYROID DISORDERS

1. **(O)**	7. **(R)**
2. **(O)**	8. **(R)**
3. **(R)**	9. **(O)**
4. **(R)**	10. **(R)**
5. **(O)**	11. **(R)**
6. **(O)**	12. **(O)**

REVIEW QUESTIONS

*The correct answers are in **boldface.***

1. **(c)** is correct. Negative feedback causes the pituitary to produce more thyroid stimulating hormone (TSH). (a) TSH does not take the place of T_3 and T_4, (b) TSH will not directly affect the metabolic rate, and (d) fat cells do not make TSH.
2. **(c)** is correct; the patient is experiencing fatigue. (a) There is no evidence in the data that the patient is overeating, (b) weight gain does not necessarily affect gas exchange, and (d) there is no evidence that the patient is experiencing depression.
3. **(a)** is correct. Tachycardia can occur if she gets too much Synthroid. (b, c) are not side effects of Synthroid; and (d) she should lose weight, not gain weight, on Synthroid.
4. **(b)** is correct. Body fluids will be radioactive. (a, c) are not necessary; and (d) exposure to even small doses of radioactivity should be minimized.
5. **(a)** is correct. Numb fingers and muscle cramps are symptoms of tetany. (b, c, d) are not symptoms of tetany.
6. **(c)** is correct. Thyrotoxicosis causes blood pressure, pulse, temperature, and respiratory rate to rise. (a, b, d) are not affected by thyrotoxicosis (peripheral pulses may be indirectly affected).
7. The correct order is (**b, c, a, d, f, e**). Airway is always a priority. Vital signs are second because the patient must be monitored for thyrotoxicosis, which could be life threatening. Surgical site is third, because physiological problems take priority, and excessive bleeding could also be life or health threatening. An analgesic is next, so the patient will be comfortable for range of motion exercises. Teaching is last; although it is important, it

does not maintain the immediate physiological integrity of the patient.

8. **(c)** is correct. Fluids will help prevent kidney stones. (a, b, d) will not help.
9. **(d)** is correct. It is the only outcome that addresses pain. (a, b, c) may all be appropriate, but they are not related directly to the nursing diagnosis.
10. **(c)** is correct. Acromegaly is caused by an excess of GH. (a, b, d) do not cause acromegaly.
11. **(b)** is correct. Buffalo hump and easy bruising are often present in Cushing's syndrome. (a, c, d) are not symptoms of Cushing's syndrome.
12. **(a)** is correct. Vital signs are important because the patient with pheochromocytoma has labile hypertension. (b, c, d) are all part of a routine assessment, but they are not as important as vital signs in this case.
13. **(c)** is correct. Addison's disease is associated with fluid loss. (a, b, d) are not relevant.

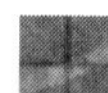 # CHAPTER 40

VOCABULARY

1. glycosuria
2. Hyperglycemia
3. Hypoglycemia
4. Kussmaul's
5. polyphagia
6. polydipsia
7. nocturia
8. peak
9. duration
10. tight

HYPOGLYCEMIA AND HYPERGLYCEMIA

1. **(O)**	5. **(O)**
2. **(R)**	6. **(R)**
3. **(R)**	7. **(O)**
4. **(R)**	8. **(R)**

LONG-TERM COMPLICATIONS OF DIABETES

1. **(E)**	5. **(G)**
2. **(B)**	6. **(F)**
3. **(D)**	7. **(C)**
4. **(A)**	

CRITICAL THINKING

1.

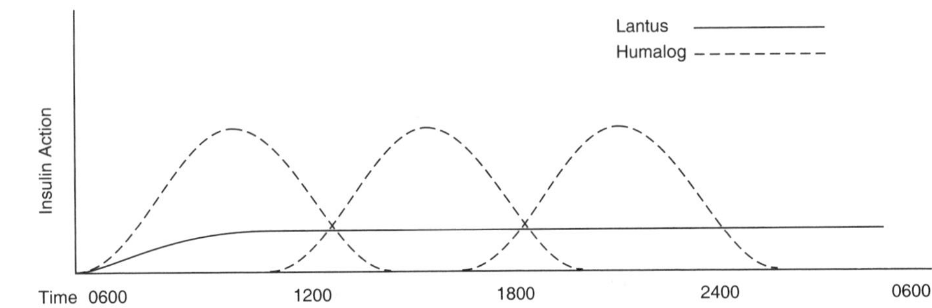

2. Keeping the blood glucose level too low can increase risk of hypoglycemia, especially in a patient who has had diabetes for some time. If autonomic neuropathy is present, symptoms of hypoglycemia may go unnoticed, making hypoglycemia even more risky. The physician should always be consulted for desired glucose range.

3. Jennie is exhibiting symptoms of hypoglycemia. You should follow hospital policy, which usually directs the nurse to check the blood glucose level and provide a quick source of glucose such as juice or glucose tablets. Notify the registered nurse according to policy.

4. It appears that the treatment has been effective; 80 mg/dL is probably okay, especially if a meal tray is to be served soon. Check to be sure her meal is on its way, and watch her for further symptoms. Consult with the physician before administering her supper dose of Humalog.

5. Common causes of hypoglycemia include skipping or delaying meals, eating less than prescribed at a meal, and more exercise than usual.

6. Because she is receiving regularly scheduled insulin, it is important to eat regularly to prevent periods during which there is insulin but not enough glucose in her blood.

7. Obesity causes insulin resistance. Losing weight has probably decreased Jennie's insulin resistance, making her insulin dose more effective.

8. Glucotrol stimulates insulin production and increases tissue sensitivity to insulin.

9. Sulfonylureas are administered 30 minutes before breakfast and 30 minutes before supper if twice-a-day dosing is ordered. This allows absorption of medication before eating.

10. Jennie has type 2 diabetes. If she had type 1 diabetes, she would not be able to take oral hypoglycemics. Obesity is also common in type 2 diabetes.

REVIEW QUESTIONS

*The correct answers are in **boldface**.*

1. (**a**) is correct. Ketones and DKA occur in type 1 diabetes. (b) Type 2 diabetes in not usually associated with ketones. (c) A patient with prediabetes would have a more normal blood glucose. (d) Gestational diabetes occurs in pregnant women.

2. (**c**) is correct. Micronase increases tissue sensitivity to insulin. (a, b, d) can all potentially raise blood glucose levels, an undesirable result.

3. (**d**) is correct. If a patient forgets a prescribed oral hypoglycemic, blood sugar levels will go up. Fatigue, thirst, and blurred vision are the only symptoms of hyperglycemia. (a, b) are symptoms of hypoglycemia. (c) is not related to diabetes.

4. (**b**) is correct; 90 to 130 mg/dL would be considered acceptable by most practitioners. (a) is too low. (c, d) are too high.

5. (**b, c, d**) are all correct. Insulin is given subcutaneously most of the time; it can be given intravenously in urgent situations, and inhaled insulin is a new route. (a) Insulin is never given orally because it would be digested.

6. (**b**) is correct. Insulin should never be given without first evaluating the blood glucose level. (a, c, d) may all be significant for the person with diabetes, but they are not immediately necessary before administering insulin.

7. (**b**) is correct. The peak action time of NPH is 6 to 12 hours after administration. (a) is the onset of NPH. (c) is the duration of long-acting insulin. (d) is incorrect.

8. (**c**) is correct. The peak of regular insulin is 2 to 5 hours. (a, b, d) are incorrect.

9. (**c**) is correct. These are symptoms of hypoglycemia. (a, b, d) are not associated with hypoglycemia. (b and d) are symptoms of hyperglycemia.

10. (**a**) is correct. Raisins contain sugar, which will raise the blood glucose level. (b, d) are protein foods and will affect the blood glucose level only very slowly. (c) is not a food.

11. (**d**) is correct. Glucagon stimulates the liver to convert glycogen to glucose, which raises the blood glucose level. (a, b, c) are all related to hyperglycemia, which would be worsened by glucagon.

12. (**a**) is correct. Obesity is a major risk factor for type 2 diabetes. (b) A viral infection may be related to type 1 diabetes. (c) Binge eating does not cause diabetes. (d) Hypertension may be a complication of diabetes, but it does not increase the risk of diabetes.

13. (**d**) is correct. Oatmeal and bread are both bread/starch exchanges. (a, b, c) are not starch exchanges.

CHAPTER 41

VOCABULARY

1. hysteroscopy
2. insufflation
3. digital rectal examination
4. gynecomastia
5. hypospadias
6. hydrocele
7. varicocele
8. libido
9. menarche
10. mammography

ANATOMY AND PHYSIOLOGY

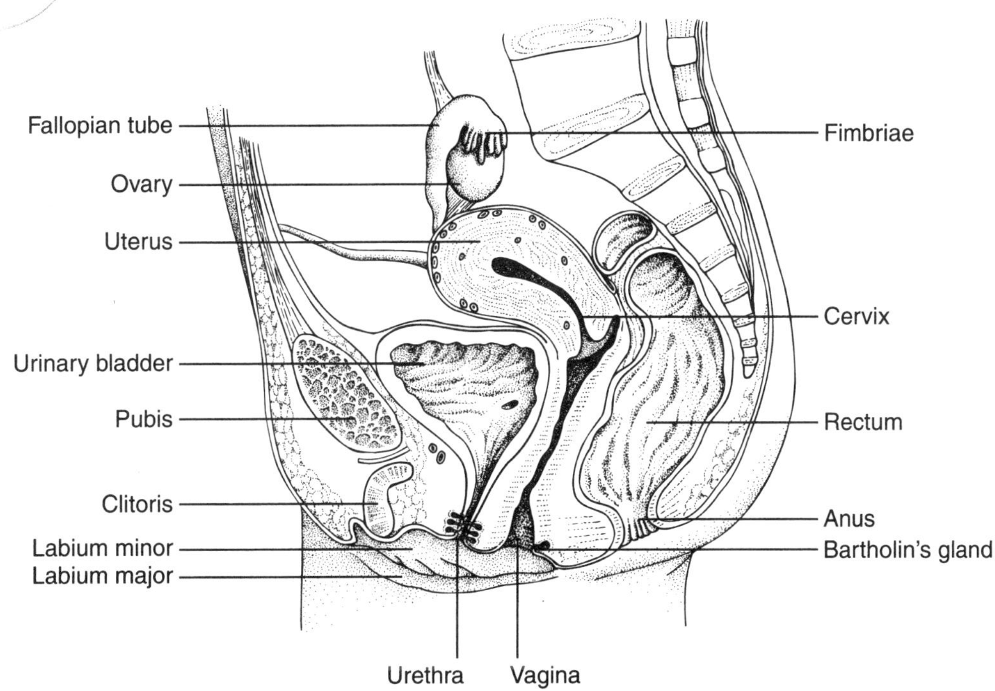

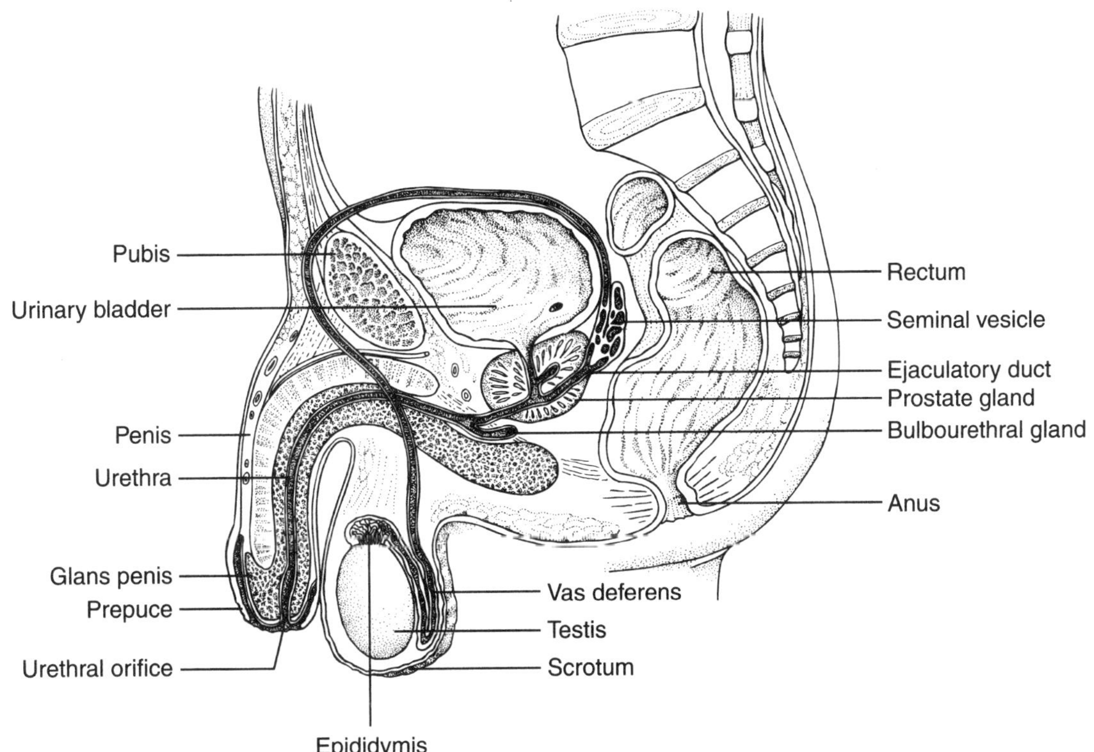

FEMALE REPRODUCTIVE STRUCTURES

1. **(E)**   5. **(B)**
2. **(G)**   6. **(A)**
3. **(F)**   7. **(D)**
4. **(C)**

MALE REPRODUCTIVE SYSTEM

4, 2, 5, 1, 3

DIAGNOSTIC TESTS

1. **(B)**   4. **(F)**
2. **(A)**   5. **(D)**
3. **(C)**   6. **(E)**

CRITICAL THINKING

1. "Even though you had prostate surgery, unless you had your entire prostate gland removed, some of the tissue will grow back, and a rectal examination is still important. We can check with your doctor to see what kind of surgery you had."

2. Examine her abdomen, and check her medical record for the report of her procedure. Most likely she had carbon dioxide (CO_2) pumped into her abdomen as part of the procedure to enhance visualization of structures. Explain to her why her abdomen is distended, and have her lie flat to decrease migration of CO_2. If there is no record of CO_2 insufflation, something may indeed be wrong, and further assessment and reporting to the nurse or physician are indicated.

3. Prepare to assist with cultures to send to the laboratory. Ask if she uses protection during intercourse. Tell her she may have to refrain from sexual activity until the source and communicability of her discharge are determined.

4. Depending on how Mr. Brown shared this initial information, you probably have a good idea how comfortable he is sharing additional information. If not, you can ask if he would like to discuss the matter further. A good question to ask might be why he is no longer sexually active. If it is not by choice, he may be experiencing erectile dysfunction from complications of diabetes. If physical problems are preventing sexual activity, inform him that there are many treatments available. If Mr. Brown wishes, talk with his physician about a consultation with a urologist or other expert.

REVIEW QUESTIONS

*The correct answers are in **boldface**.*

1. **(a)**
2. **(b)**
3. **(a)**
4. **(d)**
5. **(c)**
6. **(b)** is correct. Breast self-examination (BSE) should be done monthly. (a) is more often than necessary; (c, d) are too infrequent.
7. **(d)** is correct. Digital rectal examination (DRE) is done by a physician at a routine visit. (a, b, c) It is unreasonable to expect such frequent physician visits; testicular self-examination (TSE) can be done at home more often.
8. **(b)** is correct. A cystourethrogram involves a catheter, dye, and x-rays. (a, c, d) are not correct.
9. **(b)** is correct. The patient should empty her bladder before the Papanicolaou (Pap) smear. (a, c, d) are not necessary for Pap smears.
10. **(a)** is correct. A portion of the BSE is done while lying down. (b, c, d) are inappropriate.
11. **(c)** is correct. A charcoal swab is used for gonorrhea. (a, b, d) are used for other tests.
12. **(d)** is correct. A mammogram shows a lesion, but it cannot diagnose specifically what the lesion is. Additional tests are needed. (a, b) are not true; (c) mammogram is not the best test but is a good screening tool.
13. **(c)** is correct. Patients with metal in their bodies should avoid magnetic resonance imaging (MRI). (a) Radiation is not used with MRI, (b) MRI does not use sound waves, and (d) drugs are not injected into body cavities.
14. **(d)** is correct. Wet mounts must be viewed immediately. (a) there is not time to sit at this time, (b) is not therapeutic, (c) the wet mount needs to be delivered before spending time, and recommending her partner be tested is premature.

CHAPTER 42

VOCABULARY

1. **(C)**   6. **(G)**
2. **(D)**   7. **(A)**
3. **(B)**   8. **(F)**
4. **(J)**   9. **(H)**
5. **(E)**   10. **(I)**

BREAST SURGERIES

1. **(E)**   4. **(B)**
2. **(A)**   5. **(D)**
3. **(C)**

MENSTRUAL DISORDERS

1. **(E)**   4. **(B)**
2. **(C)**   5. **(D)**
3. **(A)**

MASTECTOMY CARE

*Errors are in **boldface**.*

You are assigned to care for Mrs. Joseph, who is 1 day postoperative following a right radical mastectomy. **You know that she is not anxious** because she had a left mastectomy a year ago and **knows everything to expect.** You listen to her breath sounds and find them clear, so it is **not necessary to have her cough and deep breathe.** You encourage her to **lie on her right side** to prevent bleeding. You use her **right arm for blood pressures** because both arms are affected and the right one is more convenient. You also encourage her to **avoid use of her right arm** to prevent injury to the surgical site. You provide a balanced diet and plenty of fluids to aid in her recovery.

It is impossible to know if Mrs. Joseph is anxious without assessing her. Most likely she is anxious because a second mastectomy probably was done for a recurrence of cancer. She needs a lot of support. A referral to Reach to Recovery or another appropriate support group would be helpful. Also, never assume that because a patient has had a procedure before, she knows everything to expect. Assess her knowledge level and teach accordingly. The incision on her chest may hurt when she coughs and deep breathes, increasing her risk of pulmonary complications. She should receive analgesics and encouragement to cough and deep breathe every hour. Lying on her right side may make elevation of her right arm difficult. She should assume a position in which her arm can be elevated on a pillow to decrease swelling. Neither arm should be used for blood pressures after mastectomies; consult with the physician about the advisability of using the left arm or possibly her legs. She should be taught to exercise her arm using exercises recommended by the institution.

CRITICAL THINKING

1. Some factors affecting her frequent yeast overgrowths may include poor nutrition, inadequate blood glucose control, overly restrictive clothing, overheating of the genital area from long periods of sitting, immune system deficiency, a strain of yeast that is resistant to her usual treatment, and antibiotic use (many young people take antibiotics regularly for acne control).

2. Some suggestions to help her prevent this problem in the future might include wearing loose-fitting skirts and light cotton underwear for bus trips, changing positions frequently, and sitting with her legs apart under her skirt, getting out and walking (if this is practical) when the bus stops, mentioning any antibiotic use to the physician, emphasizing the recurrent nature of this problem to her physician, and assessment for immune system problems if other infections are also frequent. One main area to explore with her is her blood glucose control. Find out why she is not testing often enough, and help her to plan strategies to improve testing regularity. If she is financially unable to afford the test materials, find out if there are support options available to her (the local Diabetes Association chapter or hospital diabetes clinic may be able to help you find this information). Emphasize the benefits of adequate blood glucose control for many body systems as well as this disorder.

REVIEW QUESTIONS

*The correct answers are in **boldface**.*

1. **(b)** is correct; it is not 100% effective. (a, c, d) are all true and do not indicate a need for more teaching.
2. **(c, a, d, b)** Breathing pattern takes priority because ineffective respirations can be life threatening. Ineffective tissue perfusion can be health threatening, and is second. Psychosocial problems, although important, are the last priority. Anxiety comes first because it is actual; coping is a risk in this case.
3. **(c)** is correct. A douche may wash away signs of the pathogen. (a) Better visualization is nice, but it does not help identify the pathogen. (b, d) are not true.
4. **(a)** is correct. Receiving estrogen without progestins increases risk of cancer. (b) Risk of heart disease may be associated with estrogen and progestin therapy. (c and d) may improve with HRT.
5. **(b)** is correct. Elevation of the arm reduces swelling. (a, c, d) may worsen swelling.
6. **(c)** is correct. Multiple sexual partners increase the risk of cervical cancer. (a) There is no evidence that tight underwear increases cancer risk. (b) Papanicolaou smears detect cancer early. (d) Late onset of sexual activity may reduce risk of some diseases.
7. **(a)** is correct. Her reaction shows anger over her diagnosis, a normal grieving response. (b, c, d) may be true, but there is no evidence to support them in the question.
8. **(b)** is correct. Women who have not been pregnant have higher rates of breast cancer. (a, c, d) are all associated with reduced risk of breast cancer.
9. **(a)** is correct. This therapy affects hormone function. (b, c, d) do not work by affecting estrogen.
10. **(d)** is correct. Nausea will decrease intake. (a, b, c) will not increase intake. Unpeeled fresh fruits and vegetables may be contraindicated in a patient at risk for infection due to chemotherapy, but in general, the patient should be able to eat whatever sounds good.
11. **(d)** is correct. These are signs of infection. Prompt reporting is necessary so a culture can be done and antibiotics ordered. (a and c) Another day or 2 allows time for the infection to spread. (b) May cause unnecessary concern in the patient. In addition, if she is receiving home care, it may be difficult for her to get to her physician's office.
12. **(c)** is correct. Coffee contains caffeine, which can worsen premenstrual syndrome (PMS) symptoms. (a, b, d) help PMS symptoms.

 CHAPTER 43

VOCABULARY

1. retrograde ejaculation
2. priapism
3. Phimosis
4. Smegma
5. circumcision
6. Cryptorchidism
7. orchitis
8. erectile dysfunction
9. varicocele
10. vasectomy

DISORDERS OF THE MALE REPRODUCTIVE SYSTEM

1. **(C)**
2. **(E)**
3. **(A)**
4. **(B)**
5. **(J)**
6. **(G)**
7. **(D)**
8. **(F)**
9. **(H)**
10. **(I)**

ERECTILE DYSFUNCTION

1. Medication
2. Stress
3. Hypertension
4. Transurethral resection of the prostate (TURP)
5. Heart failure
6. Multiple sclerosis

CRITICAL THINKING

1. Use the WHAT'S UP? format to assess Mr. Washington's symptoms. The most important question is what he means by "can't pass water" and how long it has been since he last urinated. If he truly can pass no urine, the situation is an emergency. You can also observe for bladder distention, but palpation may be best done by the physician because of the risk for injury. Ask if he has ever been told he has prostate problems. If it has been a long time since he urinated last or the bladder appears distended, have the physician see the patient as soon as possible.

2. In an older man, prostate enlargement is a common cause of urinary problems and inability to urinate. Benign prostatic hypertrophy and cancer of the prostate gland are two possibilities.

3. Be prepared to assist with Foley catheter insertion. It may be difficult to get past an enlarged prostate, so the physician may need to be involved. The catheter can maintain urine flow until Mr. Washington is transferred to the hospital for further diagnostic tests and possible surgery. Find out how Mr. Washington got to the urgent care center and arrange a ride to the hospital if ordered.

4. If urine flow continues to be blocked, hydronephrosis, infection, and rupture of the bladder can occur.

5. "A special scope will be inserted into your penis that will chip away the enlarged parts of the prostate gland. You will be anesthetized so you won't feel it. Afterward you can expect to have a catheter in your bladder for several days."

6. The catheter has several purposes. It allows urine to drain, places pressure on the resected gland to minimize bleeding, and provides a route to irrigate the bladder so clots can be removed. When totaling intake and output (I&O), irrigation solution should be included in the intake measurement because it is impossible to separate urine from solution in the output.

7. Bladder spasms are very painful, and the patient will inform you if they are occurring. Spasms may also cause leakage of urine around the catheter. Anesthetics and antispasmodic medications such as belladonna and opium (B&O) suppositories can help the discomfort. Irrigation of the catheter can flush out clots that can increase spasms. Relaxation exercises may also help.

8. Tell Mr. Washington that some episodes of incontinence may occur, but that they should subside in a few weeks. Teach him to do Kegel's exercises to increase sphincter tone. He should not restrict fluids because this can increase risk for urinary tract infection (UTI). A condom catheter or penile pad may help catch urine until incontinence improves. His panic could have been prevented by careful discharge teaching, letting Mr. Washington know what to expect and what to do about it.

REVIEW QUESTIONS

*The correct answers are in **boldface**.*

1. (**a, c, and f**) are all correct. (b) erectile dysfunction is not a symptom of BPH; (d, e) are signs of kidney disease.

2. (**c**) is correct. Sexual function is occasionally affected. (a) does not answer his question; (b, d) imply that dysfunction is expected, which is not true.

3. (**b**) is correct. The B&O suppository will relieve bladder spasms. (a) Demerol relieves pain but not spasms, (c) warming the solution is not recommended, and (d) notifying the physician STAT is not necessary—bladder spasms are an expected occurrence.

4. (**c**) is correct. The catheter needs to be kept free of clots so that it drains the bladder. (a) irrigation does not stop bleeding, (b) antibiotics are not normally in the irrigating solution, and (d) irrigation does not affect urine production.

5. (**b**) is correct. Kegel's exercises will help strengthen sphincter tone. (a) restricting fluids increases risk of infection, (c) reinserting the catheter will only delay the problem, and (d) incontinence may last several weeks.

6. (**d**) is correct. Asking an open-ended question will help Mr. Blaker share his concerns at his level of comfort. (a) The information provided does not support a diagnosis of impaired communication; (b) not all patients are helped by verbalizing concerns; and (c) this does not allow Mr. Blaker to identify his own concerns.

7. (**b**) is correct. The scrotum will be painful and swollen. (a, c, d) are not symptoms of epididymitis.

8. (**b**) is correct. A respiratory rate of 36 indicates respiratory distress and is the first priority. (a, c, and d) are all important and should be addressed once breathing is stabilized.

9. (**c**) is correct. Always replace the foreskin to prevent impairment of circulation and the possibility of not being able to replace it later. (a) Never leave the foreskin retracted; (b) the foreskin should be retracted if possible to wash the area; and (d) mild soap, not alcohol, should be used.

10. (**a**) is correct. Monthly TSE is one method to detect testicular cancer. (b) DRE is used to detect prostate enlargement; (c) an annual physical examination is advised, but it does not take the place of monthly checks; and (d) ultrasound is not done routinely to detect testicular cancer.

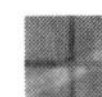 ## CHAPTER 44

VOCABULARY

1. (**D**)	4. (**E**)
2. (**B**)	5. (**A**)
3. (**C**)	6. (**F**)

INFLAMMATORY DISORDERS

1. (**A**)	4. (**E**)
2. (**C**)	5. (**D**)
3. (**B**)	

BARRIER METHODS FOR SAFER SEX

1. Latex condoms are less likely to break during intercourse than other types. Lubrication decreases the chances of breakage during use, but only water-soluble lubricants should be used because substances such as petroleum jelly (Vaseline) may weaken the condom. Condoms should never be inflated to test them because this can weaken them. Condoms should be applied only when the penis is erect. Either condoms with a reservoir tip or regular condoms that have been applied while holding approximately 1/2 inch of the closed end flat between the fingertips allow room for expansion by the ejaculate without creating excessive pressure, which might break the condom. The penis should be withdrawn after ejaculation before the erection begins to subside while holding the top of the condom securely around the penis to avoid spillage. Condoms should never be reused and should be discarded properly after use so others will not come in contact with the contents.

2. Female condoms should be applied before any penetration occurs (even preejaculation fluid can contain microorganisms). Lubrication decreases the chances of breakage during use, but only water-soluble lubricants should be used because substances such as petroleum jelly may weaken the condom. Female condoms should never be reused and should be discarded properly after use so others will not come in contact with the contents.

3. These may provide some protection for the cervix only. They are not effective barriers against sexually transmitted disease (STD) infection.

4. These may provide some barrier protection for manual and oral sexual activity. Although some groups suggest that male condoms may be split down one side and opened or rubber dental dam material may be taped over areas that have lesions to avoid direct contact with blood and body fluid, especially during sadomasochistic sexual activity; this *very high-risk behavior* is not recommended.

5. Anal intercourse is a *very high-risk activity* for transmission of many types of STDs, as well as many intestinal organisms, and is not recommended. Homosexual networks advise wearing double condoms and using water-soluble lubricants, preferably containing nonoxynol-9, to decrease the risk somewhat if engaging in this type of sexual activity.

CRITICAL THINKING

1. Misunderstandings may include the following:
   a. The mistaken idea that one blood test can diagnose all STDs
   b. Misunderstanding about the time that may be required to treat STDs (if the disease is treatable at all)
   c. Lack of understanding of the importance of interview information for diagnosing STDs
   d. Lack of understanding of the importance of physical examination for diagnosing STDs

2. The woman is an adult and has the right to make her own decisions. Unless James is her legal guardian, he has no legal right to information about her. He may be notified by a public health authority that he has been listed as a sexual contact by someone (anonymous) who has tested positive for a particular STD. However, if they have not yet become sexually intimate, he is not actually a contact. The only ethical and legal way that he can find out the information is by her choice (without coercion) to tell him.

3. Before any testing is done, both people should see the physician separately, be interviewed, be examined, and, if necessary, have samples taken for investigation. The physician should then order the tests that he or she deems necessary and counsel each patient about the test procedures, possible outcomes and treatments, and

the expected time frame for return of results. A return visit may be arranged for a time after the physician should have received notification of results.

4. No, James is not going to get his answer about whether he has a contagious STD today. Even if he is a virgin, he may possibly have contracted an STD prenatally, so he must wait for test results. Recent exposure to some STD agents may not show positive results for a long period.

REVIEW QUESTIONS

*The correct answers are in **boldface**.*

1. (**a, c, d**) are correct. Standard precautions are always appropriate, especially with possible herpes infection. Cesarean delivery may protect the baby from exposure. The obstetrician or midwife must be informed so decisions can be made for a safe delivery. (b) is incorrect. Teaching is appropriate, but reprimanding is not. (e) An antibiotic will not treat a viral infection, and would need a physician's order. (f) would protect a patient who is immune compromised, and is not appropriate in this case.

2. (**d**) is correct. A history and physical examination with diagnostic testing are the only way to diagnose an STD. (a) is untrue. (b and c) Checking for lesions and using a condom are good ideas, but will not prevent all STD transmission.

3. (**d**) is correct. Questioning a partner is only one small part of STD prevention, so if the student believes this is adequate protection, more teaching is necessary. (a, b, c) are all correct statements and do not indicate a need for further teaching.

4. (**c**) is correct. A *Chlamydia* collection kit should be set out. (a, b, d) are not used to diagnose a chlamydial infection.

5. (**a**) is correct. The ulcer should be examined for diagnosis and treatment. (b, c) may be upsetting to the patient, since the ulcer may be from something other than an STD. (d) Gentle cleaning is important, but an STD can occur at any age.

6. (**b**) is correct. The girl is asking for information to maintain health. (a, c, d) may be true, but are not supported by the data provided.

7. (**c**) is correct. Human papillomavirus causes genital warts. (a, b, d) cause other viral disorders.

8. (**c**) is correct. Urethritis causes painful, frequent urination and discharge. (a, b, d) are not symptoms of urethritis.

9. (**a**) is correct. Her pain should be assessed before intervention takes place. (b, c, d) may also be appropriate after assessment has taken place.

10.

$$\frac{2,400,000 \text{ units}}{} \cdot \frac{8 \text{ mL}}{5,000,000 \text{ units}} = 3.8 \text{ mL}$$

◼ CHAPTER 45

STRUCTURE OF NEUROMUSCULAR JUNCTION AND SARCOMERES

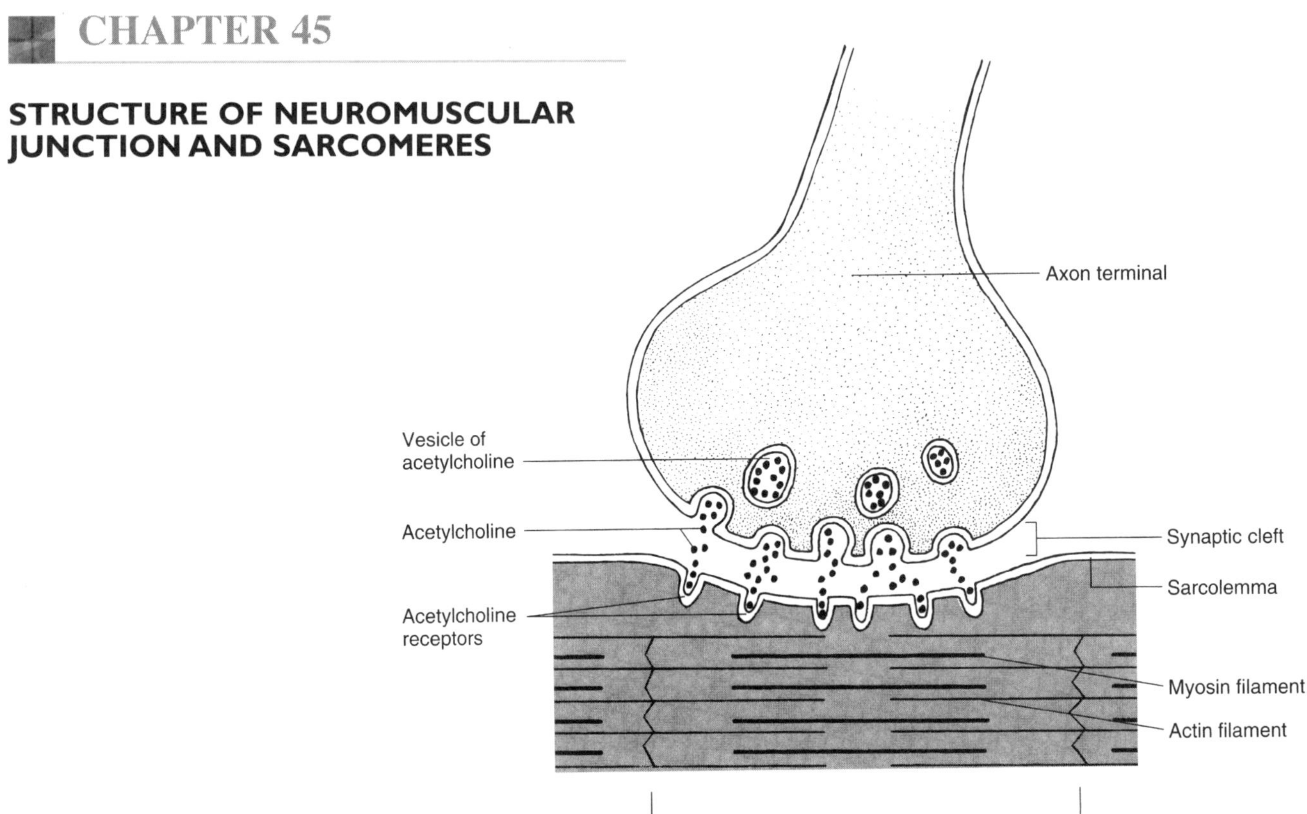

NEUROMUSCULAR JUNCTION

1. (C, E)   3. (B, D)
2. (A, F)

SYNOVIAL JOINTS

1. (E)   4. (B)
2. (C)   5. (D)
3. (A)

VOCABULARY

1. (C)   6. (F)
2. (A)   7. (H)
3. (D)   8. (G)
4. (E)   9. (J)
5. (B)   10. (I)

DIAGNOSTIC TESTS

1. (C)   7. (F)
2. (A)   8. (H)
3. (B)   9. (J)
4. (E)   10. (I)
5. (D)   11. (K)
6. (G)

CRITICAL THINKING

1. Allergies, past health, medications, surgeries, injury, cause and mechanism of injury (how injured will indicate other injuries to look for; mechanism of injury—twisting, crushing, stretching).
2. Inspection: injury, asymmetry, mobility and range of motion, swelling, deformity and limb length, ecchymosis. Palpation: skin temperature, crepitation, tenderness, sensation.
3. X-rays of his leg and any other areas of potential injury based on the history. Complete blood count (CBC) to identify loss of blood. Additional tests may be ordered based on findings.
4. Any procedures to be done, tests to be done, need to report symptoms, pain relief issues, answer any questions.

REVIEW QUESTIONS

The correct answers are in boldface.

1. (**c**)
2. (**b**)
3. (**a**)
4. (**c**)
5. (**b**)

6. (**b**) *Crepitation* is the term used for a grating sound heard in a joint. (a) A friction rub is associated with either pleural or pericardial inflammation or fluid accumulation. (c) An effusion is a collection of fluid in a space. (d) Subcutaneous emphysema is leaking air that is felt under the skin.
7. (**c**) Joint movement should immediately be stopped to prevent further joint injury. (a, b, d) would move the joint, causing possible injury.
8. (**b**) Ability to prepare food is an instrumental activity of daily living (ADL), which is part of a functional assessment. (a, c, d) are not items assessed in a functional assessment.
9. (**d**) A hematoma may develop following a biopsy. (a) does not occur from a biopsy. (b) Crackles are heard in the lungs. (c) An infection would not develop immediately, it would occur several days later.
10. (**a**) Bleeding into soft tissue is a complication of a biopsy. (b, c, d) relate to pain control.
11. (**b**) Stiff, sore joints are one of the early symptoms of rheumatoid arthritis. (a, d) are not early symptoms. (c) is not a related symptom.
12. (**b, e**) The patient should be nil per os (NPO) after midnight the night before surgery. (a) No food should be eaten after midnight. (c, d) are responsibilities of the physician.

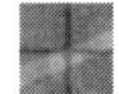 # CHAPTER 46

VOCABULARY

1. Arthritis
2. Arthroplasty
3. Synovitis
4. Arthrocentesis
5. Hyperuricemia
6. Scleroderma
7. Vasculitis
8. Polymyositis
9. Avascular necrosis
10. Replantation
11. Hemipelvectomy
12. Fasciotomy
13. Osteomyelitis
14. Osteosarcoma

FRACTURES

1. (**K**)   7 (**F**)
2. (**J**)   8. (**D**)
3. (**I**)   9. (**C**)
4. (**H**)   10. (**B**)
5. (**G**)   11. (**A**)
6. (**F**)

PROSTHESIS CARE EDUCATION

1. False—same
2. False—water
3. True
4. True
5. False—grease, prosthetist

HEALTH PROMOTION FOR PATIENTS WITH GOUT

1. purine, sardines
2. avoid
3. fluids
4. aspirin, aspirin
5. avoid
6. stress

CRITICAL THINKING

NURSING DIAGNOSIS
Impaired Physical Mobility Related to Hip Precautions and Surgical Pain

Interventions	Rationale	Evaluation
Reinforce transfer and ambulation techniques.	Activity is restricted due to hip precautions and weight-bearing limitations.	Does patient transfer and ambulate as instructed by physical therapy?
Place overhead frame and trapeze on bed; teach patient how to use it.	Patient mobility is increased and pain decreased with use of trapeze for movement.	Does patient use overbed frame and trapeze for movement?
Assess the patient for and take measures to prevent complications of immobility: Turn patient every 2 hours and check skin. Keep heels off of bed. Teach patient to deep breathe and cough every 2 hours; also teach use of incentive spirometer. Apply thigh-high elastic stockings. Give anticoagulants as ordered. Get patient out of bed as soon as possible. Ambulate patient as early as possible. Remind patient to practice leg exercises.	Immobility complications can occur if preventive measures are not used.	Does patient experience complications of immobility?

REVIEW QUESTIONS

*The correct answers are in **boldface.***

1. (**b**) Buck's traction is skin traction. (a, c, d) are examples of skeletal traction.
2. (**b**) Palming the cast to move it prevents indentations being made in the wet cast with fingertips. (a, c, d) are incorrect.
3. (**c, e**) Giving a test dose of gold is important to assess for an allergic reaction, and the patient is monitored after the test dose for an allergic reaction. (a, b, d) are incorrect.
4. (**b**) It should be wrapped in a cool moist cloth (sterile, if available) and sealed in a plastic bag. (a) It should be cool and moist. (c) It is not placed on dry ice, which is also not readily available. (d) is not readily available or moist.
5. (**d**) The morphine should be prepared now so it is ready promptly when 3 hours is up; 15 mg should be given because the pain level is at the maximum and is occurring before the minimum ordered time interval. (a) Applying ice to the cast may be helpful, but because the pain is at the maximum, it will not provide enough relief. (b) There are no abnormalities to report

to the physician at this time. (c) Removing the pillow may increase pain if swelling increases.

6. (**d**) This is a sign of hip dislocation. (a, b, c) are incorrect.

7. (**d**) Liver is an organ meat high in purines. (a, b, c) are not high-purine foods.

8. (**a**) can cause an attack of gout. (b, c, d) are incorrect.

9. (**c**) The erythrocyte sedimentation rate is a general screening test for systemic inflammation. (a, b, d) are incorrect.

10. (**a**) occurs commonly in patients with lupus. (b, c, d) are not common nursing diagnoses for lupus.

11. (**d**) A test dose is given to assess for an allergic reaction. (a, b, c) are incorrect.

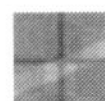 # CHAPTER 47

VOCABULARY

1. dysphagia
2. electroencephalogram
3. paresthesia
4. decorticate
5. decerebrate
6. Anisocoria
7. nystagmus
8. contractures
9. dysarthria
10. aphasia

DIAGNOSTIC TESTS

1. A myelogram is an x-ray examination of the spinal canal after injection of contrast material into the subarachnoid space. Before the procedure ask the patient about allergies to contrast media. Make sure that a consent form has been signed. Check institution policy for NPO (nil by mouth) guidelines. Following the procedure the patient is maintained on bedrest, positioned with the head elevated or according to physician's orders (based on type of dye used). Fluids are encouraged to help the kidneys excrete the dye.

2. An electroencephalogram (EEG) uses electrodes attached to the scalp to monitor the electrical activity of the brain. Before the procedure, make sure the patient's hair is clean and dry. Check with the physician for any medications to hold. After the procedure, monitor for seizures, especially if seizure medications were held. Wash the adhesive from the hair as soon as possible before it becomes hard and difficult to remove.

3. A lumbar puncture involves a needle into the spinal fluid to collect cerebral spinal fluid (CSF) for analysis. Before the procedure you may ask the physician for an order for an analgesic or sedative if the patient is especially anxious. Make sure that a consent form has been signed. Assist the patient into a side-lying position with knees flexed and back arched. Some physicians prefer the patient sitting on the edge of the bed leaning over a bedside table. Stay with the patient to offer reassurance and assist the physician with specimens. Following the procedure follow orders for 6 to 8 hours of bedrest, and encourage fluids. Monitor the puncture site for leakage of CSF. Notify the physician if a headache occurs.

4. Magnetic resonance imaging (MRI) uses magnetic energy to produce images of tissues. It is not an x-ray. Ask patients if they have any metal in their bodies (pacemakers, joint replacements, foreign bodies, tattoos)—if so they may not be able to have an MRI. Instruct the patient that he or she will be in a tunnel-like machine for 30 to 60 minutes, and that there will be banging noises. If the patient is claustrophobic, notify the physician and obtain a sedative or alternative orders. If the patient is in pain, request analgesic orders for before the procedure. No special aftercare is necessary.

5. Computed tomography (CT) produces images of layers ("slices") of tissue. It requires that the body or body part be within the scanner, which may be difficult for claustrophobic people. The physician may use contrast material. Find out if this is planned, and ensure the patient has no allergies to contrast material, iodine, or shellfish. The physician should be notified if kidney function is compromised because kidneys excrete the dye. Check institution policy to know whether the patient should be kept NPO before the procedure. If dye is used, the patient should be prepared to expect a feeling of warmth during the injection. Following any procedure using dye, fluids should be encouraged. If dye is not used, no special aftercare is necessary.

ANATOMY

Synaptic knobs
Synapse
Cell body
Nucleus
Dendrites
Axon
Myelin sheath
Schwann cell
Nucleus
Cell body
Neurolemma
Axon
Myelin sheath
Axon terminals
Dendrite
Muscle
Receptors
Parietal lobe
Corpus callosum
Frontal lobe
Occipital lobe
Lateral ventricle
Thalamus
Cerebellum
Third ventricle
Hypothalamus
Pituitary gland
Fourth ventricle
Midbrain
Brain stem
Pons
Medulla

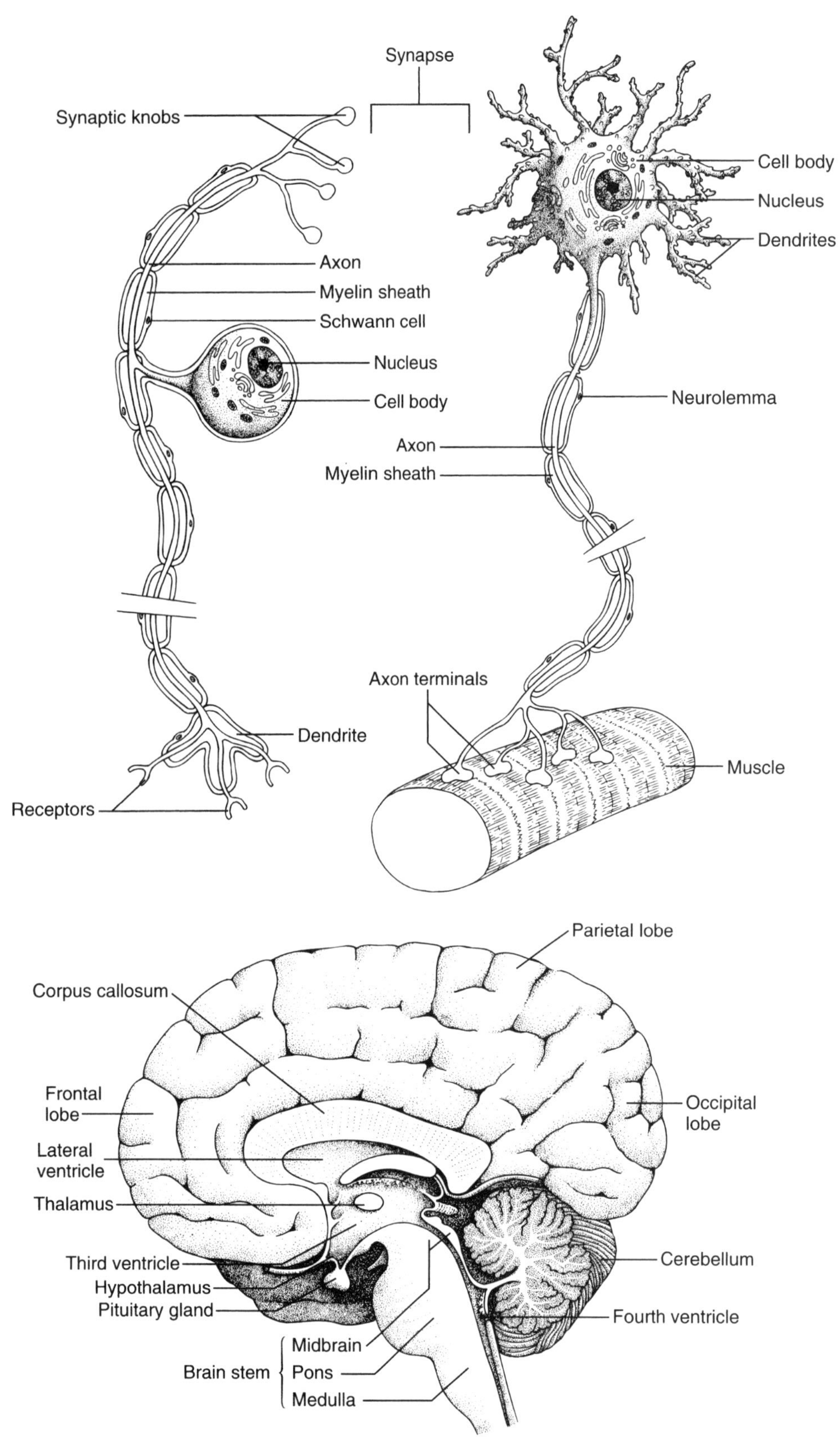

ANATOMY REVIEW

1. **(E)**   4. **(C)**
2. **(D)**   5. **(B)**
3. **(A)**

ASSESSMENT OF CRANIAL NERVES

1. **(C)**   4. **(A)**
2. **(D)**   5. **(E)**
3. **(B)**

CRITICAL THINKING

1. After checking her transfer records for previous activity level, check muscle strength in her legs and feet. Ask how she got up to the bathroom at the hospital. Then have a second nurse or aide help in dangling her at the bedside and slowly standing before attempting to ambulate. If she is unable to dangle or stand, use a bedpan or bedside commode until she becomes stronger. Document how she did and how much assistance she needed in the plan of care. Consider whether she needs an order for physical therapy.

2. Again, ask how she ate at the hospital, keeping in mind that her answers may not be reliable. Check for a gag reflex. Make sure she is sitting straight up to eat, preferably in a chair. Try small sips and bites first. Stay with her for the first meal to monitor her swallowing. Because she is weak on one side, check her mouth after each bite for pocketing of food.

3. Ask questions to assess orientation, such as the month and year, where she is, and who familiar visitors are. Check recent and remote memory. (What did you have for lunch? What is your mother's name?) Clarify her question. She may have a perfectly legitimate reason to ask for the cookies.

4. Blood pressure is affected by muscle tone. A weak arm may have a lower pressure.

REVIEW QUESTIONS

*The correct answers are in **boldface**.*

1. **(b)**
2. **(b)**
3. **(b)**
4. **(a)**
5. **(b)**
6. **(d)**
7. **(a)**
8. **(a)**
9. **(c)** is correct. The patient is positioned on his or her side to expose the spinal column for puncture. (a, b, d) are not necessary for a lumbar puncture (LP).
10. **(a)** is correct. The patient lays flat for 6 to 8 hours to prevent headache following LP. (b) The patient should drink fluids, not be NPO; (c) pedal pulses are not sig-

nificant following LP; and (d) the patient is kept flat for 6 to 8 hours, not elevated for 24 hours.
11. **(d)** correctly describes an MRI. (a) describes an electromyography, (b) describes an EEG, and (c) describes a brain scan.

CHAPTER 48

VOCABULARY

1. **(I)**   6. **(D)**
2. **(F)**   7. **(E)**
3. **(A)**   8. **(C)**
4. **(G)**   9. **(H)**
5. **(B)**   10. **(J)**

DRUGS USED FOR CENTRAL NERVOUS SYSTEM DISORDERS

1. **(B)**   4. **(E)**
2. **(C)**   5. **(D)**
3. **(A)**

ALZHEIMER'S DISEASE

1. **(C)**   3. **(D)**
2. **(B)**   4. **(A)**

CENTRAL NERVOUS SYSTEM DISORDERS

1. **(I)**   6. **(B)**
2. **(F)**   7. **(H)**
3. **(A)**   8. **(J)**
4. **(E)**   9. **(D)**
5. **(G)**   10. **(C)**

SPINAL DISORDERS

Radiating pain to the ankle, footdrop, and the inability to walk on the toes are all indications of dysfunction of a lumbar nerve root. Deltoid weakness and diminished triceps reflex indicate dysfunction of a cervical nerve root.

CRITICAL THINKING: SPINAL CORD INJURY

1. These are the hallmark signs of spinal cord injury. Loss of vasomotor control results in vasodilation. This causes hypotension. Dilated blood vessels allow more exposure of blood to the skin surface, thereby cooling the blood and causing hypothermia. Bradycardia results from disruption of the autonomic nervous system.

2. Mr. Granger no longer has full use of his respiratory muscles. Therefore, he is not able to take deep breaths.

3. (a) Cervical traction will keep his cervical spine immobile and prevent further damage to the spinal cord. (b) Administration of vasopressors may be necessary to maintain blood pressure at a level that is adequate for tissue perfusion. Intravenous fluids may be inadequate to maintain blood pressure and may result in fluid overload. (c) Loss of innervation to the bladder may result in urine retention. An indwelling catheter is used to prevent bladder rupture or urinary reflux.

4. Edema of the spinal cord, fatigue of respiratory muscles, or both are reducing Mr. Granger's already compromised respiratory function. As he feels more short of breath, he becomes more anxious, fearing that his condition is worsening. Explain to him that this is a common short-term complication of spinal cord injury. Reassure him that if mechanical ventilation is required, it will not necessarily be a permanent situation.

5. Expect that Mr. Granger will be intubated or have a tracheostomy placed to allow for mechanical ventilation. Expect the ventilation to be necessary until the spinal cord edema has subsided.

6. *Ineffective breathing pattern.* The goal is that Mr. Granger will not experience hypoxia or respiratory arrest. Monitor his pulse oximetry and respiratory pattern frequently. At the first sign of restlessness, anxiety, or shortness of breath, inform the physician.

   Impaired physical mobility. The goal is for all of Mr. Granger's care needs to be met. He will be unable to care for himself independently. Protect him from skin breakdown and other hazards of immobility. Whenever possible, give Mr. Granger choices as to how and when care will be performed. Include his significant others as much as he and they wish.

7. Mr. Granger needs simple explanations of what has happened to him and what his prognosis is. He also needs to begin to learn to direct his care. This will improve his ability to function outside of the hospital. After he is stable, he will likely be transferred to a rehabilitation facility to continue to learn self-care.

REVIEW QUESTIONS

*The correct answers are in **boldface**.*

1. (**c**) This addresses the patient's feelings and is most likely to calm her. (a and d) try to reason with a patient who is unable to reason, and may be threatening. (b) is misleading—the patient is not going to find her mother.

2. (**c**) Drowsiness is a common side effect. (a, b, d) are not common side effects.

3. (**d**) Ambulation is the best evidence that the patient with lumbar disk disease is mobile. (a, c) are good outcomes but are not related to mobility. (b) relates to cervical disease, not lumbar.

4. (**c**) Inability to move the affected leg would not be expected and should immediately be reported to the physician. (a) Incisional pain and (d) muscle spasm are common temporary results of microdiskectomy. (b) Bleeding should be monitored, but a small amount does not require immediate reporting unless it is rapidly increasing.

5. (**a**) The patient with a brain tumor is at risk for seizures. (b, c) are important interventions once the patient's safety is assured. (d) There is no reason to place the patient in isolation.

6. (**b**) A structured environment provides a quiet setting with minimal distractions. (a, c, d) could all potentiate the patient's agitation.

7. (**a**) is correct. Decreasing level of consciousness (LOC) is a symptom of increasing ICP. (b, c) Sympathetic and parasympathetic responses and (d) increased cerebral blood flow do not cause decreased LOC.

8. (**c**) Widening pulse pressure warns of increasing ICP. (a, b, d) do not occur in increasing ICP.

9. (**b**) is correct. Elevation of the head of the bed reduces ICP. (a, c, d) all can potentially increase ICP.

10. (**a, c, d, f**) can all help avoid falls. (b) Restraints are not recommended, and may increase agitation and risk of falls. (e) Assisting the patient who is at risk of falls is appropriate. Encouraging independence may be appropriate for some patients, but may not be appropriate if the patient is at risk for falling.

CHAPTER 49

VOCABULARY

1. (**B**)   4. (**D**)
2. (**C**)   5. (**E**)
3. (**A**)

DRUGS USED FOR CEREBROVASCULAR DISORDERS

1. (**A**)   4. (**B**)
2. (**C**)   5. (**E**)
3. (**D**)

CRITICAL THINKING: STROKE

1. A stroke is the infarction of brain tissue due to the disruption of blood flow to the brain. Considering Mrs. Saunders' history, the cause of her attack was most likely ischemic, the result of atherosclerosis.

2. Hemiplegia

3. Left, because her right side is paralyzed.

4. She was a smoker, she has a history of atherosclerosis and hypertension, and she is overweight.

5. Expressive aphasia

6. Her score on the Glasgow Coma Scale is 11. Symptoms of rising ICP include headache, vomiting, dilated pupil on the affected side, increasing weakness or paralysis, decorticate or decerebrate posturing, decreasing level of consciousness, increasing systolic blood pressure and respiratory rate, and increasing and then decreasing pulse rate.

7. A thrombolytic medication may have been used in the emergency room if Mrs. Saunders arrived within 3 hours of onset of her symptoms. The nurse would continue to monitor for side effects. Heparin may be ordered as an anticoagulant; antiplatelet drugs may be ordered for long-term prevention of recurrent stroke, and antihypertensives may be ordered to control blood pressure.

8. Many diagnoses fit Mrs. Saunders' situation. An example is impaired physical mobility related to flaccid right side. Measures to prevent complications related to immobility include repositioning every 1 to 2 hours, maintaining good body alignment with pillows, consulting physical therapy for exercise recommendations, range-of-motion exercises, and possibly a sling to prevent harm to her weakened shoulder muscles.

9. Reposition every 1 to 2 hours, maintain good nutrition and fluid intake, apply a pressure-reduction mattress to the bed, keep skin clean and dry, and check frequently for incontinence.

10. Because Mrs. Saunders understands spoken words, ask her if she has to go to the bathroom. Usually if a patient is attempting to get out of bed, there is a reason for it. See if she can nod yes or no in response. She may be able to point to the bedside commode or bathroom. A picture board might also be helpful.

11. Gag and swallow reflexes can both be checked. A cotton swab at the back of the throat should elicit a gag reflex. If she gags, try a small sip of water before giving her food. Be sure to follow institution policy for swallowing evaluation before giving any oral food or fluid.

12. Ask for a consultation with the speech therapy department or other swallowing expert for recommendations specific to Mrs. Saunders. Many patients do better with pureed foods and thickened liquids. Be sure she is sitting straight up, preferably in a chair, to eat. Have her tilt her head forward while swallowing. Have her swallow each bite twice. After each bite, remind her to check the right side of her mouth for food that is not noticed.

13. Involve her family in her care. Give them small tasks to do for her. Encourage them to attend physical and other therapies with her. Explain what will happen at the rehabilitation facility. Assist the family to identify resources that can help when she is discharged to home. Consult with the social worker or discharge planner to provide them with additional information.

14. Antiplatelet drugs such as aspirin or clopidogrel (Plavix).

REVIEW QUESTIONS

*The correct answers are in **boldface.***

1. (**d**) is correct. Having another staff member assist can help protect the patient from falling while the nurse assesses the patient's ability to walk. (a, b) are not safe. (c) may be true, but she may be able to walk independently if she can safely do so.

2. (**c**) is correct. Breaking a task down into simple steps helps the patient to function. (a) Performing the task for the patient and (b) telling the patient not to worry do not help the patient gain independence. (d) Having another patient demonstrate the task may further frustrate the patient, who may compare progress with the other patient. It also will not help the patient learn to do the task, which needs to be broken down into simple steps.

3. (**a**) is correct. The patient may be exhibiting unilateral neglect or homonymous hemianopsia. (b) is incorrect—there is no evidence that the patient is hard of hearing. (c) Waving fingers is rude and unnecessary in this case. (d) Using a picture board will not help if the patient cannot perceive his left side.

4. (**b**) is correct. A stroke can reduce inhibitions. (a) Punishment is inappropriate—his actions are not on purpose. (c, d) may be true, but do not address the problem.

5. (**d, e, f**) are correct. These can help prevent aspiration. (a) is incorrect—sitting upright is recommended. (b) Straws should be avoided. (c) Thin liquids are more easily aspirated.

6. (**c**) is correct. Allowing the patient to defecate on his usual schedule can help prevent incontinence. (a) If the patient is unable to detect the need to have a bowel movement, asking him will not be helpful. (b, d) Incontinence pads may be useful, and avoiding embarrassing the patient is essential, but neither will help reduce incontinence.

7.
$$\frac{62 \text{ mg} \mid 1 \text{ grain} \mid 1 \text{ tablet}}{60 \text{ mg} \mid 1 \text{ grain}} = 1 \text{ tablet}$$

8. (**b**) is correct—the stroke may be extending. (a, c, d) all delay treatment if the stroke is extending.

◼ CHAPTER 50

VOCABULARY

1. atrophied
2. exacerbations

3. neuralgia
4. ptosis
5. demyelination
6. plasmapheresis
7. fasciculations
8. anticholinesterase

PERIPHERAL DISORDERS

*Errors are in **boldface**.*

1. Miss Mary Garvey sees her physician because she has been seeing double off and on for several weeks and has been fatigued. Her physician suspects myasthenia gravis and schedules her for a **carotid ultrasound.** He confirms his suspicions with a Tensilon (edrophonium chloride) test. He explains to Miss Garvey that she has a disease that is characterized by a decrease in the neurotransmitter **norepinephrine.** He begins her on **Mastadon** and prednisone. Her nurse teaches her the importance of getting regular exercise and recommends **joining a local health and exercise club.**

   Electromyography (EMG), not ultrasound, is likely to be done. Receptor sites for the neurotransmitter acetylcholine are affected. Mestinon, not Mastadon, is an anticholinesterase drug used to reduce symptoms. (A mastadon is a prehistoric elephant.) It seems wise to recommend exercise, but individuals with myasthenia gravis become very fatigued, and rest, not exercise, is the only way to relieve it. Moderate exercise as tolerated is a better recommendation.

2. Mr. Tom Newby has a history of trigeminal neuralgia. He enters the emergency department with severe pain in his **left wrist.** The physician orders a narcotic analgesic because Mr. Newby's **third** cranial nerve is inflamed. Once the acute pain has subsided, Mr. Newby is discharged with instructions to get plenty of **fresh air** and to take his phenytoin (Dilantin) as ordered.

   Pain in the face, not the wrist, characterizes trigeminal neuralgia. The trigeminal nerve is the fifth, not the third, cranial nerve. Fresh air may aggravate pain because even a breeze on the face can cause excruciating pain.

3. Mrs. Mattie Schultz is admitted with exacerbated multiple sclerosis (MS). Her legs are becoming weaker, causing difficult walking, and she has been having difficulty swallowing. You know that **build-up** of myelin on her neurons is responsible for her weakness. You assess her for stressors that might have caused her exacerbation, such as urinary tract infection (UTI) or upper respiratory tract infection (URI). Mrs. Schultz is started on **thyroid-stimulating hormone (TSH) to stimulate her thyroid,** which will help reduce her symptoms. She is also placed on a combination of trimethoprim and trimethoprim/sulfamethoxazole (Bactrim) for the UTI you identified through your excellent assessment and on **diazepam (Valium)** for urinary retention.

   Patchy degeneration, not build-up, of myelin accounts for symptoms of MS. Adrenocorticotropic hormone (ACTH) to stimulate the adrenal cortex to secrete cortisol is given to reduce inflammation and relieve symptoms. Valium might be given for muscle spasms, but bethanechol (Urecholine) or oxybutynin (Ditropan) is given for urinary problems.

CRITICAL THINKING

1. Amyotrophic lateral sclerosis (ALS) is a nerve disease in which the nerves that stimulate the muscles to make them contract degenerate and form scar tissue. This makes it difficult for muscles to contract.
2. Nerves that control the muscles in his legs are becoming more affected. A referral for physical therapy and a cane or other walking aid might help Reverend Wilson continue to function for as long as possible.
3. He should know that ALS does not affect thinking. Therefore, as long as he can function physically, there is no reason to quit his job.
4. Muscle spasms can be relieved with medications such as baclofen (Lioresal) or diazepam (Valium).
5. Reverend Wilson's muscles that control swallowing are probably affected now. An appropriate nursing diagnosis is impaired swallowing related to muscle weakness. Because his swallowing is unlikely to improve dramatically, a good goal might be that he will not aspirate. Talk to the physician about ordering a swallowing evaluation by a speech therapist, who can recommend interventions to help prevent aspiration. Additional interventions include making sure he is sitting up straight to eat, staying with him during meals in case he has difficulty, having him swallow each bite twice, and having him avoid thin liquids. Eventually he and his wife may need to decide if they want to consider tube feedings.
6. Possible nursing diagnoses include disturbed body image, imbalanced nutrition, impaired oral mucous membranes, impaired mobility, risk for impaired skin integrity, and ineffective coping. Note that these are only possible ideas and would need to be verified with a thorough assessment.

REVIEW QUESTIONS

*The correct answers are in **boldface**.*

1. (**d**) is correct. Guillain-Barré syndrome is most likely caused by an autoimmune process. (a, b, c) are not causes of Guillain-Barré syndrome.
2. (**b**) is correct. Arterial blood gases (ABGs) monitor respiratory function. Deteriorating ABGs signal respiratory failure from weakening respiratory muscles. (a) signals kidney disease, which is not a common problem in

Guillain-Barré syndrome. (c) Bleeding and (d) electrolyte imbalances are not associated with Guillain-Barré syndrome.

3. (**d**) is correct. Tensilon is given to determine if it is effective in reducing muscle weakness. (a, b) There is no such thing as a Mestinon test or a Quinine tolerance test. (c) Pulmonary function studies might be done if respiratory muscles are affected, but would not be diagnostic for myasthenia gravis (MG).

4. (**a**) is correct. Anticholinesterase drugs reduce activity of cholinesterase, leaving more acetylcholine available to aid in muscle contraction. (b) Anticholinergic drugs will worsen symptoms. (c, d) Adrenergic drugs or beta blockers will not help.

5. (**d**) is correct. Myelin is damaged in MS. (a, b, c) are not related to MS.

6. (**b**) is correct. ACTH stimulates the adrenal cortex to release cortisol, which reduces inflammation and may induce remission. (a, c, d) are not used to treat MS.

7. (**b**) is correct. Elevating the head of the bed will reduce the workload of the respiratory muscles. (a) Antibiotics given when infection is not present can lead to resistant strains of bacteria. (c) Bedrest can increase risk of respiratory complications. (d) Suction should be done only when necessary.

8. (**d**) is correct. The patient with Bell's palsy may have difficulty closing the affected eye, and eyedrops will keep the eye lubricated. (a, b, c) are not useful for Bell's palsy. Heat, rather than ice, is sometimes used.

9. (**c**) is correct. The only way to know if nutrition is adequate without blood work is to monitor weights. Monitoring (a) meal trays, (b) intake and output (I&O), and (d) swallowing are all good interventions but will not show whether nutrition has been maintained. Serum albumin is also sometimes used to monitor nutrition status.

10.

$$\frac{30 \text{ mg} \quad \mid \quad 1 \text{ mL}}{\mid \quad 50 \text{ mg}} = 0.6 \text{ mL}$$

11. (**a**) is correct. Muscle twitchings are called fasciculations. (b) Atrophy is wasted muscles, (c) chorea is movements found in Huntington's disease, and (d) neuropathy is nerve pain.

12. (**b**) is correct. Eating uses muscles innervated by the fifth cranial nerve and is most likely to cause pain. (a, c, d) do not use the facial muscles and are less likely to cause pain. Sleeping usually relieves pain.

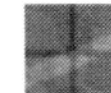

CHAPTER 51

STRUCTURES OF THE EYE

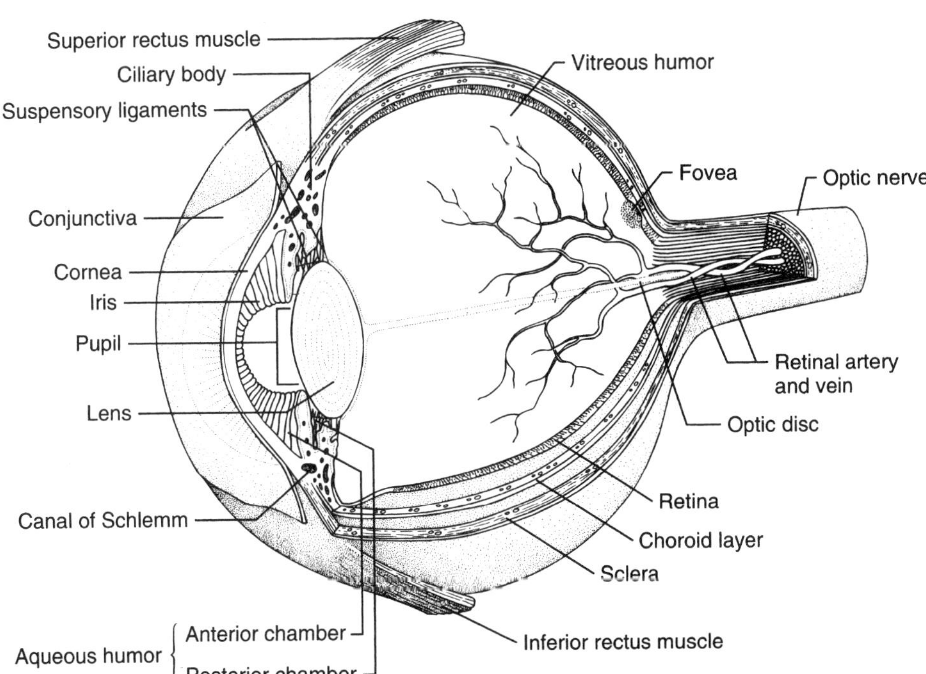

STRUCTURES OF THE EAR

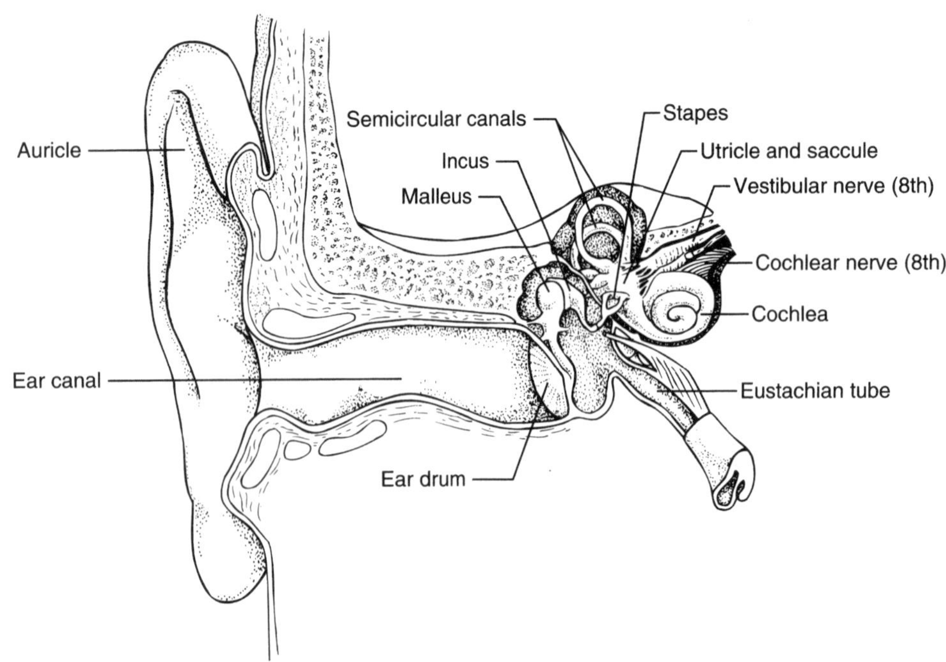

VISION

1. A	5. G
2. D	6. C
3. F	7. E
4. B	

HEARING

1. A	6. G
2. E	7. H
3. C	8. D
4. F	9. I
5. B	

VOCABULARY

Nystagmus
Definition: Constant involuntary cyclical eyeball movement.
Tropia
Definition: Deviation of eye away from visual axis.
Accommodation
Definition: Adjustment of the eye for distance to focus the image on the retina by changing lens curvature.
Ptosis
Definition: Drooping of upper eyelid from paralysis
Arcus senilus
Definition: Opaque white ring around the periphery of the cornea in aged persons from deposits of fat.

Ophthalmologist
Definition: Physician trained to diagnose and treat eye conditions and diseases.
Optometrist
Definition: Doctor of optometry who diagnoses and treats certain eye conditions and diseases.
Optician
Definition: Makes prescribed corrective lenses.

DIAGNOSTIC TESTS

Assessment Test	Purpose of Test	Normal Test Results
Snellen chart	Visual acuity	Right eye (OD) 20/20, left eye (OS) 20/20, each eye (OU) 20/20
Visual fields	Peripheral vision	Equal to examiner's
Cardinal fields of gaze	Extraocular movement	Follows in all fields without nystagmus
Accommodation	Pupillary response to near and far distance	Eyes turn inward and pupils constrict when focusing on a near object
Rinne	Differentiate between conductive and sensorineural hearing loss	Air conduction > bone conduction
Weber	Hearing acuity	Heard equally
Romberg's	Balance/vestibular function	Able to maintain standing position without loss of balance

CRITICAL THINKING

1. Eye strain from computer use
2. The nurse should ask the position of Ms. Little Thunder's computer and the lighting of the office. The nurse should also ask the size of font that Ms. Little Thunder is using.
3. The position of the bottom of the computer monitor should be 20 degrees below the line of sight and should be positioned 13 to 18 inches from the eyes. Glare should be reduced by situating the computer screen away from windows and lights. The font size should be increased if the letters on the screen appear too small.

REVIEW QUESTIONS

*The correct answers are in **boldface**.*

1. (**b**) The first distance recorded when conducting the Snellen test is the distance from which the patient can clearly read the alphabetical line on the chart. The second distance recorded is the distance from which a person with normal vision can see the same alphabetical line. (a, c) are incorrect. (d) is incorrect because normal vision is 20/20.
2. (**d**) Symmetrical eye muscle strength keeps the eyes in the same position, and the light is reflected in exactly the same place. (a) is incorrect. (b) defines accommodation. (c) defines the pupils' reaction to light.
3. (**c**) P = pupils, E = equal, R = round, R = reactive, L = to light, and A = accommodation. (a, b) are incorrect. (d) is incorrect because PERRLA is the expected finding.
4. (**a**) Visual fields test peripheral vision. (b, c, d) are incorrect because near vision is tested with a hand-held chart or by reading a book, distance vision is tested with a Snellen chart, and central vision is tested with an Amsler grid.
5. (**d**) Arcus senilis, although a physical eye finding, does not cause visual problems. (a, b, c) can lead to visual disturbances.
6. (**c**) Air conduction is heard longer than bone conduction. (a) defines bone conduction. (b) is incorrect because air conduction is more efficient. (d) is incorrect.
7. (**d, e, f**) Patients with hearing loss sometimes speak unusually loud or soft, turn to speaker to hear better or lip read, and withdraw from social situations. (a, b, c) indicate that the patient is hearing well enough to communicate.
8. (**b**) Air conduction is heard longer than bone conduction. (a) indicates the normal findings of a Weber test. (c, d) indicate abnormal findings.
9. (**c**) Ototoxic is ear toxicity. (a) Otoplasty is ear repair. (b) Otalgia is ear pain. (d) Tinnitus is ringing in the ears.
10. (**d**) Seeing halos around lights would be an important visual finding. (a, b, c) are incorrect.
11. (**a**) Darwin tubercle is a normal finding at any age. (b, c, d) are incorrect.
12. (**d**) is correct. (a) is for balance. (b) examines the tympanic membrane. (c) assesses the reflex that controls balance.
13. (**a**) Otorrhea is ear drainage. (b) Otalgia is ear pain. (c) Ototoxic is toxic to ear. (d) Tinnitus is ringing in the ears.
14. (**c**) Presbycusis is loss of high-pitched sounds due to aging. (a) Plasty is ear repair. (b) Otalgia is ear pain. (d) Tinnitus is ringing in the ears.

CHAPTER 52

VOCABULARY

1. (**E**)   4. (**F**)
2. (**D**)   5. (**B**)
3. (**C**)   6. (**A**)

ERRORS OF REFRACTION

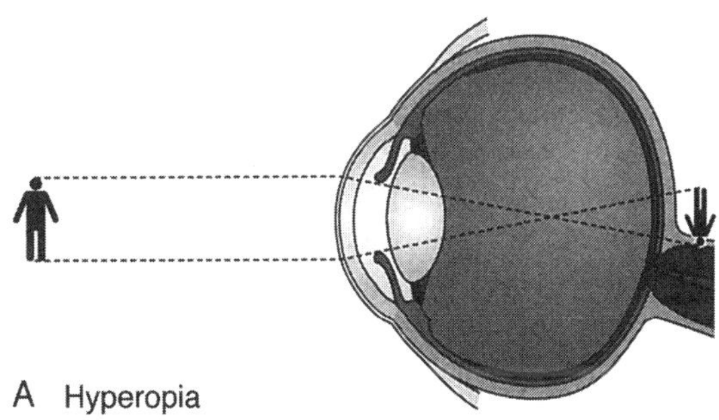
A   Hyperopia

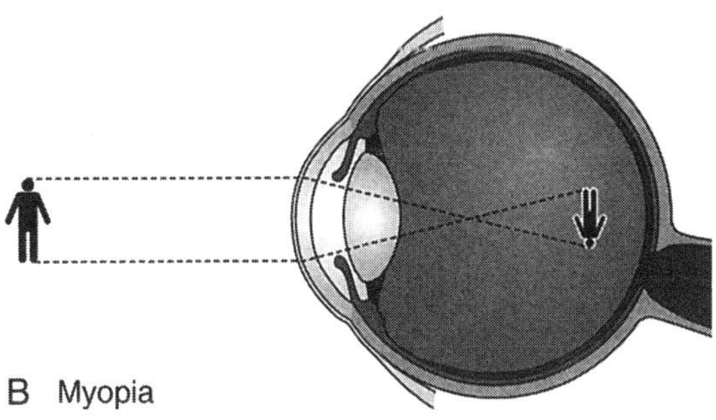
B   Myopia

PRESBYOPIA

*Corrections are in **boldface**.*

Presbyopia is a condition in which the lenses **lose** their elasticity resulting in a decrease in ability to focus on **close** objects. The loss of elasticity causes light rays to focus **beyond** the retina, resulting in hyperopia. This condition usually is associated with aging and generally occurs **after** age 40. Because accommodation for close vision is accomplished by lens contraction, people with presbyopia exhibit the **inability** to see objects at close range. They often compensate for blurred close vision by holding objects to be viewed **further away.** Complaints of eye strain and mild **frontal** headache are common.

VISUAL AND HEARING DATA COLLECTION

Macular degeneration. The patient reports slow, progressive loss of central and near vision in one or both eyes. The visual loss is described as blurred vision, distortion of straight lines, and a dark or empty spot in the central area of vision. Examination of visual acuity for near and far vision will reveal loss of vision. Use of the Amsler grid will allow the examiner to detect central vision distortion. The examiner may use intravenous fluorescein angiography to evaluate blood vessel abnormalities.

Cataract. The patient complains of difficulty seeing at night, when reading, and in bright light; increased sensitivity to glare; double vision; and decreased color vision. Visual acuity is tested for near and far vision. The direct ophthalmoscope and slit lamp are used to examine the lens and other internal structures. The lens will appear cloudy on examination, and the visual acuity may be reduced.

Hordeolum. Small, raised, lightly colored area on the palpebral border without pain.

Acute angle-closure glaucoma. The patient complains of unilateral severe pain of rapid onset, blurred vision, halos around lights, sensitivity to light, and tearing. The patient may complain of nausea and vomiting. A tonometry test will reveal increased intraocular pressure (IOP). The visual field examination may demonstrate a loss of peripheral vision.

External otitis. The patient complains of pain and may complain of pruritus. Redness, swelling, and drainage may be observed during otoscopic examination. Rinne and Weber tests may indicate conductive hearing impairment. Laboratory tests such as complete blood count (CBC), white blood cell (WBC) count, and culture may indicate infection.

Impacted cerumen. The patient may experience hearing loss, a feeling of fullness, or blocked ear. Otoscopic examination reveals cerumen blocking the ear canal. Audiometric testing, whisper voice, and Rinne and Weber tests may indicate conductive hearing loss.

Otitis media. The patient may complain of fever, earache, and a feeling of fullness in the affected ear. If purulent drainage has formed, there may be pain and conductive hearing loss. Otoscopic examination will reveal a reddened and bulging tympanic membrane. Audiometric studies and Rinne, Weber, and whisper tests will likely reveal hearing loss. Laboratory studies may indicate an elevated WBC.

Otosclerosis. The patient will have progressive bilateral hearing loss, particularly with soft low tones. The patient may experience tinnitus. Otoscopic examination may reveal a pinkish, orange tympanic membrane. Audiometric testing and the whisper voice test will show decreased hearing. The patient will hear best with bone conduction in the Rinne test,

whereas lateralization to the most affected ear will occur with the Weber test. Imaging studies will indicate the location and the extent of the excessive bone growth.

GLAUCOMA

*Corrections are in **boldface.***

Glaucoma is characterized by abnormal pressure **within** the eyeball. This pressure causes damage to the cells of the **optic** nerve, the structure responsible for transmitting visual information from the **eye** to the brain. The damage is **silent,** progressive, and **irreversible** until the end stage, when loss of **peripheral** vision occurs and eventually blindness. Once glaucoma occurs, the patient **will always have it and must follow treatment to maintain stable intraocular eye pressures.**

CONDUCTIVE HEARING LOSS

*Corrections are in **boldface.***

Conductive hearing loss is interference with conduction of **sound impulses** through the external auditory canal, eardrum, or middle ear. The inner ear is **not** involved in a pure conductive hearing loss. Conductive hearing loss is a **mechanical** problem. Causes of conductive hearing loss include cerumen, foreign bodies, infection, perforation of the tympanic membrane, trauma, fluid in the middle ear, cysts, tumor, and otosclerosis. Many causes of conductive hearing loss such as infection, foreign bodies, or impacted cerumen **can be** corrected. Hearing devices **may improve** hearing for conditions that cannot be corrected. Hearing devices are most effective with conductive hearing loss when **no** inner ear and nerve damage are present.

OTOSCLEROSIS

*Corrections are in **boldface.***

Otosclerosis results from the formation of new bone along the **stapes.** With the new bone growth, the **stapes** becomes **immobile** and causes conductive hearing loss. Hearing loss is most apparent after the **fourth** decade. Otosclerosis usually occurs **more** frequently in women than in men. The disease usually affects **both** ears. It is thought to be a hereditary disease. The primary symptom of otosclerosis is **progressive** hearing loss. The patient usually experiences bilateral conductive hearing loss, particularly with soft, **low** tones. **Stapedectomy** is the treatment of choice.

CRITICAL THINKING

1. The key symptom that this older adult is having is visual loss without pain. The nurse's examination reveals opacity of the lens, a primary indicator of cataract formation. The vision is diminished because the light rays are unable to get to the retina through the clouded lens.

2. Cataract formation is diagnosed through the eye examination. Visual acuity is tested for near and far vision. The direct ophthalmoscope and slit lamp are used to examine the lens and other internal structures. Instruct the patient that it is important for him to remain still while the health-care practitioner uses the hand-held ophthalmoscope. The slit lamp will require the patient to rest his chin and forehead against the machine while the health-care provider performs this painless test. Instruct the patient that both tests require shining a bright light into the eye, which may be uncomfortable for a few seconds.

3. Refer to Nursing Process for Patients Having Eye Surgery in Chapter 52. Areas to include in a teaching plan are disease process, surgical intervention, preoperative and postoperative restrictions, use of dark glasses, medication administration, eye protection, and activities to be avoided.

REVIEW QUESTIONS

*The correct answers are in **boldface.***

1. (**a, c, d**) Decreased distinction of colors, loss of near vision, and loss of central vision occur with macular degeneration and are tested using the Amsler grid. (b, e) are incorrect because the patient with macular degeneration may have slow loss of vision and retain peripheral vision.

2. (**b**) Myotics lower intraocular pressure by stimulating pupillary and ciliary sphincter muscles. (a) is incorrect because osmotics decrease IOP by decreasing vitreous humor production. (c) is incorrect because mydriatics dilate pupils. (d) is incorrect because cycloplegics paralyze the muscles of accommodation and can increase IOP.

3. (**c**) Dilated pupils cannot protect the eye from the sun by constricting. (a, b, d) are incorrect.

4. (**d**) A stapedectomy involves removing or replacing part or all of the stapes with a prosthesis. Otosclerosis is the hardening of the stapes, so a stapedectomy is the treatment of choice. (a) is incorrect because a myringotomy is an incision made in the tympanic membrane to drain out fluid or suction the inner ear. (b) is incorrect because a myringoplasty is reconstructive repair of a perforated tympanic membrane. (c) is incorrect because a mastoidectomy is the excision of mastoid cells.

5. (**a**) There are no specific medicines to relieve dizziness; however, antihistamines are helpful for some patients. (b, c, d) are incorrect.

6. (**a**) Hearing aids amplify sound and are most useful with conductive hearing loss. Hearing aids are less useful when nerve damage is also present. (b, c, d) are incorrect.

7. (**d**) is correct. (a, b, c) are incorrect.

8. (**a**) These three symptoms are known as the triad of symptoms of Ménière's disease. (b, c, d) are incorrect.

9. (**b**) The labyrinth is involved with balance and equilibrium. Avoiding sudden movements can help prevent dizziness. (a, c, d) are incorrect.

10. (**d**) is correct. (a, b, c) are incorrect.

11. (**c**) Blurring of vision is the first symptom of cataracts due to the clouding of the lens. (a, b, d) are incorrect.

12. (**c**) is correct. (a, b, d) are incorrect.

13. (**c**) Sudden onset of acute pain could indicate increased IOP, bleeding, or detachment; all could lead to permanent eye damage. (a, b, d) are important nursing interventions with lesser priority.

14. (**b**) The intraocular pressure increases as the aqueous humor is prevented from flowing from the anterior to the posterior chamber. (a, c, d) are incorrect.

15. (**c**) is correct. (a) occurs in detached retina; (b) lens opacity is usually found with a cataract; and (d) occurs in Ménière's disease.

16. (**b**) Coughing, sneezing, bending over, and vomiting all increase intraocular pressure and put the patient at risk of hemorrhage. (a, c, d) do not directly increase IOP.

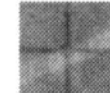 **CHAPTER 53**

INTEGUMENTARY STRUCTURES

1. (**E**)	6. (**C**)
2. (**D**)	7. (**H**)
3. (**G**)	8. (**A**)
4. (**B**)	9. (**F**)
5. (**I**)	

VOCABULARY

1. (**E**)	4. (**C**)
2. (**A**)	5. (**D**)
3. (**B**)	

PRIMARY SKIN LESIONS

1. (**B**)	5. (**F**)
2. (**E**)	6. (**C**)
3. (**H**)	7. (**D**)
4. (**A**)	8. (**G**)

DIAGNOSTIC SKIN TESTS

1. (**B**)	3. (**A**)
2. (**D**)	4. (**C**)

CRITICAL THINKING

1. Left-sided paralysis; immobility; confusion; nothing by mouth and lack of adequate nutrients being provided to maintain healthy tissue; diaphoresis causing skin excori-

ation and breakdown; and thin build, which provides less padding and greater pressure on blood vessels, resulting in ischemia and tissue necrosis.
2. Approximately 170 calories per 1000 mL of 5% dextrose, which is far less than the recommended daily caloric intake.
3. Risk for impaired skin integrity: Assess skin every 4 hours; keep linens and clothing clean and dry; place on turning schedule every 1 to 2 hours; keep skin dry; avoid massaging reddened or bony areas. Consider a pressure-relieving device or mattress for his bed.

Impaired mobility: Place on turning schedule every 1 to 2 hours; perform active or passive range-of-motion; encourage patient to participate in activities of daily living.

Imbalanced nutrition, less than body requirements: Assess patient's daily fluid, caloric, and nutrient needs; consult dietitian; request referral to speech therapist for swallowing studies; provide fluids and nutrition as ordered (tube feedings, hyperalimentation).

REVIEW QUESTIONS

The correct answers are in **boldface.**

1. (**d**) is correct.
2. (**c**) is correct.
3. (**b**) is correct.
4. (**a**) is correct.
5. (**c**) is correct.
6. (**d**) is correct. (a, b, c) are younger and have more moisture and elasticity.
7. (**a**) is a bluish color resulting from a decrease in tissue oxygen. (b) is a reddish color. (c) is a yellowish color. (d) is a pale color.
8. (**c**) results in the decreased ability to maintain warmth. (a, b, d) do not affect warmth.
9. (**d**) provides protection for a skin tear. (a) is used for a deep or infected wound. (b) is used for deeper pressure ulcers. (c) is used to fill in a deep wound.
10. (**c**) Petechiae indicate a clotting problem, so the physician must be informed immediately. (a, b, d) are not of use because this is a clotting problem.

 **CHAPTER 54**

VOCABULARY

1. (**O**)
2. (**N**)
3. (**M**)
4. (**L**)
5. (**K**)
6. (**J**)
7. (**I**)
8. (**H**)
9. (**G**)
10. (**F**)
11. (**E**)
12. (**D**)
13. (**C**)
14. (**B**)
15. (**A**)

BENIGN SKIN LESIONS

1. (**C**)
2. (**E**)
3. (**D**)
4. (**F**)
5. (**A**)
6. (**B**)

PLASTIC SURGERY PROCEDURES

1. rhinoplasty
2. face lift
3. blepharoplasty

CRITICAL THINKING

1. Diabetes, immobility, pressure, hypotensive period that resulted in ischemia, poor initial circulation indicated by need for femoral-popliteal bypass.
2. Sacrum: stage III. Heel: stage II.
3. Turning every 2 hours relieves pressure, but this is not frequent enough to prevent ischemia in the high-risk patient because ischemia begins to develop in 20 minutes. Elevation of the right foot relieves pressure and is very helpful. Sheepskin is used for comfort only; it does not relieve or reduce pressure, so it is not effective in preventing or treating pressure ulcers. Nursing staff can implement more frequent turns without an order and initiate a care plan for impaired skin integrity.
4. The patient is at high risk for pressure ulcers, and sheepskin provides only comfort, not pressure relief, which the patient requires. An order for a pressure-relief device should be requested, such as a special air mattress or bed.

REVIEW QUESTIONS

The correct answers are in **boldface.**

1. (**c**) is correct. Shear can result from pulling a patient up in bed, leading to tissue injury and a pressure ulcer. (a, b, d) help prevent pressure ulcers.
2. (**a, d, e**) are correct. Patting the skin dry prevents injury to skin. Short nails and gloves prevent scratching. (b, e) are incorrect. If the patient is confused, medications should not be left at the bedside. A transparent dressing is generally not recommended for a rash.
3. (**a**) is correct. A nonocclusive dressing should be used on an infected wound. (b, c, d) are occlusive dressings that are contraindicated for infected wounds.
4. (**b**) is correct because it describes light red (blood-tinged) drainage. (a, d) There is no indication of infection or pus. (c) There is not a large amount.
5. (**b**) is correct. Because the wound is not infected, gentle flushing produced by a needleless syringe is desired. (a, d) are pressure flushing techniques for infected wounds. (c) will cause further tissue damage.
6. (**a**) is correct. This describes basal cell carcinoma, and should be reported immediately. (b, c, and d) are incor-

rect—any care of the lesion should be ordered by the physician.

7. (**b, a, d, c**)
8. (**a**) is correct. A fungal infection has most likely developed due to the use of the antibiotics. (b, c, d) do not fit the description.

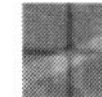 # CHAPTER 55

VOCABULARY

1. (**F**)
2. (**D**)
3. (**C**)
4. (**A**)
5. (**E**)
6. (**B**)

CRITICAL THINKING

1. The most likely cause of this change is the effect the electrical current had on the bones in the forearm. Remember that the bones offer the most resistance to electrical injury. This type of burn can develop worsening symptoms from the inside out. Mr. Patel is experiencing ischemia. His burn needs to be reevaluated.
2. Further assessment: Check his left arm and use it as a basis for comparison for changes in the right. Check the size of the discoloration. Measure the circumference of the right forearm. Check his right brachial pulse. Also, recheck his right leg and foot for assessment changes.
3. Elevate his right arm, and make sure that the dressing is not binding. Contact the RN or physician immediately. An escharatomy may be necessary to relieve pressure. Further debridement may be necessary.

REVIEW QUESTIONS

The correct answers are in **boldface.**

1. (**d**) is correct. This burn has damaged all the skin layers. (a, b, c) are incorrect.
2. (**d**) is correct. These are signs of an infection, which is a common cause of death in burn patients. The physician must be notified immediately. (a) removing the dressing will not help, (b) an occlusive dressing can worsen the infection, and (c) an antibiotic must be ordered by the physician.
3. (**d**) is correct—stage III is rehabilitation, and exercises will be used to return the patient to optimum function. (a, b, c) are more appropriate for stages I and II.
4. (**c**) is correct—inhalation injury is a priority concern in a home fire. (a, b, d) are important once respiratory status is stabilized.
5. (**b**) is correct—clothing must be removed because it can hold heat in and continue the burning process. (a, c, d)

may be appropriate based on assessment, after clothing has been removed and process stopped.
6. (**a**) is correct—circulation is a concern with any burn, but especially with a circumferential burn. (b) numbness and tingling are signs of circulatory impairment and are not normal. (c, d) may be appropriate, but are not priorities.
7.

$$\frac{100 \text{ mL}}{1 \text{ hour}} \times \frac{1 \text{ hour}}{60 \text{ minutes}} \times \frac{15 \text{ gtt}}{1 \text{ mL}} = 25 \text{ gtt per minute}$$

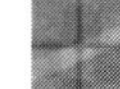 # CHAPTER 56

VOCABULARY

1. Coping
2. cognitive
3. Psychopharmacology
4. Electroconvulsant therapy
5. milieu
6. insight
7. Orientation
8. affect

DEFENSE MECHANISMS

1. Denial
2. Rationalization
3. Reaction formation
4. Compensation
5. Repression
6. Displacement or transference
7. Projection
8. Restitution
9. Avoidance
10. Conversion reaction

CRITICAL THINKING

1. Dirty hair, clothing, and personal hygiene are not normal. Neither is morbid obesity. A good way to open up communication related to the subject is to ask if she would like you or an assistant to help her with a bath. If her state of cleanliness is bothersome to her, she will most likely welcome the help and maybe even share information as to why she has been unable to bathe. On the other hand, if she refuses help or says she doesn't need a bath, further assessment of her ability to care for herself is warranted.
2. It should become fairly obvious whether Mrs. Jewel knows where she is and whether she is oriented to person and time during routine data collection. If you have any doubts, ask specific questions such as "Where are you? Why are you here? Who is this sitting over here?" (Point to a family member if one is in room.) "What

year is it? Who is the President of the United States?" (Or other questions to which most people should know the answers.)

3. During routine data collection, listen carefully to Mrs. Jewel's responses. Document any irrational or inconsistent responses.

4. For recent memory, ask questions such as what she ate for breakfast, or ask about a news event in the last week that everyone should have heard about. For remote memory, ask questions about her younger years, such as where she lived, the name of her grade school, or the year she got married.

5. There is no special questioning needed to assess communication ability. Simply pay attention to her responses to routine questions. Document unusually fast or slow speech, stuttering, inappropriate volume, or difficulty getting ideas across.

6. *Affect* is the outward expression of emotion. If this expression does not match what Mrs. Jewel is telling you, or if it is inconsistent with her situation, her affect is inappropriate. For example, it would be unusual to be laughing about being in the hospital.

7. Asking her to explain a proverb (such as "a stitch in time saves nine") will help determine if she has good judgment. In addition, you might ask her what she would do under certain circumstances, such as if her blood sugar was low. Keep in mind that her response might reflect both judgment and knowledge.

8. *Perception* is the way a person experiences reality. Pay attention to her responses to your questions. For example, if she stopped taking medication for her diabetes because some voices in her head told her to do so, her perception is faulty. Normal responses are based on reality.

REVIEW QUESTIONS

*The correct answers are in **boldface.***

1. (**d**) is correct. Close friends and relationships are a sign of mental health. (a, b, c) may all be healthy behaviors.

2. (**b**) is correct. Blaming is a type of projection. (a, c, d) do not necessarily involve blaming others.

3. (**c**) is correct. It is important to establish a therapeutic relationship for psychotherapy to be effective. (a, b, d) are not helpful for the patient with mental health problems.

4. (**b**) is correct. The patient may be disoriented following electroconvulsive therapy (ECT). Maintaining safety is a primary goal during this time. (a) Restraints are inappropriate, (b) the patient should not be discharged until he or she is oriented and safety is ensured, and (d) oxygen is not standard treatment following ECT.

5. (**d**) is correct. A stressor must be defined by the patient. (a, b, c) Although surgery, divorce, and loss of a job would seem stressful to most people, it is important to

allow the patient to identify for herself or himself what is stressful.

6. (**b**) is correct. An MRI is used to rule out physiological problems. (a, d) MRI does not measure neurotransmitters or electrical activity. (c) MRI is a diagnostic test, not a treatment.

7. (**b**) is correct. Helping the patient identify stressors is most helpful. (a) does not help the patient work through the problem. (c) It is impossible to eliminate stress. (d) Giving advice is not appropriate.

8. (**c**) is correct because it reflects the question back to the patient. (a) Giving approval is not therapeutic. (b) Asking "why?" may be threatening. (d) may discourage a potentially good decision.

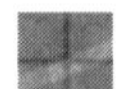 ## CHAPTER 57

VOCABULARY

1. alogia
2. codependence
3. phobia
4. obsession
5. bipolar
6. psychosomatic or somatoform
7. schizophrenia
8. delirium tremens
9. Addiction
10. Anhedonia

CRITICAL THINKING

1. Remain calm, and keep your distance. Ask, "Who told you what I am up to?" If his answer is not in touch with reality (such as, the voices in his head told him), then gently say, "Mr. Joers, I know the voices seem real to you, but I can't hear them. The surgeon wants to fix your broken hip this morning, so I need to check your blood pressure. It will just take a minute." If the night nurse is still on the unit, consider having him or her assist, since it will be a familiar face to Mr. Joers.

2. This depends on several factors. He will need to be reasonably cooperative in order to complete preoperative care. Check to see if his consent form has been signed. If he is disoriented or psychotic, then he will not be able to legally sign. See if he has a legal guardian who can give consent. It is possible that surgery will need to be delayed until he is more stable.

3. The stress of admission to the hospital, fear and anxiety related to pain, and impending surgery. Also, medication schedules are sometimes disrupted during transfers from one institution to another.

4. Check his medication record to see if any medications that might help are due to be given. Be sure to consult physician orders for medications to give or hold prior to surgery. Notify the RN and/or the surgeon of Mr. Joers'

symptoms. Based on his response to your interventions, be prepared to share your opinion about whether he is cooperative enough to be able to proceed with surgery. If there is a family member who has a close, trusting relationship with Mr. Joers, consider calling him or her in to assist with his care.

5. If Mr. Joers is psychotic, he will not be oriented to the fact that he has a broken hip. His gait also is affected by his Parkinson's disease. He is at risk for danger to himself or others. He will need 1:1 supervision to be sure he does not try to get out of bed or otherwise further harm himself. In addition, his paranoia may pose a danger to staff if he perceives that staff is trying to harm him.

REVIEW QUESTIONS

*The correct answers are in **boldface***

1. (**a**) is correct. This amount of sleepiness is unusual. (b) Tolerance can occur, but this amount of sleepiness is not an expected response. (c) It is unsafe to get the patient up if he is difficult to arouse. (d) is not an independent nursing action.

2. (**c**) is correct. Drinking alcohol before work could impair judgment and cause harm to patients. (a, b, d) are all reasonable and safe responses to anxiety.

3. (**c**) is correct. This response lets the patient know what is real, then distracts with a walk. (a, d) do not correct her misperception, and (b) is not kind or respectful.

4. (**b**) is correct. Fluctuations in sodium affect metabolism of lithium. (a, c, d) are not known to affect lithium.

5. (**c**) is correct. Pill counts, although unreliable at times, are the most reliable source of data of the responses given. (a) The patient or (b) significant other may not provide accurate or truthful data, and (c) refills may or may not have been taken.

6. (**a**) is correct. Group support is one of the most effective treatments for alcoholism. (b) Drugs may be used during acute withdrawal but are not ideal for long-term therapy. (b) ECT is not a treatment for alcoholism. (d) Reducing alcohol consumption is not successful for most people.

7. (**d**) is correct. Speaking to other staff so that the patient cannot hear may be interpreted personally by the patient. (a, b, c) are therapeutic for the patient with schizophrenia.

8.
$$\frac{150 \text{ mg} \quad\big|\quad 5 \text{ mL}}{\big|\quad 100 \text{ mg}} = 7.5 \text{ mL}$$

9. (**a**) is correct. It shows the patient is able to sort what is true and what is not. (b, d) show hopeless thoughts, and (c) it is not healthy for one's own feelings to be dependent on another person's behavior.

10. (**c**) is correct—it may take 2 to 4 weeks for an antidepressant to be effective. (a, b) are not appropriate. (d) can cause a dangerous drug interaction.